Introduction to Applied Pharmacoeconomics

Notice

Introduction to Applied Pharmacoeconomics

F. Randy Vogenberg, Ph.D., R.Ph.
Director and National Practice Leader
Actuarial Sciences Associates, Inc.
(an AON Consulting Company)
Wellesley, Massachusetts

Deans' Professor of Pharmacy Management
Philadelphia College of Pharmacy
University of the Sciences in Philadelphia
Philadelphia, Pennsylvania

McGraw-Hill
Medical Publishing Division

New York St. Louis San Francisco Auckland Bogotá Caracas
Lisbon London Madrid Mexico City Milan Montreal
New Delhi San Juan Singapore Sydney Tokyo Toronto

McGraw-Hill

A Division of The ***McGraw-Hill*** *Companies*

INTRODUCTION TO APPLIED PHARMACOECONOMICS

1 2 3 4 5 6 7 8 9 0 DOC/DOC 0 9 8 7 6 5 4 3 2 1 0

ISBN 0-07-134846-8

This book was set in Times Roman by Keyword Publishing Services.
The editor was Steve Zollo.
The production supervisor was Phil Galea.
Project management was provided by Keyword Publishing Services.
The cover designer was Aimee Nordin.
R.R. Donnelley & Sons was the printer and binder.

This book is printed on acid-free paper.

Cataloging-in-Publication data is on file for this title at the Library of Congress

Contents

Contributors

Edward P. Armstrong, Pharm.D., BCPS, FASHP (3)
Associate Professor
College of Pharmacy
University of Arizona
Tucson, Arizona

K. C. Carriere, Ph.D. (2)
Associate Professor of Statistics
Department of Mathematical Sciences
University of Alberta
Edmonton, Alberta

Amy Grizzle, Pharm.D. (3)
Assistant Director
Center of Health Outcomes and Pharmacoeconomic Research
University of Arizona
Tucson, Arizona

Gireesh V. Gupchup, Ph.D. (10)
Assistant Professor of Pharmacy
University of New Mexico Health Science Center
Albuquerque, New Mexico

David Hawkins, Pharm.D. (9)
Professor and Chair of Pharmacy Practice
Mercer University
Southern School of Pharmacy
Atlanta, Georgia

Rong Huang, M.Sc. (2)
Ph.D. Candidate in Statistics
Department of Mathematical Sciences
University of Alberta
Edmonton, Alberta

Jay Jackson, Pharm.D. (9)
Outcomes Research Fellow
Mercer University
Southern School of Pharmacy
Atlanta, Georgia

Patty J. Keys, Pharm.D. (6)
Assistant Professor of Pharmacoeconomic Research
Wayne State University
Detroit, Michigan

Stephen J. Kogut, M.B.A., R.Ph. (13)
Ph.D. Candidate
Program in Pharmacoepidemiology and Pharmacoeconomics
University of Rhode Island
Kingston, Rhode Island

E. Paul Larrat, Ph.D., M.B.A. (10, 13)
Associate Professor of Epidemiology
College of Pharmacy
University of Rhode Island
Kingston, Rhode Island

Lon N. Larson, Ph.D. (1)
Professor of Pharmacy, Social and Administrative Sciences
College of Pharmacy
Drake University
Des Moines, Iowa

Patricia Marshik, Pharm.D. (10)
Assistant Professor of Pharmacy
University of New Mexico Health Science Center
Albuquerque, New Mexico

Susan K. Maue, Ph.D. (8)
Senior Managing Consultant
Navigant Consulting, Inc.
Palm Harbor, Florida

William W. McCloskey, Pharm.D. (4)
Associate Professor of Clinical Pharmacy
Chairman, Department of Pharmacy Practice
Massachusetts College of Pharmacy and Health Sciences
Boston, Massachusetts

Patrick D. Meek, Pharm.D. (5)
Assistant Professor
School of Pharmacy
University of Wisconsin
Madison, Wisconsin

Sanjay Merchant, M.S., M.B.A. (11)
Doctoral Candidate
University of Maryland
Baltimore, Maryland

Peter Mok, Pharm.D. (12)
Director of Pharmaceutical Care
Whitney M. Young, Jr. Health Center
Albany, New York

C. Daniel Mullins, Ph.D. (11)
Associate Professor
University of Maryland
Baltimore, Maryland

Eleanor M. Perfetto, Ph.D. (13)
Executive Vice President and COO
QualityMetric, Inc.
Lincoln, Rhode Island

Richard Segal, Ph.D. (8)
Professor and Chair
College of Pharmacy
University of Florida
Gainesville, Florida

Linda Simoni-Wastila, B.S.Pharm., Ph.D. (7)
Senior Research Associate
Co-Director, Doctoral Training Program in Alcohol Services Research
Brandeis University
Waltham, Massachusetts

Amy Steinkellner, Pharm.D. (5)
Director, Clinical Services
ProVantage Health Services, Inc.
Brookfield, Wisconsin

Daniel Touchette, Pharm.D., M.A. (6)
Assistant Professor of Pharmacy Practice
Pharmacoeconomics and Outcomes Research
Oregon State University College of Pharmacy
Oregon Health Sciences University
Portland, Oregon

F. Randy Vogenberg, Ph.D., R.Ph. (12)
Director and National Practice Leader
Actuarial Sciences Associates, Inc.
(an AON Consulting Company)
Wellesley, Massachusetts

Deans' Professor of Pharmacy Management
Philadelphia College of Pharmacy
University of the Sciences in Philadelphia
Philadelphia, Pennsylvania

Preface

Purpose

Drugs and related technology are now in the forefront of US health care policy discussion around the future of our market-driven health care system. Pharmacoeconomic and outcomes research are important tools for health care practitioners to understand and use in their patient care practice settings. The purpose of this book is to provide an understanding of these tools so that they can be applied and information generated by researchers in the field may be translated by practitioners to advance the quality of patient care outcomes.

This book explores the commonly used pharmacoeconomic evaluations, applying these evaluations into drug and disease decision-making, common barriers to conducting evaluations, and modeling versus patient-based evaluations for outcome assessments. Chapters in this text present pharmaceutical economics in the context of how it is applied in the marketplace setting. Case studies are used to illustrate applications or barriers and facilitate an integrated learning approach to this topic.

A main purpose for an introductory textbook is to acquaint the reader with various methods and issues in pharmacoeconomic and outcomes research. Both the opportunities and challenges are identified, along with the issues that need to be addressed in this field of evolving patient care research. Pharmacists, pharmacy students, and other health care professionals will find this useful in their undergraduate or graduate study programs as well as for application in their patient care practice settings.

Organization

Each chapter builds on the subject matter of previous chapters while providing references for additional reading to explore topical areas presented in this book. The book is divided into thirteen chapters to facilitate teaching on a quarterly or semester system. Depending on need, chapters can be used individually to supplement graduate coursework or individualized learning by health care professionals.

Chapter 1 reviews pharmacoeconomics in the context of our rapidly changing US health care delivery system. Defining what is pharmacoeconomics, why the US system is inefficient, and how pharmacoeconomics can increase efficiency are highlights of this chapter.

Chapter 2 explores the considerations required in conducting pharmacoeconomic research. Traditional approaches and methods are explored in addition to discussing the various end products of pharmacoeconomic research. Strengths and weaknesses of the various methods are described with an eye toward optimizing their application in practice.

Chapter 3 deals with patient-based outcomes research and the role of various types of outcomes research in patient practice settings. Issues of efficacy versus effectiveness, quality of life instruments, applications of outcomes research, and differences between pharmacoeconomics and outcomes research are contained in this chapter.

Chapter 4 reviews the principles of drug literature evaluation and its application to patient care practice settings. Understanding information resources, pharmacoeconomic literature evaluation, and considerations that need to be taken into account by health professionals in reading this literature are clearly described in this chapter.

Chapter 5 takes a different perspective on pharmacoeconomics by using the payer or employer viewpoint. Perspective is an important element in any pharmacoeconomic evaluation and these payer perspectives are increasingly important for practitioners to understand.

Chapter 6 identifies, discusses, and explores issues with variables in pharmacoeconomic research. There are many approaches and perspectives to consider in conducting a pharmacoeconomic evaluation that must be accounted for in the methodology. This chapter addresses those variables with a practical emphasis for the researcher.

Chapters 7 through 10 provide a disease- and/or drug-specific application to pharmacoeconomic research. Specific issues, opportunities, or challenges in conducting pharmacoeconomic and outcomes research in select therapeutic areas are discussed with one or more case examples. Chapter 7 looks at mental health, Chapter 8 is on gastrointestinal disease, Chapter 9 covers cardiovascular disease, and Chapter 10 details respiratory diseases. Generalists and specialists will find these illustrative chapters insightful on how to apply pharmacoeconomics to a given contemporary clinical topic area. In addition, the case examples presented provide students and practitioners with practical insights into conducting these types of pharmacoeconomic research by experts in those fields.

Chapter 11 looks at the evolving requirements and standards for pharmacoeconomic research. Aside from Federal guidelines, existing or new requirements of other organizations or countries from pharmacoeconomic research is important to students of this topic.

Chapter 12 is both a review and a practical application of pharmacoeconomic and outcome methods in typical practice settings. How to bring together the science, rigor, and practicality of pharmacoeconomic research into a typical practice setting is explored. Examples for practitioners and different presentation methods are presented in this chaper.

Lastly, Chapter 13 looks at current and evolving Federal requirements in the field of pharmacoeconomics and outcomes research. The role of government in this area has been increasing, not only due to its financial support, but because of its place in fostering as well as disseminating pharmacoeconomic research.

Each chapter and its accompanying charts and tables and/or graphs are intended to assist the reader in better understanding the topic while illustrating key aspects of the text. References and additional reading information are also provided to allow the reader to explore the topical areas at their leisure.

Audience

Although this textbook is written primarily for those in the field of pharmacy or drug technology assessment, students in health services administration and other health-related professions, such as medicine, nursing, physician assistants, social work, and dietetics, would also find it helpful.

Others who can benefit from an understanding and application of pharmacoeconomics include academics, providers of health care, decision-makers in insurance companies, employee benefit managers, health care professionals, government policy-makers, and consumers.

Acknowledgments

I gratefully acknowledge the valuable input from each of the authors and from other experts in this expanding field of research with whom this book was discussed. I received a number of valuable and constructive suggestions from practitioners, all of whom are involved in the application of pharmacoeconomics to patient care. Their timely input was found valuable in the final development and editing of this contemporary textbook.

I appreciated the opportunity to work with Stephen Zollo, Medical Editor at McGraw-Hill, and thank him for his key role in facilitating the preparation of this textbook.

Lastly, I want to acknowledge the support of co-workers at Actuarial Sciences Associates and my family, without which I could not have completed this task.

F. Randy Vogenberg, Ph.D., R.Ph.

CHAPTER

1

US Health Care System and Pharmacoeconomics

Lon N. Larson

Keeping a child healthy requires more than periodic physical examinations and vaccinations; it requires good playgrounds, schools, parents with jobs, crime-free neighborhoods, and counseling about drugs, tobacco, and reproduction.

David Eddy[1]

INTRODUCTION

Background and Objectives

The US health care system and pharmacoeconomics—are they a marriage made in heaven, or the odd couple? While the US health care system is notoriously inefficient, pharmacoeconomics (economic evaluation) aims to improve efficiency. Efficiency is the focal point of this chapter. What is it and why is it important? Efficiency can be briefly defined as using resources (inputs) in a way that generates the greatest possible benefit (output). When a system is inefficient, it means that the same level of resources could be used differently and generate more benefit—simply, we are not getting our money's worth. Pharmacoeconomics can help resolve this problem; quoting from one of the classic articles on economic evaluation, "The underlying premise of [pharmacoeconomics] is that for any level of resources available, society (or the decision-making jurisdiction involved) wishes to maximize the total aggregate health benefits incurred."[2]

Pharmacoeconomics is particularly relevant when managing the health of a group or population. This includes any organization that uses pooled resources to pay for health services, such as managed care organizations, government programs (e.g., Medicaid), and insurance plans. Each of these organizations has limited resources available to it (evidenced by the negative reaction to premium increases or tax increases), and each wants to "get the most" from these resources; the most "what"? The performance—or quality—of these organizations is best measured by the collective health status of its members, using indicators that incorporate length of life and its quality.[3] Thus, the goal of these organizations is to use its pool of available resources to maximally improve the health of its members. This is also the purpose of "pharmacy management at the population level"; [4] a phrase used to describe the activities and services (e.g., formularies, prior authorization, prescribing guidelines) that are designed to influence prescribing and drug use for a population or group.

However, the quest for efficiency is not painless. Doing more and better pharmacoeconomic evaluations is not enough. It also requires a change in attitude. As we shall see, efficiency requires that we realize that resources are limited and change our attitudes about patient care accordingly. Providers have to weigh the best interests of the individual patient against the interests of the population or group. Health care services will have to be rationed; that is, services with potential benefit to patients will be withheld because those resources can generate more benefit in other endeavors.

The US health care system and pharmacoeconomics is a marriage made in heaven, when one views pharmacoeconomics as a necessary, but not necessarily sufficient, ingredient in increasing efficiency. On the other hand, they are an odd couple, if efficiency is seen as an unwelcome intruder that is associated with a loss (access to unlimited health care for some individuals) rather than a gain (improved health status of the population).

The purpose of this chapter is to help the reader understand why pharmacoeconomics is an integral part of today's health care system and practice of pharmacy. After reading this chapter, the reader should be able to: (1) explain the resource allocation dilemmas facing the US health care system, and (2) explain the usefulness of pharmacoeconomic evaluations in resolving those dilemmas.

The chapter is organized in three sections. They address the following questions:

- What is pharmacoeconomics? We begin with a brief explanation of pharmacoeconomics; it is intended to help the reader visualize a pharmacoeconomic evaluation so as to better understand its role and importance in the health care system. Pharmacoeconomics is defined, costs and consequences are briefly described, and a cost-effectiveness ratio is explained. (As indicated by the objectives, this chapter is not a thorough review of the principles and methods of economic evaluation.)

- Why is pharmacoeconomics important? This section provides background information on the economic aspects of the health care system that make pharmacoeconomics so important. Society is spending too much for health services—the health care system is inefficient; in this section, we explore why.
- How can pharmacoeconomics increase efficiency? In this section we explore how pharmacoeconomics can add rationality to the health care system. Using the results of pharmacoeconomic evaluations is discussed from three differing views of efficiency in health care. This section discusses rationing and the conflict between the individual patient and population in allocating health care resources.

Definitions

Before beginning, a few definitions, as used in this chapter, may help the reader:

- Benefit: the value or utility of a therapy or activity; a synonym for consequences and output.
- Consequences: the outcomes of a therapy on the health state of the patient, potentially measured as life years saved, quality-adjusted life years (QALYs), a clinical indicator, or less commonly, in dollars.
- Cost: the value of resources consumed.
- Cost-effectiveness: a generic term for economic evaluation; also refers to a specific method of analysis (along with cost-utility analysis).
- Cost-effectiveness ratio: cost-per-unit of effect; ratio of incremental (additional) cost to incremental effectiveness; cost is the net burden on health care resources; effectiveness is a measure of the desired outcome.
- Economic evaluation: the comparison of the costs and consequences of two or more alternative courses of action; although pharmacoeconomics is a subset of economic evaluation, they are used as synonyms in this chapter
- Efficiency: the relationship between inputs and outputs; producing the most benefit from a given level of resources.
- Health insurance: used generically to refer to third-party payment programs, including managed care organizations and government programs (Medicare, Medicaid).
- Pharmacoeconomics: economic evaluations applied to drug therapy or pharmacist services.
- Population: those who pool their resources to buy health services—synonyms in this chapter are "group" and "community."

WHAT IS PHARMACOECONOMICS?

Economic evaluation is formally defined as the comparison of the costs and consequences of two or more alternative courses of action.[5] Costs are the resources consumed to perform an activity or implement a decision, while consequences are the outcomes—positive and negative—of that action or decision. Economic evaluations assess efficiency—the relationship between outputs (consequences) and inputs (costs). Their ultimate purpose is to enable the decision maker to better allocate pooled or community resources. Cost-effectiveness analysis is commonly used as a synonym for economic evaluation, although cost-effectiveness analysis is also a type of method, along with cost-utility and cost-benefit analyses. Pharmacoeconomics is the application of economic evaluation methods to drug products and pharmacist services.

To clarify the nature of a pharmacoeconomic evaluation, we will briefly describe the components of a cost-effectiveness ratio of a medical therapy (e.g., drug therapy). Costs, for our purposes here, refer to the therapy's effects on health care resources. (Potentially other types of resources are affected, but we will limit ourselves to those in the health care system.) In looking at the health care costs of a therapy, five elements may be relevant.[6] First, is the resources used in producing the therapy itself; for instance, with drug therapy, these may include the drug product, and the supplies and personnel time consumed in preparation, administration, and monitoring. A second element is the health care resources used in treating the side effects of the therapy. Thirdly, if an illness is prevented by the therapy, the avoided costs (resources saved) are calculated and included as savings. Fourthly, if a diagnostic or referral process is involved, the costs that result from information obtained (e.g., information or recommendation from a pharmacist) are included. Finally (and this one is contentious), if life is extended by the therapy, the costs of health care services consumed during the additional years of life should be included. The net sum of these elements is the net cost of the therapy; it includes health care resources consumed as well as those saved. In other words, it is the therapy's overall effect on health care resources. This is the "cost" in a cost-effectiveness ratio.

Two of the ways consequences are expressed in economic evaluations are effectiveness and utility; these relate to cost-effectiveness analysis and cost-utility analysis. Effectiveness refers to the objective of the therapy or service. Commonly, effectiveness is measured in "years of life saved" (i.e., the number of lives saved multiplied by the average remaining life expectancy of the patients). However, if an analysis deals with one condition, a clinical indicator can be used as the measure of effectiveness, if it captures all important outcomes. Utility, the second measure of consequences, adjusts length of life for its quality. Utility values are preferences for health states, ranging from 0 (death) to 1 (normal health). When utility is multiplied by years of life, the result is quality-adjusted life-years, or QALYs. With a measure like QALYs, comparisons can be made across conditions. Recently a task force, charged with developing recommendations to improve the quality of economic evaluations, specified QALYs as the preferred measure of consequences.[7]

A cost-effectiveness ratio (or cost-utility ratio) includes the incremental or additional gain in health status that the therapy produces compared with the next most effective alternative; this is the denominator of the ratio. The numerator is the incremental or additional cost of the therapy, compared with the alternative. As an example, when a therapy is said to cost $30,000 per QALY, this figure is the additional resources required by the therapy for each additional QALY that it generates.

WHY IS THE HEALTH CARE SYSTEM INEFFICIENT?

Society is spending too much on health services; we are not getting our "money's worth" from our health care expenditures. This statement summarizes the conclusions of several health economists and policy experts.[8–11] It is a remarkable statement, indicating a serious situation; it implies that resources are not producing as much utility or benefit as they are capable of producing. In 1997 national health expenditures amounted to nearly $4000 per person (or $16,000 for a family of four).[12] Most families do not realize they have spent this much; but they have. Some of the spending is visible, such as out-of-pocket expenses for services and insurance; some is less visible—taxes for Medicare and Medicaid; and finally some is virtually invisible, i.e., reduced wages to offset the employer's portion of the insurance premium. Health care costs may be well hidden, but they are real. The consensus is that health care spending is not generating a commensurate benefit. This section explores why this is the case—why we spend too much for health services. Several ideas are discussed: the difference between the perceived and the actual importance of health services as a contributing factor to health status; the imperfect nature of the health care marketplace, especially the effects of insurance; hiding costs through employer-sponsored insurance and deceiving ourselves into thinking that health care resources are unlimited; and a further explanation of the economic concept of efficiency.

Health Services vs. Health Status

We often hear statements like, "You can't put a price on good health," or "When you have your health, you have everything." Certainly, good health is important in enjoying life and fulfilling one's aspirations. Placing a high value on health (i.e., health status) is understandable. However, should a similarly high value be placed on health services as well? The answer has implications for health care spending. Realistically, the answer is "no"; yet our behavior in using health services indicates we believe the answer is "yes."

Two models of health status provide different perspectives of the benefits or value of health services.[13] In one model, health is narrowly defined as the absence of disease, and health services, with the stated purpose of preventing and treating disease, are the primary determinant of health status. This model is intertwined with society's deep-seated faith in the powers of medical technology and biomedical research. We are fascinated by medical technology; newspapers and broadcast media carry stories, almost daily, of the latest results in medical research. We tend to believe that modern medicine can cure anything; and if not now, then soon. As George Annas states, "We have become modern believers in faith healing, faith based not in a Supreme Being, but in Supreme Science."[14] This model guides our use of health services; we believe that life can be prolonged and/or health status restored if the appropriate types and quantities of health services are consumed.

The second model involves a broader view of health status and its determinants. In this model, health status encompasses physical, mental, and social functioning. (These dimensions are commonly measured in health-related quality-of-life instruments.) Health is more than the absence of disease. Health status is seen as having multiple causal or contributing factors. These include heredity or genetic predisposition; toxins or hazards in the physical environment; personal behaviors, such as smoking and dietary habits; one's socioeconomic status and social environment including social support; and finally health services. The debate continues as to the relative importance of each of these in determining health status, but many experts are convinced that health services are not as important as some of the other determinants.[15,16] This multicausal view of health status more accurately portrays reality; yet, it is not the one that governs our use of health services.

Further, we behave as if health status and well-being were synonymous. They are not. As mentioned above, health status is the level of functioning—physical, mental, and social. Well-being, in contrast, may be thought of as happiness, fulfillment, and satisfaction with life. Certainly health status contributes to well-being, but many other factors do so as well. Examples are economic prosperity, spiritual growth, meaningful relationships, and intellectual discovery. A long, disease-free life is not necessarily a fulfilled one. The statement by Eddy that introduces this chapter emphasizes this point: the well-being and development of children is influenced by many factors other than medical care services.

To conclude, we tend to overestimate the value of health services as a determinant of health status and well-being. Consequently, we justify the intensive and relentless use of health care services to fight death and disease. However, there is more to life than health, and there is more to health than health services. Yet, as we shall see later, we have built a financing system that allows—even encourages—us to prescribe and consume health care services congruently with our misperceptions.

The Imperfect Health Services Marketplace

A frequently quoted figure when discussing health care spending is the proportion of GDP spent on health care. (Gross domestic product or GDP is the value of goods and services produced by a nation.) For the United States in 1997, the figure was about 13.5%.[17] No one knows the "correct" or ideal amount to spend on health services. The proportion in the United States is often portrayed as too high. The proportion of GDP spent on health services has grown over the decades—in 1960 and 1980, it was 5.1 and 8.9%, respectively—and it is higher in the United States than in other developed countries.

Generally, we are not concerned about the proportion of our nation's economy spent on a specific good and service. For instance, the proportion of GDP spent on personal computers, golf course green fees, or athletic shoes (as well as many others) is not newsworthy nor a public policy issue. This is because in a market economy, customers (who are assumed to be knowledgeable) are spending their money among various goods and services according to their preferences. Their money is limited, but their wants are unlimited, so they spend their resources in such a way that achieves the maximum utility or satisfaction for them. Meanwhile, several suppliers are competing with each other to meet the needs of these customers. Those that succeed in this are profitable. Customers are price-sensitive because their overall utility or satisfaction is diminished if they buy higher-priced products that provide no more utility than less-expensive alternatives. Thus, producers have an incentive to produce their goods and services as inexpensively as possible. This is how normal markets operate.

Health care is not a normal market for a couple of reasons. First, most health services are "demanded" by a physician and not by the customer or patient. Given the complexities of human physiology and modern medical and surgical therapies, relying on the advice of an expert(s) is understandable. The physician's recommendations are supposed to reflect the patient's best interests. A couple of barriers stand in the way of physicians acting in each patient's best interests. One is the uncertainty that accompanies many medical procedures; even experts disagree on the results or outcomes of a given procedure.[18] Medical care is gray; it is not black and white. This is seen quite vividly in the variations in physician practice patterns. The second barrier is the personal interests of the physician; human beings have trouble ignoring their own interests. Oftentimes, the physician who recommends the service is also the supplier (e.g., surgeons recommending surgery). In a fee-for-service environment, the physician's interests may be better served by doing more; while in a capitation environment, doing less is encouraged.

The second factor that makes the health care marketplace abnormal or imperfect is the presence of insurance, especially employer-sponsored insurance. (Here, the term insurance encompasses all third-party programs, private and public.) With insurance, the cost-consciousness of patients and physicians is diminished, perhaps to the point of being eliminated. Unlike the normal market where the customer is spending his or her own money, an insured patient is spending from a pool of resources, into which many individuals contribute. Employers and employees contribute to the pool of employment-based insurance, and taxpayers contribute to the Medicare or Medicaid pools. Spending others' resources is easier than spending one's own. In buying health services, we demand (in an economic sense) the best, regardless of price—cost is no object. In contrast, when purchasing goods or services with our own money, we search for value, comparing price and benefits, and make a choice, given our preferences and given our resources. This last phrase, "given our resources," is important. When using our own resources, we realize they are limited (e.g., if we have only enough money for a lower-priced car, we don't demand a high-priced luxury car). For health services, in contrast, the resources available for spending appear to be unlimited, and patients seek—and providers provide—care accordingly.

Insurance also affects the behaviors of providers in ways that do not promote efficiency. Physicians control the use of about 80% of health care spending; for example, they order lab tests, prescribe drugs, and admit to hospitals. With insured patients, physicians are able to recommend or prescribe any diagnostic and treatment procedure, knowing that the patient will not be harmed financially. In prescribing drugs, for example, if the patient has insurance, the physician need not be concerned about the price of the drug; the physician does not need to worry that the prescription will go unfilled or the family's other bills will go unpaid because of the high price of the prescription. Secondly, insurance can also affect the cost-consciousness of providers in producing their services. Since patients are not price-sensitive (from their viewpoint, all providers charge the same), they do not "price-shop" among providers. Consequently, providers have less incentive to produce their services as inexpensively as possible. This adverse effect of insurance is especially pronounced with usual and customary or cost-based reimbursement. With cost-based reimbursement of hospitals, insurance provided the means to finance the dissemination of medical technology; this coincided nicely with society's love affair with technology.

Not only does insurance hide the costs of a particular service, the method of paying premiums in the United States has allowed us to also hide the cost of the premiums.[19] Premiums for private insurance are paid largely by employers. Most persons with private insurance have group policies through their places of work; a few persons have individual policies, which they pay the entire premium themselves. Employees pay a relatively small portion of the premium; hence, to the employee, health insurance appears to be free—a benefit from his or her employer. Such is not the case. In reality, the employer's costs of employee health benefits are recouped through higher prices to its customers or through lower wages to its employees; economists suspect the latter is more prevalent. An employer is concerned about its total labor costs, whether a dollar is spent for benefits or salary is not a major concern. Thus employees end up paying the premium through lower wages, but do not realize it.

So what? What are consequences of hiding health costs through employer-sponsored benefits? It further reduces the cost-consciousness of participants in the system. With the costs of health insurance hidden, services appear to be free. Consequently, it is easy to expect the most and the best health services, because no apparent cost is associated with them. We are appalled when we hear of a patient being refused a particular treatment by an insurance company or managed care organization; many believe it is wrong to not provide a potentially beneficial treatment. With our system of financing, it is harder to accept limits or rationing in health coverage. We do not see resources as limited; we believe we can have it all—but the reality is that resources are limited and choices have to be made.

Medical Necessity vs. Efficiency

As has been described above, health insurance, especially employer-sponsored health insurance, increases the demand for health care services. If all the services being used are medically necessary, is this a problem? In a word: yes. The reason is that providing all medically necessary services does not take the cost of services into account, only their effects. Consequently, we demand or use too many services—the "too many" services are those which yield benefits less than their cost. In other words, the resources could generate more benefit if used in a different manner.

As the quantity consumed of a good or service increases, the additional benefit or value of each successive unit consumed diminishes. In economics, this is referred to as diminishing marginal utility; the marginal or additional benefit of each unit consumed is less than the benefit gained from the previous one. The concept is easy to imagine with shoes; one pair is essential, a second is quite nice (some might even say essential), but it provides less benefit (i.e., utility or satisfaction) than the first pair. Similarly, the third pair provides less benefit than the second; and so on. Let us look at a hypothetical situation:

Units consumed	1	2	3	4	5	6
Benefits (per unit) ($)	22	20	16	8	2	−2
Cumulative benefits ($)	22	42	58	64	66	64

Instead of shoes, imagine these are the units of a particular health service consumed by a person during a year. (They could be tests of cholesterol levels; physician visits; or pharmacist-conducted drug regimen reviews.) Two or three of them are very beneficial in maintaining the patient's health status; a couple of others provide less benefit; and finally, in this example, one causes iatrogenic disease and has a negative benefit.

In deciding the optimum level of use, let us consider three situations. If the goal is to provide all medically necessary services, the patient would receive five units because each of them provides benefit. However, from an economic perspective, this is not enough information to determine if this is the optimal level of use. The economist also wants to know the cost; i.e., the value of the resources consumed in producing the benefit. For simplicity, let us assume that a unit costs \$20. In this case, \$20 is the value of resources consumed to produce the unit and also the price charged to a customer. The five units consume \$100 worth of resources and generate \$66 worth of benefits. Intuitively, most of us recognize that this is not a wise use of resources. Secondly, let us consider a patient with insurance, where the patient has to pay \$5 for each unit and the insurance pays the rest. Now the patient consumes four units, because each of the first four generates benefits greater than the apparent or out-of-pocket price; in total, resources worth \$80 produce \$64 in benefits. Again, this is not a wise use of resource. In the third situation, the patient pays the market price (i.e., the value of the resources used to produce it). The patient purchases two units, because at this point the benefits received from the last unit purchased are equal to the costs of that unit; it is also the point where the difference between total benefits and total costs is greatest. (If the cost or price fell to \$16, then three units would be consumed.) From an economic perspective, this is the efficient level of consumption.

So what if the health care system is inefficient? Virtually all of the units consumed in our example are medically necessary; they provide benefit to the patient. The problem is that those resources could be spent elsewhere and derive more benefit. When resources are used inefficiently, the maximum level of benefit or well-being is not being obtained. As an example, in 1970, about 7% of GDP was spent on health care and a similar proportion on education; in 1994, the proportion spent on health care had grown to 13.6%, while education remained at about 7%.[20,21] Is this an efficient use of resources? Does this maximize well-being? Given the distortions of the health care marketplace, there is room for doubt.

In summary, the health care marketplace is not like other markets: someone other than the ultimate customer makes the purchasing decision and insurance distorts the incentives facing providers and patients, resulting in more services being used, at higher prices, than would be the case in a competitive marketplace. Managed care is intended to counteract these imperfections (other than employer-paid premiums). For instance, paying providers by capitation (a specified amount per member per month), rather than fee-for-service, is designed to change the financial incentives facing providers. Working with a few "preferred" providers is an attempt to inject price competition and cost-consciousness among suppliers. Developing practice guidelines is one way to deal with the cost-dulling effects of insurance on the prescribing patterns of physicians. The role of pharmacoeconomics in the quest for efficiency is the focus of the next section.

HOW CAN PHARMACOECONOMICS INCREASE EFFICIENCY?

Given that the health care system is inefficient, how can pharmacoeconomics help correct this situation? This section discusses three alternative views of the role of efficiency in clinical (patient care) decisions. Pharmacoeconomic evaluations play a different role in each. One view is that efficiency is irrelevant and perhaps immoral in patient care decisions. This view posits that such decisions should be based only on effectiveness, and cost should not be a factor. A second view is "efficiency in treating individuals." Here, pharmacoeconomic evaluations are used to quantify costs and consequences of alternative therapies. Given the intangibility of opportunity costs in our system, it is difficult to say that any incremental benefit is not worth its associated costs. The third view is "efficiency in treating populations." Here the focus shifts from the individual patient to the entire population (those pooling their resources); resources are accepted as limited, and opportunity costs are more visible. Potentially beneficial services may be withheld from patients because the services are too costly for the benefit generated. In other words, those resources could be more beneficial for the health of the entire population if used in another endeavor. We now explore each of these views in more detail.

"Efficiency is Irrelevant (or Immoral)"

One view of efficiency in health care is that it should not be a consideration in patient care. In this view, the individual patient should receive what is best for him or her, regardless of cost. As detailed in the previous section, our system of paying for health care services has enabled us to adopt this view. Health care costs are hidden; we have deceived ourselves into believing health care resources are unlimited. Withholding or denying beneficial treatments because of cost is viewed by many practitioners and patients as immoral. The (erroneous) assumption that underlies this outlook is that resources are unlimited, and so no one is harmed by allowing individual patients unlimited use of services. But the reality is that resources are limited, and further, with pooled resources, one person's consumption of resources from the pool affects the others who contribute to the pool. In this view, there is no meaningful role for pharmacoeconomic evaluations in clinical decisions; they are seen as a detriment to quality of care.

"Efficiency in Treating Individuals"

A second view of efficiency in health care may be labeled, "efficiency in treating individual patients." In recent years, with the emphasis on cost containment and growth of managed care, this perspective has begun to supplant the perspective of irrelevance/immorality; how much is arguable. In this view, no beneficial therapies are withheld from patients, but costs and effectiveness are considered in choosing specific agents. If only one therapy is available, the tendency is to use it, regardless of its costs. The focus of concern remains the individual patient being treated. This role assumes that health care resources are unlimited (no potentially beneficial therapy should be denied), but it also assumes that resources should not be "wasted"; that is, expensive therapies should not be used when less expensive, but equally effective ones are available.

In this situation, pharmacoeconomic evaluations are used to elucidate and quantify the benefits and costs of alternative drugs, for the purpose of deciding which therapy to use in treating a particular condition. The desire is to use the most cost-effective therapy, but as we shall see, deciding which alternative is the best choice is not necessarily easy. Let us assume that three options are available to treat a condition; each has been compared to a placebo or do-nothing option, and their respective cost, effectiveness (as measured by an appropriate clinical indicator for that condition), and cost-to-effectiveness (C/E) ratios are:

- Option A: 25 units of effect; cost of $300 per patient; C/E ratio 12.0
- Option B: 20 units of effect; cost of $150 per patient; C/E ratio 7.5
- Option C: 15 units of effect; cost of $150 per patient; C/E ratio 10.0

Which option is the most cost-effective? In comparing B and C, we find that B produces more effect for the same cost; consequently, choosing B over C is relatively easy and subject to little disagreement. Moving to the comparison of A and B, the decision becomes more difficult. Option A produces more effect, but it also costs more. Option B has a lower cost-to-effectiveness ratio; it produces a unit of effect less expensively than does A. Does this—in and of itself—make B the preferred choice? Not necessarily.[22] The question that must be answered is: Is the incremental effect of A compared with B worth its incremental cost? In this case, the incremental effect of A is 5 units (25 minus 20), and the incremental cost is $150 ($300 minus $150). Expressing the question differently: Is $30 a reasonable amount to pay for an unit of improvement on this particular clinical indicator? If so, A should be chosen; if not, then B is the choice. The answer to this question is a value judgment; pharmacoeconomic analysis cannot provide the solution.

The decision becomes a bit easier, if comparisons are possible. To this end, it would be helpful if the improvement on this disease-specific clinical indicator could be extrapolated (via modeling, perhaps) to a more general measure of outcome (e.g., years of life saved, or QALYs gained). In this way, the results presented above can be compared with the cost-effectiveness of therapies for other diseases. For instance, if the 5 units of improvement result in an additional month of life, the incremental cost per life-year gained is $1800; however, if the result is 1 day of life, the incremental cost per life-year gained is $54,000. In either case, the decision of whether a year of life is worth $1800 or worth $54,000 is a value judgment.

One solution is for society (or other decision-making entity) to explicitly state the value that it places on a unit of health; in other words, to set a maximum incremental cost-effectiveness ratio that is considered acceptable.[23] This establishes what a unit of health is worth, and any therapy that produces health at or below that cost is deemed worthwhile. Continuing the above example, if $50,000 is set as the value of an additional year of life, then B is chosen, because A is too costly; but if the cut-off is $60,000, then A is the choice. A potential problem with this decision rule is that a health budget can increase as new therapies are developed that have cost-to-effectiveness ratios below the maximum. (The other way to use economic evaluations in allocating resources is to work within an overall spending limit or budget; this is discussed later.)

Again to reiterate a key point, setting a limit—whether in the form of a maximum cost-effectiveness ratio or an overall budget—requires a value judgment; analysis cannot provide the answer. In a society accustomed to focusing on the needs of individual patients and viewing costs as irrelevant in patient care decisions, it is difficult to say that any incremental benefit is *not* worth its additional cost. The results, however, are expensive—and inefficient.

"Efficiency in Treating a Population"

The third view of efficiency in health care may be labeled, "efficiency in improving the health of a population." (Again, population refers to those who pool their resources to purchase health services.) Two significant differences contrast this view from the others. First, its focus is the health of the group, rather than individual patients. In an article written several years ago but still relevant today, Howard Hiatt used a shared community pasture as an analogy for health spending.[24] Each user increased the size of his herd, and as long as the pasture could support the increased numbers, each user prospered. But each continued to increase the size of his herd, and eventually the pasture was overgrazed and ruined. With pooled resources, each individual acting in his or her own best interest may inadvertently produce negative consequences for the community. Pooling funds to buy health services is similar to the pasture.

Secondly, this view accepts the economic fact that resources are limited. The reality of limited resources is seen in the unwillingness of premium-payers and taxpayers to continuously pay more for health services. Consequently, this view emphasizes using resources efficiently so they yield the most benefit for the population. In this situation, with the recognition of limited resources and the focus on the health of the population, pharmacoeconomic analysis is a valuable tool in allocating those resources. Let us assume that a health care organization (managed care plan or Medicaid program) has a budget—a set amount of money—for services. Let us say the budget is $4000 and can be used to buy the therapies shown in Table 1-1. The table presents hypothetical cost and effectiveness data for six therapies, each used to treat a different condition. For simplicity, we will assume that each of the six was compared with a do-nothing alternative (the data are incremental data, compared with an alternative with no effectiveness and no cost). The effectiveness of all six treatments is expressed in a general, overall health status measure (again, hypothetical), labeled "health-related well-being," abbreviated "HrWb." If the goal of the organization is to maximally improve the health of its members, how should the money be spent? This becomes the question addressed by pharmacoeconomic evaluation.

Several criteria could be used in deciding how to spend the budgeted sum. For instance, priority could be given to the therapies that have the most effect on patients (i.e., those with high per-patient HrWb); if so, therapies 1, 2, and 3

TABLE 1-1.

Hypothetical Cost and Effectiveness Data for Different Therapies

	Per patient			*Total C/E*		
Therapy	*HrWb*	*Cost*	*Patients*	*HrWb*	*Cost*	*Ratio*
1	25	$300	5	125 units	$1500	12.00
2	20	$150	10	200	$1500	7.50
3	15	$150	6	90	$900	10.00
4	12	$100	15	180	$1500	8.33
5	9	$120	12	108	$1440	13.33
6	7	$50	20	140	$1000	7.14

Notes:
Each therapy treats a different condition.
Data are incremental (compared with do-nothing alternative).
C/E, cost-effectiveness; HrWb, health-related well-being.

would be chosen. In total, they cost $3900 and generate 415 units of HrWb. Alternatively, the decision could be based on the number of affected patients and therapies 6, 4, and 5 chosen, representing a total cost of $3940 and a benefit of 428 HrWb units. However, to get the most benefit from the budget, therapies should be selected by their cost-effectiveness ratios. If therapies with the lowest ratios are selected until the budget is reached, the maximum output is obtained. This is the approach used in the Oregon Medicaid program's effort to ration care.[25] Using this rule in our example, therapies 6, 2, and 4 are selected; they cost $4000 and generate 520 HrWb units. In sum, to achieve the maximum output from a given level of resources, cost-effectiveness or pharmacoeconomic data are essential.

This view of efficiency also recognizes that every therapy has an opportunity cost; that is, when resources are used for one activity, other opportunities for using those resources are foregone or lost. The health of the community is improved by moving scarce resources away from "high cost, low benefit" services to "low cost, high benefit" ones. From this perspective, some services or therapies may not be used for some conditions, even though they may benefit the individual patient, because the health of the community can be better served by spending those resources in some other fashion. Cost containment programs (formularies, practice policies) are not merely means to avoid waste, but rather means to improve quality (i.e., population-based outcomes). The health of a community is not served well by allowing individuals unlimited use of services. The efficient use of pooled resources mandates that some services are not provided, although they may be beneficial to the individual patients. Rationing—defined as denying potentially beneficial services to individuals—is necessary to improve the health of the community.

David Eddy presents a vivid example of these concepts and the relationships among them.[26] A health maintenance organization (HMO) was faced with how to use a new radiographic contrast medium; it was more expensive than its competitor, but it was associated with fewer adverse reactions. Given the potential use in the HMO, the new agent represented an additional expenditure of $3.8 million per year. The benefits derived from its use consisted of 1000 fewer patients with mild reactions; 100 fewer cases of moderate reaction; and about 40 fewer cases of severe reaction. The savings which would result by preventing these events were estimated to be $0.3 million, so the net cost was estimated at $3.5 million. The question facing the HMO was: Is the new agent "worth it"? Even though the cost exceeded the savings, health status was improved; and the ultimate purpose of health services is to improve health, not save money. At this point, the HMO was in a spot similar to that described above, where one option represents additional health, but also additional costs. To provide a comparison, the benefits that could potentially be obtained from other uses of the net cost were estimated. For instance, the $3.5 million, if spent on breast cancer screening for women aged 50 to 65, was estimated to prevent 35 deaths from breast cancer; or if used in a cervical cancer screening program,

100 cervical cancer deaths could be prevented. These figures illustrate the opportunity cost of the new contrast medium.

A dilemma, which is beyond the scope of this chapter, arises as to how the savings are spent. When a beneficial therapy is withheld, are the savings spent in some other health-producing endeavor? Or are they put in the coffers of the organization as retained earnings or profits? For some, this is particularly problematic with for-profit organizations. The relevant point here is that the resources devoted to the new contrast medium could be used in other more productive ways. This was shown through an analysis of cost and effectiveness data, and was not merely one person's opinion. Economic evaluations are capable of improving the health of the population!

Limitations

Using cost-effectiveness data to allocate resources efficiently for the benefit of the population is not without barriers or problems. Some of them are mentioned briefly here. The intent is not so much to diminish the potential benefits of pharmacoeconomic evaluations in allocating resources, but rather to alert the reader that these analyses are not a perfect, nor easy, solution to inefficiency in health care.

A couple of barriers are methodological, and others are ethical. Methodologically, it requires that all therapies be measured in the same unit of effectiveness. Secondly, the results of economic evaluations are most useful if relatively specific therapy-condition pairs are specified. If the condition-therapy pairs are too general or broad, too many exceptions arise. On the other hand, specific pairs require many analyses, each of which requires updating and revising as new knowledge is gained about a pair. Ethically, economic evaluation is a utilitarian approach to allocating resources.[27] Utilitarianism seeks the greatest good for the greatest number, but other considerations may be important in allocating or rationing health resources. For instance, equity or need may be regarded as a relevant variable in allocating resources; those with more need may justifiably have a higher priority for care than those who are less in need of care. For instance, although they are equal in additional effectiveness, is it more important for someone to get from a quality of life of 0.7 to 0.8 than someone to get from 0.9 to 1.0? Also, age (or other variables) may be relevant considerations in allocation decisions. For instance, saving the life of a newborn which results in 75 QALYs is the same output as adding 1 QALY to each of seventy-five 80-year-old persons; but are they really equal?

Regardless of the barriers, Eddy makes the point—quite convincingly, I believe—that we need not wait for the perfect data and the perfect analysis.[28] Rather, economic evaluations can be used immediately to improve the allocation of resources. In addition to the contrast medium cited above, he presents the case for moving resources away from treating high cholesterol in those with less risk of coronary heart disease and moving the resources to treating high cholesterol among those with greater risk. Similarly, the health of the population is improved if mammography resources are moved away from women in their forties to those older than fifty.[26]

Summary: Pharmacoeconomics and Pharmacy Practice

Today and in the future, health professionals must consider two factors in prescribing or recommending drug therapy that have not traditionally been considered. First, that resources are limited, and they must be spent wisely (efficiently); secondly, that health professionals are responsible for the health of a population, and not just their individual patients. In other words, the opportunity costs of their drug therapy decisions must be considered. Pharmacoeconomics can help clarify and quantify these factors.

REFERENCES

1. Eddy DM: *Clinical Decision Making: From Theory to Practice*. Boston: Jones and Bartlett, 1996, p. 126.
2. Weinstein MC, Stason MB: Foundations of cost-effectiveness analysis for health and medical practices. *New Engl J Med* 1977;296:716.
3. Eddy DM: op. cit., p. 279.
4. Bailit H: Impact of managed care on pharmacy practice and education. *Am J Pharm Educ* 1995;59:396.
5. Drummond ME, O'Brien B, Stoddart GL, et al.: *Methods for the Economic Evaluation of Health Care Programmes*, 2nd edn. New York: Oxford University Press, 1997.
6. Weinstein MC: Principles of cost-effective resource allocation in health care organizations. *Int J Technol Assess Health Care* 1990;6:93.
7. Weinstein MC, Siegel JE, Gold MR, et al.: Recommendations of the panel on cost-effectiveness in health and medicine. *JAMA* 1997;276:1253.
8. Reinhardt UE: Rationing health care: what it is, what it is not, and why we cannot avoid it. In: Altman SH, Reinhardt UE, eds, *Strategic Choices for a Changing Health Care System*. Chicago: Health Administration Press, 1996, p. 63.
9. Fuchs VR: *The Future of Health Policy*. Cambridge: Harvard University Press, 1993.
10. Aaron HJ: *Serious and Unstable Condition: Financing America's Health Care*. Washington, Brookings Institution, 1991.
11. Eddy DM: op. cit.

12. Levit K, Cowan C, Braden B, et al.: National health expenditures in 1997: more slow growth. *Health Affairs* 1998;17(6):99.
13. Evans RG, Stoddart GL: Producing health, consuming health care. *Soc Sci Med* 1990;31:1347.
14. Annas GJ: Faith (healing), hope, and charity at the FDA: the politics of the AIDS drug trials. In: Henderson GE, King NMP, Strauss RP, et al., eds, *The Social Medicine Reader*. Durham: Duke University Press, 1997, p. 375.
15. Kindig DA: *Purchasing Population Health: Paying for Results*. Ann Arbor: University of Michigan Press, 1997.
16. Adler NE, Boyce WT, Chesney MA, et al.: Socioeconomic inequalities in health: no easy solution. In: Henderson GE, King NMP, Strauss RP, et al., eds, op. cit., p. 109.
17. Levit K, Cowan C, Braden B, et al.: op. cit.
18. Eddy DM: op. cit., p. 308.
19. Reinhardt UE: op. cit.
20. Kindig DA: op. cit., p. 20.
21. Levit K, Cowan C, Braden B, et al.: op. cit., p. 100.
22. Doubilet P, Weinstein MC, McNeil BJ: Use and misuse of the term "cost effective" in medicine. *New Engl J Med* 1986;314:253.
23. Karlsson G, Johannesson M: The decision rules of cost-effectiveness analysis. *PharmacoEconomics* 1996;9(2):113.
24. Hiatt HH: Protecting the medical commons: who is responsible? *New Engl J Med* 1975;293:235.
25. Eddy DM: op. cit., p. 130.
26. Eddy DM: op. cit., p. 199.
27. Williams A: QALYs and ethics: a health economist's perspective. *Soc Sci Med* 1996;43:1795.
28. Eddy DM: op. cit., p. 279.

C H A P T E R

2

Traditional Paradigms in Pharmacoeconomics: Consideration for Cost-Effective Designs

K. C. Carriere
and
Rong Huang

INTRODUCTION

Pharmacoeconomics describes and analyzes the costs of drug therapy to health care systems and society. It identifies, measures, and compares the costs, and consequences of pharmaceutical products and services, with its research methods related to cost-minimization, cost-effectiveness, cost-benefit, cost-of-illness, cost-utility, decision analysis, and quality of life assessments. The main purpose of this chapter is to describe the traditional paradigms in phamacoeconomics to aid in drug efficacy and cost-effective studies in a cost-efficient manner.

Pharmacoeconomical analysis employs important tools for examining the impact of drug therapy and related medical interventions. One such tool is the use of optimal experimental designs and the majority of drug studies are done in randomized controlled trials (RCTs). An optimal design is a technique designed to assist a decision maker in identifying a preferable choice among many possible alternatives. Health benefits and resources used by competing health care programs are to be summarized effectively for policy makers to determine programs that accomplish a given objective at minimum cost. However, many of the statistically optimal designs that are available in the literature to help obtain valid scientific findings have certain undesirable features from a clinical and practical perspective.[1,2] In this chapter, we summarize the merits and limitations of the tools that are employed to compile and analyze the actual costs and benefits attributed to specific drug therapies.

Among the many RCT designs in medical, clinical, and pharmaceutical research, the most useful and popular design is crossover design. Many of the studies planned or conducted in support of the efficacy claims for new drugs are designed as crossover experiments.[3] For example, in a survey of numerous studies on the effects of antianxiety drugs on human performance, 68% of the studies used the crossover approach.[3]

Crossover designs are especially popular in pharmaceutical clinical trials for comparing the efficacy of several noncreative treatments. In such designs, several treatments are applied in successive periods to each experimental unit in a serial arrangement. This successive administration with different treatments has the desirable effect of providing one's own control. For example, consider the traditional 2×2 design, which is the simplest two-period two-treatment (denoted as A and B) design. Subjects are randomly assigned to the treatment sequences AB and BA. Data are then obtained over two periods on two treatments, with two observations per subject. In other words, in AB sequence, each subject receives treatment A during the first period, and treatment B during the second period; the subject's response is measured separately during each period. Generally, crossover designs have been the most feasible design of choice, when recruiting study subjects is expensive or if the response is expected to show high variability among study subjects.[4] Also, budget limitations may suggest that it is less costly to treat a subject already in the study for an additional period(s) than to recruit another subject into the study. Furthermore, experimental units may be so scarce that using them repeatedly is the only option, especially with a set time limit. Each subject in the study may require a special training period for the experiment; experimenting on the already trained subjects will save time compared with recruiting new subjects. Lastly, the investigators may have a special interest in the successive application of treatments so as to observe changes or trends over time.

Given these compelling reasons to use crossover designs, there are however concerns with how the data were analyzed and which model was used. Most of these concerns are caused by the residual or carryover effect that results from treating the same subject repeatedly.[5] Thus, the effect of a treatment in a given period can be carried over to influence the responses in subsequent periods. Often, the residual effect of a treatment may be ignorable after two periods. However, the residual effect between the responses of experimental units over two consecutive treatment periods may not be assumed negligible. Indeed, the main attraction of crossover designs requires that the residual effects from treatments be equal so that they can provide efficient within-subject estimators of direct (short-term) treatment effects by removing between-subject variations.[4,6] We note here that, statistically, the presence of residual effects does not invalidate the use of crossover designs. Rather it is the inequality of the residual effects of each test treatment that must be deliberated carefully. If the residual effects are equal for the treatments being tested, then it is statistically the same as to say that the residual effects do not exist.[5] Figure 2-1 shows the various interactions of treatment effects over time.

Apart from the methodological issues concerning how to best model the biological and chemical interactions of the treatment effects, ethicists in general apparently have less of a problem with crossover (self-controlled) designs than with completely randomized or parallel-group designs.[7] This is even more so when a trial involves treatments for patients with life-threatening conditions such as coronary artery disease. In parallel-group studies, a group of patients randomly allocated to a placebo group receives a placebo or ineffective treatment for one or more periods of time; thus, the use of such a design may seem unethical. Completely randomized designs are not as efficient, as they are not capable of providing within-subject estimators of treatment effects.

We organized this chapter in the following order. We first discuss some traditional pharmacoeconomic methodologies. Then, we discuss the statistical models for crossover designs, by separating fixed effects from random effects. Optimal designs satisfying certain criteria will follow. Next, we discuss some popular designs, that are not necessarily statistically optimal and suggest ways to maintain balance between these two notions of optimality. Other statistical issues with crossover designs will also be discussed, solutions of which are being currently developed by various investigators.

SOME TRADITIONAL PHARMACOECONOMIC METHODOLOGIES

Cost-Benefit Analysis (CBA)

CBA is a type of clinical economic evaluation of the outcomes from a program or intervention. The outcomes are measured in monetary terms by net benefits (NB = total benefits − total cost) or benefits-to-cost ratio (BCR = total benefits/total cost). Cost-benefit analysis can be conducted for a single or multiple interventions to provide foundations for decision making to achieve the desired objectives. Based on the CBA, determination on whether an intervention should be implemented and, if so, which intervention should be chosen, can be made accordingly. A complete CBA can be summarized in

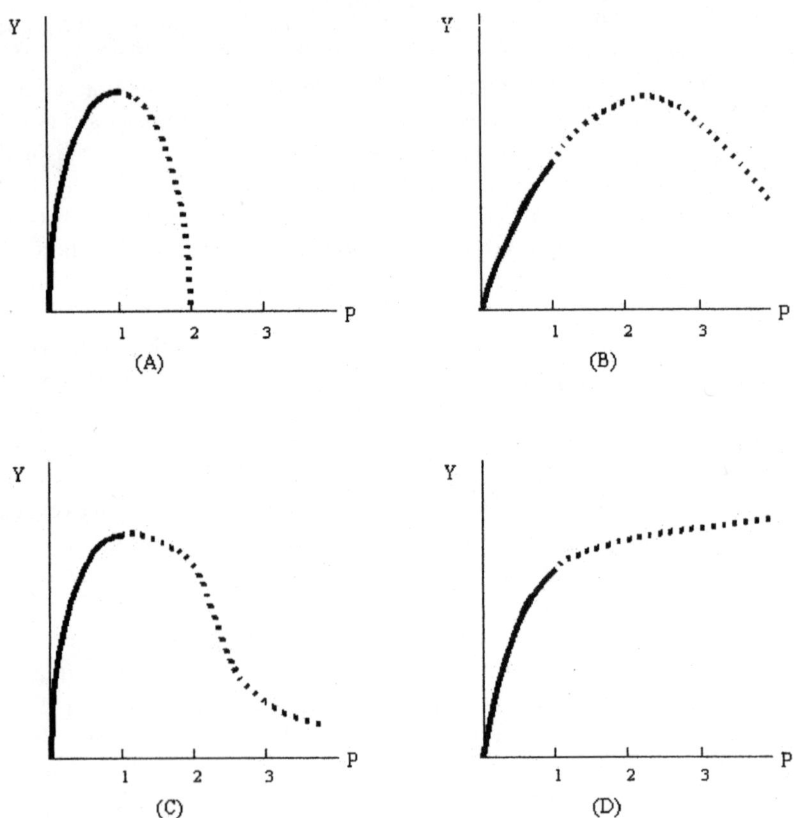

Figure 2-1. Used by permission from Bootman J, Townsend RJ, McGhan WF: *Principles of Pharmacoeconomics*, 2nd edn. W Harvey Whiteney Books Company; 1996:63. Possible patterns of treatment effects against the treatment periods separating the residual treatment effects (dotted line) and the treatment effects (solid line). Figure 2-1A portrays the ideal pattern of treatment effects; the treatment effect given in a period reaches its peak when the treatment effect is to be measured, and the residual effect gets washed out completely in the next period. Figure 2-1B portrays a poorly planned experimental situation where the treatment effect is measured before it reaches its peak. Figure 2-1C displays a pattern combining the possibilities of the uncertain treatment effects and the uncertain experimental situations shown in Figures 2-1A and 2-1B; the treatment effect is measured when it reaches its full potential but the effect of the treatment washes out rather slowly. Figure 2-1D illustrates that the treatment has a lasting and curative effect; crossover design is not a good experimental tool for such situations.

several steps, but these steps are rather basic in that all other analyses should follow as well, with slight modifications.

The first step is to state the program or the intervention to be evaluated. Such detailed questions as what are the objectives; what physician services or hospital services are involved in this program; what experiment designs are being applied for this program, etc. should be answered in advance. Also, the perspective from which the analysis is conducted is an important consideration. The cost savings or benefit may have different values from different perspectives, as a cost for one perspective may be a benefit from another perspective. For instance, staying for rehabilitation may be a benefit for rehabilitation centers, especially when they have unoccupied beds, but it is a cost for health insurers. Multiple perspectives may be included in an analysis, such as analysis from the perspective of society (combination of perspectives of patients, those of insurers, etc.). All alternatives have to be identified, with specific objectives defined for the program. A well-defined problem usually narrows the selection of alternatives.

In the second step, all resources of relevant costs and benefits have to be identified and evaluated in monetary terms. The net benefits or benefit-to-cost ratios is calculated, based on which choice of the intervention with optimum value of net benefit or benefit-to-cost ratio is followed. Investigators would like to include all costs and benefits, direct costs and benefits, indirect costs and benefits, and intangible benefits. Practically, investigators will evaluate as many benefits and costs as possible in monetary terms to obtain the net benefits and benefit-to-cost ratios.

In the third step, benefits are identified and valued. The results from step 2 are adjusted by a discount rate because the monetary values at present depreciate over time. The importance of doing adjustment increases if the positive return takes a long time.

Finally, a sensitivity analysis is needed. In practice, investigators have to estimate the values for some factors involved in the CBA—for instance, the discount rate. Will the conclusion of CBA change with the variation of the values of those factors being considered? Attention should be given to appropriately estimating those values if the conclusions change, or one should state clearly that the conclusions are sensitive to the values of those factors considered.

Cost-Effectiveness Analysis (CEA)

CEA is a method for comparing the health outcomes (effectiveness) and the net costs from a program or an intervention against other alternatives with similar health outcomes. Unlike CBA, CEA measures health outcomes in real terms not in monetary term, such as mortality, disability, or quality of life. The health outcome concerned in CEA is a single dimensional health measure. The net costs from a program or intervention are the costs for providing the program and for committing the resources for treatments after subtracting the non-health benefits from the program measured in monetary terms. Decision makers would choose the intervention that is most effective and least expensive. The basic steps for CEA are identical to those for CBA, except for a few minor modifications. In step 2, CEA evaluates the health outcomes in real terms instead of in monetary terms. In step 3, CEA requests not only to adjust for the monetary outcomes by a discount rate but also to adjust for the health outcomes in some circumstances. The adjustment of health outcomes depends on what the health outcomes are and how the values of the health outcomes change with time. The interpretation of the results from CEA will depend on the incremental cost-effectiveness ratio defined by the additional cost of an alternative relative to its additional effectiveness, or the original net costs and effectiveness.

Cost-Minimization Analysis (CMA)

CMA is a technique designed to identify the preferred choice among possible alternatives with equivalent outcomes or consequences by examining the cost associated with each of those alternatives. CMA can be regarded as a CEA when the outcomes from all interventions in the analysis are equivalent. The intervention with the least cost is the choice of decision makers. Again, the procedure of conducting a CMA follows very similarly that for CBA.

All traditional pharmacoeconomical analysis methods have a common goal in attempting to achieve the optimal outcomes most effectively and most economically. However, no specific designs have been considered. We must recognize that these approaches can lead to vastly different results on possible benefits and conclusions, unless a suitable statistical design is employed to optimize the experimental conditions. Various external influences on the experiment must also be appropriately controlled. In the next section, we examine various treatments of these external influences to the outcome using the popular crossover designs.

STATISTICAL MODELS FOR CROSSOVER DESIGNS

Models for the Fixed Effects

The most widely read statistical paper on the use of the crossover experiment in clinical trials was published in 1965.[6] Under the assumption of an additive relationship of these effects, the responses can be modeled as:

$$\text{Response} = \text{overall mean} + \text{period effects} + \text{sequence effects} \\ + \text{direct treatment effects} + \text{residual treatment effects} \\ + \text{some random effects}$$

The sequence effects are the effects analogous to column effects in a simple Latin square design; they exist in crossover design experiments in addition to direct and residual treatment effects.[8]

Some designs cannot accommodate all these effects. For example, the traditional two-period two-sequence two-treatment design cannot accommodate sequence effects in the presence of an unequal carryover effect.[5] The sequence and the carryover effects are, therefore, tested by the same test statistic in the traditional design; the test statistics for other effects in the model are highly dependent on whether or not the model includes the sequence or the carryover effects.[8]

Models for the Random Effects

"Some random effects" specified in the models above have at least three components.[9] The first can be attributed to random subject effects, which are due to random fluctuations among subjects; the second to within-subject serial correlations among repeated measurements; and the third to the random measurement errors within subjects.

This implies that each response is

$$\text{Response} = \text{true value} + \text{noise}$$

where the noise (error) may consist of

$$\begin{aligned} \text{noise} &= \text{variation between subjects} + \text{variation within subjects} \\ &\quad + \text{measurement error} \\ &= V_1 + V_2 + V_3 \end{aligned}$$

in estimating the true value using the models discussed above. Without differentiating specific model structures for fixed effects, there have been at least six different considerations in modeling approaches for estimating the parameters of main interest (e.g., direct and residual treatment effects), mainly depending on how the noise components have been treated:

(a) no subject effects and independent error model (V_3)
(b) no subject effects and dependent error model ($V_2 + V_3$)
(c) fixed subject effects and independent error model (V_3)
(d) fixed subject effects and dependent error model ($V_2 + V_3$)
(e) random subject effects and independent error model ($V_1 + V_3$)
(f) random subject effects and dependent error model ($V_1 + V_2 + V_3$)

One usual approach is (c) above, where the subject effect is assumed fixed and the experimental error is independent with zero mean and a common variance.[4]

However, when the response is measured on the same subject, introducing dependence among within-subject experimental errors is appropriate. To address such concerns, some investigators considered a random subject effects model.[1,5,6] In such a model, the subject effect and the measurement error are assumed to be mutually independent and normally distributed. The model (e) above is one of the most common models in the literature for repeated, longitudinal, or correlated data.[1,5] Note that these variance component models implicitly assume a priori that the correlations are positive. Under such model assumptions the model parameters are estimated using the generalized least squares method.[5] Simplicity is the major reason for the popularity of this approach in modeling repeated measures and, thus, correlated data. The error structure of model (e) involves two parameters—within-subject correlation and the variance of the measurement error. Depending on the prior information and the distribution about the data, Bayesian[9] or nonparametric methods[10] can also be used for the analyses.

As a possible model for serial correlations, a stationary first-order autoregressive (AR(1)) covariance structure can be used that also has two parameters (the variance of the measurement error and serial correlation in within-subject measurement). The correlation is the greatest for measurements from two adjacent periods; it decreases as the time between the two treatment periods increases. This can be accommodated by model (b), (d), or (e).

A modified AR(1) covariance structure with random subject effects has also been considered in the crossover data analyses with baseline measurements.[11] This structure is similar to the stationary AR(1) process, but observed at times $1, 2, 2 + w$, and so on; a fixed constant washout period w (typically larger than 1) between the two treatment periods is used to better fit the model.[11] In other words, if there is an intercorrelation between measurements on the same experimental unit, the correlation between measurements from before and after the treatment application in a given period is expected to be higher than the correlation between measurements from the treatment period and the baseline period. The baseline period has a washout period w following the period in which the treatment is given. If the washout period is long enough and approaches infinity relative to the treatment period, the covariance between a measurement (baseline or post-treatment) in the treatment period and a measurement in the baseline period immediately following the treatment period is equal to the variance between subjects, while that between the baseline period and the subsequent treatment period is zero. This model has been considered in the context of accommodating (b).[11]

We extend the current state of literature to include the results under model (f) with random subject effects and dependent error, where the dependency in measurements within subjects and the measurement errors will be accommodated by an autoregressive error model.

OPTIMAL TWO-TREATMENT DESIGNS

The optimal design, among a class of all designs, is the one that maximizes information by minimizing errors in the model.[5] By translating the model error into statistical power and cost, the optimal design is the one that allows investigators to conduct the experiment with maximum possible power at the minimum possible cost. Many investigators have worked at finding optimal designs for certain repeated measurement experiments.[12–14]

As optimal designs are constructed with a specific model in mind, there are various optimal designs even within the class of two-treatment designs. They are dependent upon the specific model assumptions such as the assumed error structure and the effects that are included in the model. As a result, designs which are optimal under certain model assumptions are not optimal under other models. Some optimal designs can be actually poor designs.[5,12,15]

We further note that most optimal designs may lack some practical (clinical) requirements in an experimental situation. Most such examples of some statistical optimal but practically poor designs are found especially in medical, pharmaceutical, and clinical trials where the experiments are done on human subjects. As with many other factors in such trials, the determination of an appropriate number of periods is usually based upon practical considerations. Planning a large number of periods, which means that the patients will be followed up in several experiments in many predetermined future time periods, is not feasible in practice.[1,3] Consequently, of all the RM designs, a small number of periods (two or three) two-treatment designs have been the most popular and practical to use.

One useful terminology that we will frequently use in describing designs is first defined. For two-treatment experiments, a design is defined to be dual balanced if it includes a set of two sequences where it allocates an equal number of subjects to each set of sequence (known as a sequence and its dual), where the treatments planned for one sequence are the opposite of its dual for each period.[5,12] For example, in a two-treatment experiment to compare treatments A and B, patients randomly assigned to an AB sequence will receive treatment A in the first period and treatment B in the second period. In its dual sequence BA, patients will receive treatment B in the first period and treatment A in the second period, and there are an equal number of patients allocated AB and BA sequences. Similarly, in a three-period experiment, subjects allocated an ABB sequence will receive treatment A in the first period and treatment B in the second and third periods, while subjects assigned its dual sequence BAA will receive treatment B first and treatment A in the next two periods. The number of subjects in the ABB sequence is the same as in the BAA sequence. Consideration of dual-balanced designs simplifies the estimation and testing of hypotheses considerably. In repeated measurements designs, the possibility of subject dropouts and noncompliance should also be taken into consideration. We will deal with this possibility in our discussion of optimal designs.

We will consider the following designs under the more general model given in (f) earlier. Specifically, we used the model accommodating random subject effects under an autoregressive error model.

DESIGN I : AB, BA
DESIGN II : AB, BA, AA, BB
DESIGN III: AA, BB
DESIGN IV : ABB, BAA
DESIGN V : AAA, BBB
DESIGN VI : ABB, BAA, AAA, BBB
DESIGN VII : ABB, BAA, AAB, BBA
DESIGN VIII : ABB, BAA, ABA, BAB

All the designs we consider are dual-balanced designs; that is, we assume that if *n* number of subjects are allocated in one sequence, there is a dual sequence that has an equal number of subjects allocated. Some features or problems of the designs listed above are noteworthy.

Two-Period Designs

DESIGN I is the optimal design only under no carryover effect.[5] For this design to be useful, the assumption of no residual effects is crucial or baseline measurements must be available.[6] The reason is that in the presence of unequal residual effects, the treatment effect contrast uses the first period of measurements only and, therefore, the design does not utilize the main advantage of within-subject comparison of treatment effects in crossover designs.[5,6] Further, it does not use the data obtained in the second period. In other words, the popular two-sequence design suffers from the lack of estimability on statistical grounds. The unbiased estimator for the direct treatment effect contrast from DESIGN I using the first period data only is not more efficient than the estimator from a completely randomized design, since the within-subject variations are not removed. Also, failure to use the readily available information (second period data) has been a major drawback in a two-period two-sequence crossover design when the residual effects cannot be assumed to be non-existent. To alleviate the problems in the traditional two-period design, Grizzle[6] suggested that a test of no residual effect be done at a higher significance level if the assumption of equal carryover effects is in doubt. If rejected, the estimator of the direct treatment effect contrast should be based on the first period data only. However, the problems of inadequate power in testing for equal carryover effects was shown in Grizzle's method.[3] Others found that the amount of carryover effects that makes completely randomized designs preferable is quite substantial and thus unlikely to exist.[16] Also, some investigators claimed that the criticism should be limited to two-period designs only and recommended the continuing use of repeated measurement designs with or without the assumption of equal residual effects for its own merit.[1] Another recommendation to resolve the problem of lack of power found in tests of equal carryover effects is to use baseline measurements.[5]

DESIGN II is the universally optimal design. It contains two additional treatment sequences where subjects are given the same treatments in both periods.[5,12] Although statistically optimal, this design has not received much attraction in practice. The optimal DESIGN II for two-period experiments in the presence of residual effects will assign an equal number of subjects to each of the four treatment sequences: AB, BA, AA, and BB. However, despite the number of researchers supporting this design on the basis of statistical optimality, clinicians have been reluctant to use subjects twice with the same treatment whose efficacy is unknown. Also, if there are no (i.e., equal) carryover effects, then the two-sequence (AB and BA) design is optimal and use of large numbers of subjects for the AA and BB sequences will be highly inefficient.[5] Therefore, a modification to this statistically optimal design to produce a completely symmetric design has been considered[5] by allowing unequal allocation of subjects to AA and BB sequences that is disproportionately smaller than that to AB and BA sequences. Such designs have been constructed so that their efficiencies are not affected much by uncertain presumptions about the absence of residual treatment effects. Therefore, the resulting designs are relatively robust.[5] For example, allocating 70% of the subjects to AB and BA sequences and only 30% to AA and BB sequences results in fairly high efficiency (e.g., 0.89 for direct treatment effect contrast when the within-subject correlation is 0.75), and is preferable to the two-sequence design.[5] That is, the modified design is not perfect, but it can perform to at least 89% of what the optimal design can offer.[5] When there are no carryover effects, the optimal allocation is the two-sequence design. Equal allocation to all four sequences in the absence of carryover effects would result in an efficiency of only 0.57 for the same situation relative to the optimal design.[5] However, even in this situation, allocating 70% of the subjects to AB and BA sequences results in a moderately high efficiency of 0.74.[5]

DESIGN III is the parallel group two-period two-treatment design. Quite naturally, DESIGN III is the optimal design, if the primary parameter of interest is in estimating the residual effects, but the worst in estimating the direct effect of test treatments.

Three-Period Designs

For three-period designs, there are eight possible sequences to consider: AAA, AAB, ABA, ABB, and their duals. To keep the experiment manageable, Carriere[1] considered the four designs enumerated earlier as DESIGNs IV, VI, VII, and VIII. We consider here DESIGN V; i.e., the three-period parallel group design. DESIGNs IV–VIII are three-period two-treatment designs that are found to be optimal by one or more investigators. Having one more period also opens up other possibilities such as an increased number of treatment sequences and an increased chance of having large dropouts and noncompliance. For example, one can consider the entire eight treatment sequence design. However, such a design may suffer from missing data problems and difficulties in following the subjects according to the protocol, due to ethical, experimental, administrative, and other reasons.[1,3] Problems of noncompliance are often found in a planned, controlled clinical trial. For example, consider the situation where the treatment sequences such as ABA and BAB are to be used. Some patients may develop a strong preference for one treatment over another after being treated with two distinct treatments. At the third period, they may not comply to the trial protocol; they may request the other unplanned treatment or they may simply drop out. These issues must be taken into consideration in constructing truly optimal designs. We first review the properties of the three-period designs listed above.

DESIGN IV is the universally optimal design under an equicorrelated covariance structure within the class of all three-period designs for estimating the direct treatment effects.[13,15] Under a first-order autoregressive error model with fixed subject effects, however, the optimal design depends on the value of the autoregressive coefficient.[17] For a positive autoregressive coefficient, it has been shown that DESIGN IV remains "nearly" optimal among three-period designs, except for values of the autoregressive coefficient close to 1 or 1.[17]

DESIGN V is the parallel group three-period two-treatment design, that has not been found to be optimal under the usual model (c); however, this may be because most work to date has been concerned with positive correlations in within-subject measurements. Our work will not restrict the correlation to positive. These two sequences appeared first in Kershner,[18] when he considered various three-period designs under several possible models; the treatment sequences AAA or BBB are seen to gain their usefulness under a model that includes both the first- and second-order residual effects.

DESIGN VI is a combination of DESIGNs IV and V. Therefore, this design will gain strength if the model being considered is that of equal correlation error with no or fixed subject effect and a second-order residual effect is expected.

DESIGN VII was considered by Carriere.[1] She recommended the DESIGN VII as a "nearly" optimal three-period design that maintained balance between statistical power and clinical factors. Carriere[1] observes that, in three-period designs, there is essentially no difference and almost no loss in efficiency if the sequences beginning with AA and BB are included. Including these, however, is helpful for experiments where a high level of dropouts and noncompliances appear inevitable after the second period. The relative performance of the various three-period designs has been shown to depend on the nature of the residual treatment effect[1] as much as it does on the form of the error structure.[17,18] The rather widely publicized[8,13,15] optimal three-period DESIGN IV is optimal under a very narrow class of model assumptions, namely in the absence of residual effects or in the presence of only the first-order residual effects.[1] DESIGN VII can be modified to be statistically nearly optimal to the universally optimal DESIGN IV. DESIGN VII was in fact better than DESIGN IV under other models when multiplicative or second-order residual effects were considered and performed very competitively under various models.[1] Here, the second-order residual effects are the treatment effects that last up to two periods beyond the treatment period. Also, Carriere[1] highlighted the fact that it will reduce to be the universally optimal DESIGN II when the third period suffers from severe dropouts and noncompliance. DESIGN VII is also shown to be the optimal design when the autoregressive coefficient is moderately negative. Under the autoregressive error model, when the autoregressive coefficient is high (0.4), the universally optimal design allocates subjects to AAB and BBA sequences.[17] Carriere[1] suggested an unequal allocation of subjects with a much smaller number of subjects to AAB and its dual. Her suggestion which was primarily based on what is desirable in practice applies to the optimal design under no subject effect with the first-order autoregressive error model; the optimal design was found to be DESIGN VII, with over 90% of the subjects allocated to the sequence AAB and its dual.[15]

DESIGN VIII was considered by Ebbutt,[19] fully acknowledging its statistical inferiority. Undesirability of using the sequences ABB and BAA alone in three-period designs has been discussed by Ebbutt,[19] who preferred the use of ABB, ABA, and their duals to DESIGN IV, while admitting the statistical inferiority of the chosen design. His rejection of the use of the sequences AAB and BBA does not seem well justified, as discussed by Carriere.[1] Unless carefully designed, even the multi-period designs may not be well protected against a large proportion of dropouts or the curtailment of the experiment after the second period, in which case the investigator can be left with data from the problematic two-period design.[1]

None of the three-period designs are protected against the severe dropouts in the third period, except DESIGN VII and DESIGN VI.

Multi-Period Designs

Multi-period designs extending more than three periods were also extensively constructed, but most of these are dual-balanced designs for comparing two treatments.[4,12,13,17] For example, under an equicorrelated error model the design consisting of the sequences ABBA, AABB and their duals is universally optimal for four-period design.[15] This design is optimal under an autoregressive error model only when the autoregressive coefficient is less than or equal to 0.42;[17] when it is higher than 0.42, only ABBA and its dual are used in the optimal design.[17]

COST-EFFICIENCY COMPARISONS

One major reason for using repeated measurement designs may be the possible cost savings. As mentioned earlier, most often the cost of recruitment of a subject is more expensive than the cost of treatment of a subject already in the trial.[4] However, as there are rather wide selections of possible optimal designs, which vary from one model assumptions to another, it is only natural to question the implication of these model assumptions on costs. In order to appreciate the economics of the various crossover designs, we performed relative cost comparisons to that of completely randomized and parallel group designs. The experimental costs were separated into two components: S_0 for the cost of recruiting a new subject and S_1 for the cost of treating a recruited subject in a given period. For ease of comparisons, these costs will be assumed here to be the same for both the crossover designs with n subjects and the completely randomized designs with m subjects. Thus, the total costs for the trial are

$$\text{Cost} = \text{cost for recruiting subjects} + \text{cost for treating subjects}$$

and equivalently

$$S_{CO} = snS_0 + psnS_1 \quad \text{and} \quad S_{CR} = 2mS_0 + 2mS_1$$

with subscripts CO and CR denoting crossover and completely randomized experiments, respectively. The relative costs defined as

$$R = S_{CO}/S_{CR}$$

will be examined upon selecting the n and m subjects in such a way that the treatment effects are estimated with equal precision.

Brown[3] compared the two-period designs and concluded that the cost of the crossover experiments relative to the completely randomized experiments depends on two ratios: the ratio of between-subject variation to within-subject variation and the ratio of the cost of treating a patient for one period relative to that of recruiting the patient into the study.[3] A large recruiting cost (small S_1/S_0) and a large variation between subjects argue against the completely randomized experiment and favor the crossover experiment.[3] However, these early results are based on the assumption that the residual effects are nonexistent, which leads to the conclusion that crossover experiments should not be used when there are unequal carryover effects.[3] Furthermore, none of the available recommendations that was meant to resolve the practical and statistical problems in two-period design appeal to clinicians, when coupled with the necessary assumption of no carryover effects. This fact motivates the need for a new investigation of the extent of cost savings possible in crossover designs under a more general model as given in (f) for various designs.

Tables 2-1 and 2-2 illustrate the cost-efficiency comparisons in two- and three-period designs, respectively. The values tabulated are the relative cost of crossover designs to completely randomized designs. If the goal is to compare with parallel group designs, one can simply divide the relative cost of a design by that of parallel group DESIGNs III and V for two- and three-period experiments, respectively. In both situations, note that R approaches 0 (large savings possible by using crossover or repeated measurement design) as S_1/S_0 approaches 0 (large recruiting costs), as the level of autoregressive coefficient increases to be positive, and as the between- and within-subject variation ratio

TABLE 2-1.

Relative Cost of Two-Period Designs to Completely Randomized Designs for Two-Treatment Clinical Trials

	Autoregressive coefficient				
S_1/S_0	*−0.8*	*−0.4*	*0*	*0.4*	*0.8*
(a) DESIGNs I and III					
1/10	0.56	0.32	0.30	0.32	0.56
1	0.94	0.55	0.50	0.55	0.94
10	**1.33**	0.77	0.70	0.77	**1.33**
(b) DESIGN II					
1.10	0.26	0.16	0.13	0.11	0.12
1	0.45	0.27	0.21	0.19	0.20
10	0.63	0.37	0.30	0.27	0.29

The entries correspond to the efficiencies when the ratio of between- and within-subject variance is 1.

Adapted from Bootman J: *Pharmacoeconomics*, 2nd edn. New York: McGraw-Hill; 1996.

TABLE 2-2.

Relative Cost of Three-Period Designs to Completely Randomized Designs for Two-Treatment Clinical Trials

	Autoregressive coefficient				
S_1/S_0	*−0.8*	*−0.4*	*0*	*0.4*	*0.8*
(a) DESIGN IV					
1/10	0.09	0.06	0.05	0.05	0.05
1	0.16	0.11	0.09	0.08	0.08
10	0.23	0.15	0.13	0.12	0.11
(b) DESIGN V					
1/10	0.32	0.30	0.30	0.32	0.53
1	0.54	0.51	0.50	0.53	0.90
10	0.27	0.19	0.16	0.14	0.13
(c) DESIGN VI					
1/10	0.14	0.10	0.09	0.08	0.08
1	0.24	0.17	0.15	0.13	0.14
10	0.34	0.25	0.21	0.19	0.19
(d) DESIGN VII					
1/10	0.06	0.06	0.05	0.05	0.04
1	0.11	0.10	0.09	0.08	0.07
10	0.15	0.14	0.13	0.12	0.10
(e) DESIGN VIII					
1/10	0.11	0.08	0.07	0.06	0.05
1	0.19	0.13	0.11	0.10	0.09
10	0.15	0.14	0.13	0.12	0.10

Note: See footnote to Table 2-1.

gets large. The numbers in bold face in Table 2-1 indicate the situations where completely randomized designs may be the best economically.

In the more traditional DESIGN I, under the no residual effect assumption, and restricted to the situation of a positive within-subject correlation, Brown[3] concluded that the crossover designs are favored, perhaps, unfairly. Our investigation on this design under a more general model indicates that the cost is an increasing function in S_1/S_0, and became non-competitive when the cost for treatment administration exceeds that for recruitment. Note also that our comparison does not assume an equal carryover effect, as in Brown.[3] Under an unequal carryover effect, the direct treatment effect contrast uses only the first period. This is reflected in the relative cost comparison, with the increasing cost being associated with the increasing autoregressive coefficient in absolute value. The parallel group DESIGN III produced essentially identical results to those in DESIGN I, because in the two-period DESIGNs I and III in the presence of residual effects, the treatment effect contrast use only the first-period data. This can also be observed in Carriere and Reinsel,[5] by setting the autoregressive coefficient at zero.

DESIGN II was constructed as the universally optimal design among all two-period designs, where less popular sequences AA and BB are used. We find that its optimality remains unchanged under the model (f) and also when compared with the completely randomized designs. The cost savings increase with decreasing treatment costs relative to those of recruitment. Our investigation demonstrates that an overwhelming level of cost savings is attainable by the use of crossover designs in many situations, even in the presence of unequal residual effects under the usual model of (b), (c), or (e). This is seen readily by setting the autoregressive coefficient at zero.

Table 2-2 compares the five three-period crossover designs under the autoregressive error model with random subject effects. In general, Table 2-2 indicates that use of the three-period design will result in great cost savings, contrary to what others have suggested, even when the within-subject correlation is negative. Among these, DESIGN VII suggested by Carriere[1] maintained its strengths overall. Recall that when the autoregressive coefficient is zero, the universally optimal design is known to be DESIGN IV. The results for DESIGNs IV and VII for zero autoregressive coefficient are shown as identical when we reported rounded numbers at the third decimal points. In fact, the relative costs for DESIGN IV were slightly smaller than those for DESIGN VII, as seen in Carriere.[1] DESIGN VII's superiority is followed by DESIGN IV, DESIGN VIII, DESIGN VI, and then DESIGN V. Except when the autoregressive coefficient is extremely large even in DESIGN V, crossover designs are shown to be excellent in saving the cost involved. Again, we find that designs including sequences that have AA and BB in the first two periods are better than others, because of the presence of residual effects. Crossover designs seem to be the design of choice, even when the within-subject correlation is negative.

In summary, large recruiting cost and large between-subject variance are the factors determining the cost savings from crossover experiments. We also considered the case when recruiting subjects in a crossover design was twice as costly as that in completely randomized experiments, but the impact was rather minimal. Cost savings of these designs relative to those of parallel group designs is evident by comparing the two- and three-period designs to DESIGNs III and V, respectively.

In general, crossover designs performed much better than the completely randomized designs or the parallel group designs. When the correlation is negative, the cost savings are heavily dependent on the factor S_1/S_0. That is, when the recruitment costs are much smaller than the treatment costs, negative within-subject correlation in the repeated measurements appears to have significant implications for the use of crossover design. However, in situations where recruitment costs outweigh treatment costs, crossover design seems to be the design of choice even when the within-subject correlation is negative. This finding reinforces the recommendation of using the statistically "nearly" optimal DESIGN VII with sequences ABB, BAA, AAB, and BBA, balanced with optimal statistical and practical considerations,[1] which appears to be the optimal design under the model with random subject effects and an autoregressive error model.

SUMMARY

The objective of investigating theoretically optimal designs is to provide a tool for identifying efficient and practical devices for the experiment.[2] However, the practical factors that have not been considered in construction of optimal designs have generally eliminated their ready adoption by practitioners. Some designs that are optimal under certain model assumptions are not optimal under other models. In fact, some were found to be poor designs in practice. This chapter reviewed some practically desirable crossover designs with special application to pharmacoeconomic drug testing trials. Particular attention was given to the cost-effectiveness of some selected designs under a general model allowing one extra noise component than that typically considered. In repeated measurement designs, there can be three sources of random variations, while optimal designs have mainly considered one or two components only. Our goal has been to examine and verify the optimality of some of the popular designs.

Cost savings and statistical power of the crossover designs have been examined. For two-period experiments such comparisons were made in 1980.[3] However, the findings are limited because the investigation was limited to a situation with no residual effects for the traditional two-period two-sequence two-treatment design; this design is optimal only when there are no residual effects.[1] Therefore, the earlier results and recommendations apply only to two-period experiments when the residual effects can be safely assumed nonexistent.

We examined the eight designs under the model that includes random subject effects and the serial correlation with the measurement error term. One of the primary objectives has been to investigate if the efficiency of crossover designs can be maintained under the model that allows for a negative correlation between measurements within subjects. Concern has developed over the use of crossover designs when a negative within-subject correlation is possible.

Clinicians have been advised that crossover designs should not be used in such a situation.[7]

We once again concluded that the benefit of using crossover designs is tremendous. This was found even when the correlation is negative, especially when the cost of recruiting a new patient exceeds that of treating each patient. However, we note that the comparisons made are from a purely statistical point of view without considering other possible clinical factors.

In many clinical and pharmaceutical trials, crossover designs continue to be the most useful designs of choice in spite of criticisms raised by many authors.[20–22] When the problems of two-period designs become apparent, other possibilities are available. Such an alternate regulatory strategy includes adopting extended multi-period designs. However, planning a large number of periods, which implies that the patients will be followed up in several experiments in many predetermined future time periods, is not feasible in practice. Consequently, some optimal two- to four-period designs have received considerable attention in the literature.

For two-period experiments, not many options are possible.[1–3] The best strategy seems to adopt the dual-balanced design with an unequal allocation as discussed by Carriere and Reinsel[5] with or without baseline measurements.

For three-period experiments, several recommendations are given for optimal designs that differ depending upon various inclusions of experimental and other effects in the model. The common feature of an optimal (statistically as well as clinically) design appears to be the design that includes a sequence that has AA and BB in the first two periods. This finding is in general accord with the available results[1,2] that were concluded under considerations slightly different from the current one. We find DESIGN VII to be "nearly" optimal under various models. The variety of models studied so far includes consideration of multiplicative treatment effects, presence of second-order residual effects, and a negative within-subject correlation in responses.[1,2,5]

ACKNOWLEDGMENTS

This work was funded in part by a grant from Natural Sciences and Engineering Research Council of Canada. The first author is a National Health Scholar with the National Health Research and Development Program of Health Canada (6609-2120-48) and a Heritage Senior Scholar with the Alberta Heritage Foundation for Medical Research (AHFMR). The second author is funded in part by a Studentship award from the AHFMR.

REFERENCES

1. Carriere KC: Crossover designs for clinical trials. *Stat Med* 1994;13:1063–1069.
2. Carriere KC: Regulatory affairs in biotechnology: optimal statistical designs for biomedical experiments. *Biotechnology Annual Review*, Volume 4, MR El-Gewely, ed. 1998;215–238.
3. Brown BW: The crossover experiment for clinical trials. *Biometrics* 1980;36:69–79.
4. Hedayat A, Afsarinejad K: Repeated measurements designs I. In: Jones J, ed., *A Survey of Statistical Design and Linear Models*. New York: North-Holland, 1975.
5. Carriere KC, Reinsel G: Investigation of dual-balanced crossover designs for two treatments. *Biometrics* 1992;48:1157–1164.
6. Grizzle JE: The two-period changeover design and its use in clinical trials. *Biometrics* 1965;21:467–480.
7. Cleophas TJM, Tavenier P: Fundamental issues of choosing the right type of trial. *Am J Therap* 1994;1:327–332.
8. Kershner RP, Federer WT: Two-treatment crossover designs for estimating a variety of effects. *J Am Stat Assoc* 1981;76:612–618.
9. Grieve AP: A Bayesian analysis of the two-period crossover designs for clinical trials. *Biometrics* 1985;41: 979–990.
10. Koch GG: The use of non-parametric methods in the statistical analysis of the two-period change-over design. *Biometrics* 1972;28:577–584.
11. Wallenstein S, Fleiss JL: The two-period crossover design with baseline measurements. *Comm Stat Theory Meth* 1988;17:3333–3343.
12. Laska EM, Meisner M, Kushner HB: Optimal crossover designs in the presence of carryover effects. *Biometrics* 1983;39:1087–1091.
13. Cheng C, Wu C: Balanced repeated measurements designs. *Ann Stat* 1980;8:1272–1283.
14. Cochran WG, Cox GM. *Experimental Designs*, 2nd edn. New York: Wiley, 1957.
15. Laska EM, Meisner M: A variational approach to optimal two-treatment crossover designs: Application to carryover-effect models. *J Am Stat Assoc* 1985;80:704–710.
16. Willan AR: Using the maximum test statistic in the two-period crossover clinical trial. *Biometrics* 1988;44:211–218.
17. Matthews JNS: Optimal crossover designs for the comparison of two treatments in the presence of carryover effects and autocorrelated errors. *Biometrika* 1987;74:311–320.
18. Kershner RP: Optimal 3-period 2-treatment crossover designs with and without baseline measurements. *Proc Biopharmaceut Sec Am Stat Assoc* 1986;152–156.

19. Ebbutt AF: Three-period crossover designs for two treatments. *Biometrics* 1984;40:219–224.
20. Fleiss JL: On multiperiod crossover studies—letter to the editor. *Biometrics* 1986;42:449–450.
21. Fleiss JL: A critique of recent research on the two-treatment crossover design. *Controlled Clin Trials* 1989;10:237–243.
22. Jacobs P. Economic dimensions of the healthcare system. In: *The Economics in Health and Medical Care*, 3rd edn. Gaithersburg, MD: Aspen, 1991:47–48.

C H A P T E R

3

The Role and Use of Outcomes Assessments

Amy Grizzle
and
Edward P. Armstrong

BACKGROUND: GROWING INTEREST IN OUTCOMES RESEARCH

Factors Leading to Outcomes Research

The current "outcomes movement" originated in the 1950s and 1960s in response to the rapid growth in hospitals, physicians, and medical technology in the United States. Health insurance plans that freely reimbursed medical expenses contributed to this explosion in health care costs. Within two decades of the creation of Medicare, US health care costs rose from 4% to over 11% of the gross national product.[1]

These changes in health care systems prompted third-party payers to re-evaluate reimbursement practices. During this time, there was growing concern regarding the quality and outcomes of medical care. Investigation revealed unexplained variability in medical practice (e.g., use and frequency of medical procedures and medications) across the United States. These geographical variations were not accompanied by differences in patient outcomes.[1] In other words, increased use (and cost) of medical technologies in some areas was not producing improvements in patient care. These variations became widely publicized and eventually came under the scrutiny of health care regulators, third-party payers, the media, and the general public. One researcher, Wennberg, concluded that variations in medical practice occur due to a lack of consensus regarding the indications for medical procedures.[2] Furthermore, he found that decisions to use a particular intervention were rarely based on the knowledge of anticipated outcomes.

Response to Rising Health Care Costs

Much attention was focused on cost-containment strategies in the 1980s. Methods for reducing health care costs included the use of generic drugs, development of formularies, therapeutic substitution, fixed fees for services, shortened hospital stays, and the use of less expensive procedures and medications.[3]

Outcomes research became the focus of medical evaluation largely because of the costly variations in utilization that resulted from such a lack of consensus in the medical community. Additionally, a discipline of health economics surfaced in which models were developed to assist decision makers in this process of selecting drugs and therapies. The goal was to find treatments that enabled the goals of therapy to be met at the lowest possible cost.

In summary, the factors contributing to the rise of outcomes research include:

- the unexplained variation in medical practice due to insufficient information about the effectiveness of common medical treatments;
- the need to control the escalating cost of health care; and
- the trepidation that cost-containment activities would lead to sacrifices in the quality of health care.

DEFINITION

Outcomes research is the field of study describing the ultimate (final) health events that occur as a result of a condition or its treatment.[4] Stated differently, outcomes research is the process by which health care interventions are evaluated in order to measure the extent to which a goal of therapy can be reached.[3] The outcomes movement is described not as a new type of clinical study but rather as a new emphasis on the traditional study methodology. Outcomes identified in the literature as relevant for patients include economic, clinical, and humanistic outcomes.[4] Outcomes have been broadened beyond the traditional clinical measures to include those that are financial (encompassing resource utilization and cost of care) and those that are more patient-focused (such as quality of life (QoL), symptom control, functional status, activities of daily living, knowledge, behavior, and satisfaction).

One classic list of outcome measures comprised the five Ds: death, disease, disability, discomfort, and dissatisfaction.[5] Several of these Ds reflect a patient's QoL, which is one measure of focus when evaluating patient-centered (or humanistic) outcomes. Addition of a sixth D (dollars) produces a comprehensive list of measures to assess outcomes of medical interventions.[6]

The types of outcomes typically measured can generally be grouped into three categories:[7]

- clinically-based outcomes
- patient-based outcomes
- cost-based outcomes.

Clinical Outcomes

Traditional medical evaluation centers around the assessment of clinical outcomes, such as

- reduction in blood pressure
- cure rate for breast cancer
- healing time for duodenal ulcers
- prevention of migraine headache.

While these measures remain important indicators of treatment success, outcomes research has shifted the focus from solely evaluating clinical outcomes. For example, although blood pressure reduction is a treatment goal, the true outcome desired is a reduction in cardiovascular events, such as myocardial infarction. Outcomes research has brought attention to the ultimate treatment goal, minimizing intermediate endpoints as a definition of treatment success. Obviously, for conditions such as cardiovascular disease, where the ultimate outcome (prevention of myocardial infarction) is not immediately measurable, intermediate endpoints serve as a surrogate for the treatment goal. Wherever possible, however, clinicians and researchers should emphasize final outcomes experienced by patients as the true measure of an intervention's value.

Patient-Based Outcomes

Patients should play an integral role in making medical decisions and judging the results of treatment. After all, it is the patient being treated—not the organ, disease, or condition. Too often, interventions are aimed only at achieving clinical endpoints, such as a lowering of blood glucose or cholesterol level. Although these clinical endpoints may be a sound measure of disease progression, they are not reflective of the ultimate goal of therapy—improving the patient's overall health and well-being.

Measuring patient-centered outcomes addresses the need to evaluate medical treatments based on the attributes important to patients. Patient outcomes include measures such as

- impact of asthma on patient QoL
- post-surgical pain assessment
- patient preference for oral compared to intravenous therapy
- satisfaction with amount of information provided
- functional status following myocardial infarction
- impact of Parkinson's disease on activities of daily living.

These patient-centered measures will be described in more detail in another section.

Economic Outcomes

Economic outcomes point to the health care resources utilized to produce a particular health outcome. These resources include items such as prescription medications, physician visits, and pharmacist and nursing time to prepare and administer medication, laboratory tests, hospital stays, surgical procedures, etc. Additionally, costs associated with adverse events and treatment failures are considered economic outcomes. Indirect costs such as work loss can also be included when assessing the economic impact of interventions.

Examples of economic outcomes include:

- decreased length of hospital stay for patients with catheter-related sepsis
- reduction in visits to the emergency room for patients with asthma
- prevention of skilled nursing facility placement for patients with Alzheimer's disease
- decreased nursing time to administer intravenous antibiotics for infection
- reduction in adverse drug effects requiring additional treatment
- improvement in days lost from work due to back pain.

Economic outcomes can be measured in several ways. Units of resource use may be collected and assigned a monetary value based on costs or charges of a specific institution or from national averages. This method of data collection is useful because costs from various sources may be substituted, making the results more generalizable to other practice settings. Medical resource use can be determined via patient self-report (patient questionnaires or interviews), prospective physician reports, medical charts, or billing records. Although more labor intensive, chart review is typically more accurate than self-report due to recall bias. Prospective collection is desirable, but takes longer to complete than a retrospective assessment of resource utilization. Medical chart review is very effective when dealing with a single provider or medical system whereby all medical services are recorded. When patients have multiple providers it becomes very difficult to ensure that all resource use has been identified and captured. Computerized records simplify the chart extraction process, but still require computer programming support and can be labor intensive depending on the data structure and format. Proper collection and costing of medical resource data requires careful and thoughtful consideration.

Outcomes measurement must take into account economic considerations while recognizing that acceptable clinical and humanistic outcomes are also important objectives. The true value of health care interventions, programs, and policies can be assessed only if all three dimensions of outcomes are measured and considered.

DIFFERENCE BETWEEN PHARMACOECONOMICS AND HEALTH OUTCOMES RESEARCH

Health outcomes research is a broad term encompassing a variety of possible endpoints resulting from treatment. These outcomes could include measures such as morbidity, mortality, quality of life, cost, etc. Pharmacoeconomics refers to that subset of outcomes research dealing specifically with economic and/or humanistic outcomes of drug therapy.

One could view pharmacoeconomics as a key outcomes management tool since it goes beyond traditional clinical measures of efficacy to include effectiveness and efficiency issues. The tools of pharmacoeconomics enable decision makers to understand the true total costs of medical interventions and provide information to assist in the improvement of patient care.

PATIENT-CENTERED OUTCOMES

Quality of Life

Patient QoL should be an important criterion in determining the success of medical interventions. Although there is no standard definition for QoL, several authors have attempted to describe its meaning. For example, Cramer and Spilker define QoL within the framework of the World Health Organization (WHO) definition of health.[8] The WHO defines health as "a state of complete physical, mental and social well-being and not merely the absence of disease or infirmity."[9] Cramer and Spilker broaden this definition to include other aspects of one's personal life that affect health through stress, anxiety, or other emotions. Schron and Shumaker define QoL as "a multidimensional concept referring to a person's total well-being including his or her psychological, social, and physical health status."[10] While QoL evaluation includes all aspects of a patient's life, such as the quality of the living environment, work conditions, relationships, etc., health-related QoL refers specifically to those areas influenced by personal health. Because only health outcomes will be discussed, the term QoL will be used to refer to health-related QoL throughout this chapter.

An exhaustive review of QoL taxonomy, methodology, instruments, analysis techniques, etc., is beyond the scope of this chapter. Entire books have been authored on the subject for those who desire more in-depth study.[11–15] Instead, the basic types of QoL instruments and how they are used as outcomes measures will be discussed.

Measuring QoL offers a way of evaluating and monitoring treatment effects that are important to patients. Commonly measured dimensions of QoL include:[16]

- physical functioning
- social and role functioning
- mental health
- general health perceptions.

QoL instruments are typically used to collect and quantify this information. Quality of life questionnaires can be divided into different categories, the two most common being generic (or general) and disease-specific.[17] Another method to quantify patient QoL is via utility (or patient preference) measurement. These three approaches to measuring patient QoL (generic, disease-specific, and utility measures) are discussed below.

Generic QoL instruments

Generic instruments are designed to assess QoL across all patient populations, regardless of disease, treatment, or patient demographics. Examples of commonly used generic questionnaires include:

- Medical Outcomes Study (MOS) Short Form-36
- Quality of Well-Being Scale
- Sickness Impact Profile.

Generic instruments are very popular in part because they are widely used and accepted by the research, medical, and regulatory communities. Although comparisons may be made between patients with different conditions, generic instruments may lack sensitivity to capture changes in patient outcomes. For example, a patient suffering from rheumatoid arthritis may experience great improvement in hand dexterity following drug treatment. Generic instruments are designed to measure broad domains of QoL applicable to many patients (such as physical functioning, role functioning, mental health). Although this improvement in hand dexterity may greatly impact the patient's QoL, the questions posed in the generic questionnaire may not be specific or detailed enough to demonstrate this important life change.

Disease-specific QoL instruments

The above example leads us to the purpose of disease-specific instruments: to provide greater detail regarding distinct outcomes resulting from a particular health condition or disease. A disease-specific instrument for rheumatoid arthritis should include an assessment of hand dexterity, and would probably detect the QoL improvement experienced by the patient. Because disease-specific instruments focus on particular conditions, they do not afford the opportunity to compare QoL impacts among patients with different diseases. Additionally, disease-specific questionnaires do not typically evaluate the overall impact of interventions on QoL.[18] For this reason, it is advisable to include both a generic and a disease-specific instrument in studies evaluating treatment alternatives.[19]

Utility-based instruments

Utility is a measure of value or worth placed on a particular health state or condition.[20] Utility is measured on a scale from 0 (death) to 1 (perfect health) and is generally based on the preferences of society or people at risk for the health state being evaluated. Utility measures are necessary for calculating quality-adjusted life years (QALYs), a common outcome used in cost-utility analysis. QALYs incorporate both quantity and quality of life, and can be a key outcome in diseases where treatment can greatly affect patient functioning and well-being (e.g., cancer).[19] For example, consider a drug that extends a patient's life by 10 years, but causes undesirable adverse effects during these extended life years, such as nausea, depression, and headaches. An alternative medication may also extend life by 10 years in the absence of untoward effects. Without incorporating QoL, these treatment interventions would be considered equal; i.e., they both add 10 years of life. Because quantity and quality of life are both important considerations, QALYs are a valuable outcome in many instances.

There are various methods for measuring utility, the most common of which include:[21]

- visual analogue scale
- standard gamble
- time trade-off

Visual analogue scale Measuring utility on a visual analogue scale (or rating scale) is the simplest of the three methods discussed. A visual analogue scale looks like a thermometer, marked from 0 (death) at the bottom to 100 (perfect health) at the top (Figure 3-1). The respondent is given a description of a health state and is then asked to mark a line on the scale representing how they feel about that health state relative to the endpoints (death and perfect health).

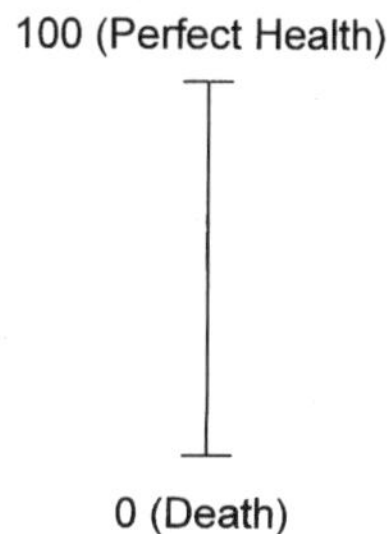

Figure 3-1. Visual analogue scale.

Multiple health states can be evaluated and placed on the rating scale, reflecting the patient's preference for the conditions compared with one another as well as death and perfect health.

Standard gamble The standard gamble poses a choice between two alternatives: choice A—living in health state i (a chronic condition between perfect health and death) with certainty; choice B—taking a gamble on an intervention with an uncertain outcome (Figure 3-2). The respondent is told that the intervention has a probability of p to restore perfect health, and a probability of $1 - p$ to result in immediate death. The subject chooses between this gamble or remaining in a health state less desirable than perfect health. The probabilities are varied until the respondent is indifferent between the choices A and B. For example, if a subject is indifferent between the alternatives when the probability $(p) = 0.60$, the utility of the health state i is 0.60.

Time trade-off Like the standard gamble, the time trade-off offers a choice between two alternatives; but instead of choosing between a gamble and certainty, the respondent is asked how much time they are willing to trade to remain in perfect health. Figure 3-3 represents the time trade-off for a chronic

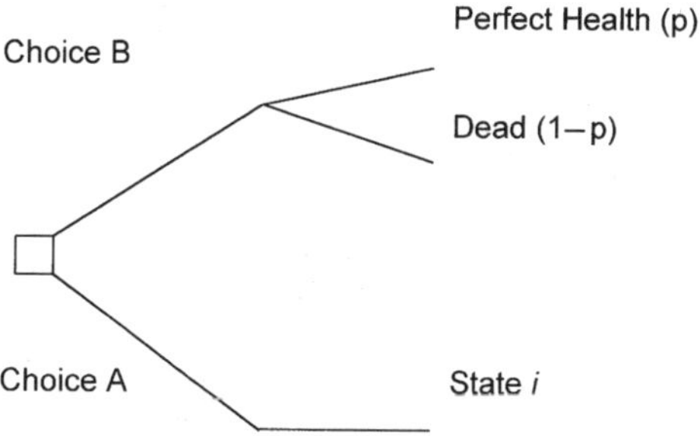

Figure 3-2. Standard gamble for a chronic health state, where $i =$ chronic condition; $p =$ probability of achieving perfect health.

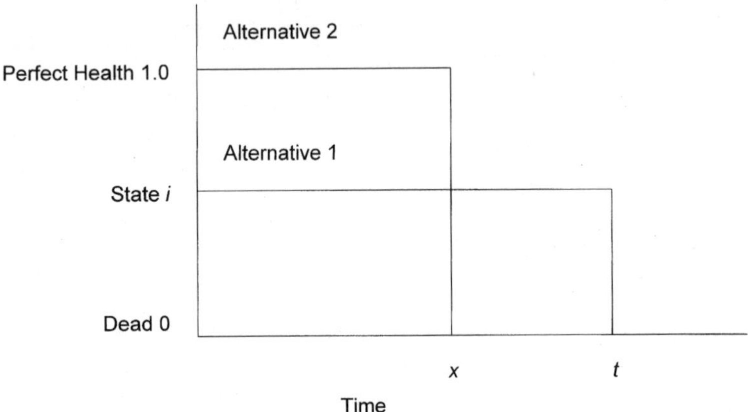

Figure 3-3. Time trade-off for a chronic health state $hi = x/t$, where i is the chronic health condition, t is the amount of time spent with the chronic condition, and x represents the time when the respondent is indifferent between the two alternatives.

condition. To determine the preference or value (h) for a particular health state, the respondent is given a choice of living for a specified time (t) in health state i (chronic condition between perfect health and death), or perfect health for time x. Times x and t are followed by immediate death. Time x is varied until the subject is indifferent between the choices ($hi = x/t$). In other words, the respondent is indifferent when he feels that living a certain amount of time with a chronic disease is the same as living x amount of time in perfect health. For example, a subject may indicate that having severe depression for 10 years is the same as having perfect health for 4 years. Therefore, the value of that health state (severe depression) would be 0.4 ($hi = 4/10$).

Patient satisfaction

The concept of outcomes assessment has been broadened to include patient satisfaction as a further indicator of quality in the assessment of medical care.[22] Satisfaction measures are commonly used in clinical settings to gauge physician and/or institution performance. Despite the wealth of literature addressing patient satisfaction, there is still debate regarding the best methods for assessing such a subjective outcome. Use of these measures should encourage patients to become involved in the decisions regarding their medical care. Outcomes research has shown that patients make very different treatment choices when given accurate, unbiased information about the risks and benefits of an intervention; i.e., patients vary in the values they place on treatment alternatives and potential outcomes. Again, patient satisfaction measures are a tool that can be used to enrich the patient–provider relationship and open the lines of communication.

EFFICACY VS. EFFECTIVENESS

The distinction between efficacy and effectiveness is an important one when examining outcomes. Efficacy relates to how well a treatment or intervention performs under ideal circumstances, e.g., within the framework of a randomized controlled clinical trial. Effectiveness refers to performance in a real world setting, when factors such as compliance and patient selection may not be closely monitored. When assessing outcomes, it is preferable to use measures of effectiveness if possible. This is more reflective of the true outcomes that will be experienced once a therapy or service is approved and in use. Effectiveness data are not always available, as is the case during drug development or soon after drug approval. In this instance, efficacy data may be used as a proxy for effectiveness information. Sensitivity analysis can then be employed to estimate the impact of differences in outcomes that might be attributed to differences between efficacy and effectiveness.

APPLICATIONS OF OUTCOMES RESEARCH

Outcomes research can provide a wealth of information and can be used for several purposes. Outcomes data are useful in evaluating the effectiveness of health care interventions. As previously mentioned, adding patient-centered and economic outcomes to the traditional assessment of clinical outcomes provides a comprehensive assessment of treatments or services. Giving patients and providers more information on which to base treatment decisions will result in improved care and patient satisfaction. In addition to assessing new interventions, outcomes information can be used to evaluate improvement after policy changes have been implemented. Repeated assessment is necessary to ensure that benefits are maintained and therapy goals are being achieved. Outcomes data may also be used to support and understand research conclusions. This is the type of information that health care providers and third-party payers need to make decisions regarding patient care and policy development. Formulary committees are beginning to incorporate outcomes measures (such as cost-effectiveness and QoL) in their decision-making process. With third-party payers assuming more authority for drug purchases, pharmaceutical companies now need to provide additional evidence of drug benefits, including better cost-effectiveness ratios and improvements in QoL compared with competitors. Outcomes research, therefore, becomes an important aspect of new product development, as pharmaceutical companies need to demonstrate more than clinical benefits. Outcomes research can provide valuable information and have a great impact on health care decisions. Finding appropriate uses will be the key to its value in medical decision making.

FUTURE ROLES OF OUTCOMES RESEARCH

Ellwood has suggested that the outcomes movement will continue to grow and develop, relying on four existing techniques.[23] First, Ellwood suggests that a greater reliance on treatment guidelines and standards will lead to greater consistencies in physicians' practices and measurement techniques. The MOS was a first attempt to create standardization in the way outcomes are defined and measured; it was a 2-year observational study designed to assess the impact of specific aspects of medical care on patient outcomes. The aims of the study included (1) establishing a relationship between variations in patient outcomes with differences in health care systems, clinician training and practice style, and amount of resource utilization, and (2) developing more practical tools for routine assessment of patient outcomes. The MOS included such outcomes as clinical endpoints; physical, social and role functioning; patient perceptions of their general health and well-being; and satisfaction with treatment. Valuable information was learned about the impact of various chronic diseases on patient functioning and well-being. Government support of outcomes research has been demonstrated by mandating the Agency for Health Care Policy and Research (AHCPR) to determine outcomes associated with selected disease areas that impact the large patient population supported by the government. The AHCPR has created inter-disciplinary research teams to examine the effectiveness and appropriateness of medical interventions that affect the survival, health status, and QoL of patients. Results from large studies such as these will help pave the way in selecting standard outcomes to assess specific conditions, and in recommending appropriate methodologies.

Secondly, Ellwood suggests a systematic approach to measuring patient outcomes (such as well-being and QoL) at routine intervals will assist physicians in adopting these practices and incorporating these measures in the medical decision-making process. Integrating QoL measures, for example, into routine medical examinations would enhance physician awareness and provide opportunities for conversations with patients based on the impact of treatment in their daily lives. Customary use of these measures would also help physicians habitually consider patient-based outcomes when selecting or evaluating treatment options. Additionally, this attention to patient well-being could certainly enhance the physician–patient relationship. Educating physicians in the administration and interpretation of QoL and functional status tools would be the key factor to successfully implementing these types of outcome measures in routine practice.

Thirdly, Ellwood suggests that pooling clinical and outcomes data on a large scale will broaden the scope and use of outcomes information. Using an epidemiological approach could assist in achieving these goals of expanding the usefulness of outcomes research. This would include attempting to collect longitudinal data on large groups of patients, and improving and maintaining large computerized databases. Currently existing disease management strategies could serve as a model for applying guidelines to large groups of patients. In essence, the goal is to achieve an optimal outcome in the greatest number of people possible.

Finally, Ellwood suggests outcomes data will be analyzed and disseminated based on the information most appropriate to the concerns of each decision maker. This is critical if outcomes data are to be incorporated in the decision-making process. The perspective of individual decision makers (such as federal government, hospitals, managed care organizations, etc.) must be addressed in order to impact the way care is provided.

The future of outcomes research depends on the successful implementation of these steps described by Ellwood. They should provide a framework for continuously evaluating and improving patient outcomes in light of medical advancements, changing patient expectations, and resource allocation needs.

EXAMPLES OF OUTCOMES STUDIES

Outcomes research covers a broad range of study types and methods for evaluating the success of medical interventions. A variety of outcomes can be assessed in determining the value of procedures, therapies, and services. The following section provides an overview of some different types of outcomes that have been included in research studies. Several studies from the literature have been selected and summarized briefly to show how different interventions can best be evaluated. The review is not meant to be exhaustive, but rather to give a flavor of the breadth of this field of study. Additional detail regarding study methodology, target population, sample size, etc., is included in Table 3-1.

TABLE 3-1.

Examples of Outcomes Studies in the Medical and Pharmacy Literature

Author
Year
Title
Study type
Population
Sample size
Time period
Outcomes measured
Results expressed as
Primary study results

Case Study 1

The impact of clinical pharmacy services on the care of hospitalized patients was evaluated in a study by Bjornson et al.[24] Clinical pharmacists participated in two of five medical teams and in one of three surgical teams. The authors compared teams that received pharmacy services with those having no clinical pharmacist support. Outcomes evaluated included:

- hospital length of stay
- mortality
- drug cost per hospital admission

One-year data showed that clinical pharmacists had a positive impact on patient outcomes. Teams receiving pharmacy services reported shorter hospital stays, lower drug cost per hospital admission, but no difference in mortality compared with teams without pharmacist involvement. Using pharmacist salaries and estimating time spent in providing clinical services to the medicine and surgery teams, the cost-benefit of the program was calculated. Pharmacist participation resulted in savings of $377 per admission, with a benefit:cost ratio of 6.03:1 (i.e., for every dollar spent on clinical pharmacy services, $6.03 was saved) leading to a net annual return on investment of nearly $151,000. The authors concluded that clinical pharmacist involvement in health care teams was cost-effective and provided beneficial outcomes for the hospital.

CASE STUDY 1

Cost-benefit analysis (CBA) of the effect of pharmacists on health care outcomes in hospitalized patients

All in-patients cared for by general medical or surgery team
3081
1 year
Length of stay, drug cost per admission, mortality
Cost savings, benefit:cost ratio
Clinical pharmacists shorten patient length of stay, lower drug cost per admission, and have no effect on mortality rates. Pharmacists saved $377 per admission, with a benefit:cost ratio of 6.03:1.
Bjornson et al.[24]

Case Study 2

A cost-benefit analysis (CBA) was performed to evaluate the impact of a *Hemophilus influenzae* type b (Hib) vaccination program for small children in Spain (Jimenez et al.[25]). The number of children requiring vaccination was estimated along with the costs and savings associated with providing this program. Outcomes (which are all converted to dollars in CBA) measured in the study included:

- (Costs): cost of program, including costs for vaccine dose, storage, nursing training and administration time, adverse reactions caused by vaccine.
- (Benefits): savings associated with cases of disease prevented by vaccination program.

With an average incidence of 15 cases of invasive disease per 100,000 children, the program would prevent 219 cases of disease and 8 deaths over a 5-year period. Programs costs were estimated at $19.3 million. Program savings were estimated at $17.3million, with a net program cost of approximately $2 million. These figures yield a benefit:cost ratio of 0.89, meaning that for every dollar spent on the vaccination program, $0.89 were regained (a loss of $0.11 per dollar). The authors concluded that a universal vaccination program would be cost saving for annual incidence rates greater than 20 cases of invasive disease per 100,000 children. Furthermore, decreasing the cost per vaccine dose could result in cost savings for areas with lower incidence rates.

CASE STUDY 2

Cost-benefit analysis (CBA) of Haemophilus influenzae *type b vaccination in children in Spain*

All children aged 1 or under in Spain

383,883

5 years

Cost of vaccine program, cost savings of cases prevented

Benefit:cost ratio

Program costs exceeded benefits by about $2 million, resulting in a benefit:cost ratio of 0.89:1. For areas of Spain experiencing > 20 cases per 100,000, the program would be cost saving.

Jimenez et al.[25]

Case Study 3

Direct medical charges were measured to examine the effect of diabetes on medical resource use in the year following myocardial infarction.[26] Resource use was compared between patients with and without diabetes and included the following outcomes:

- total medical charges, including:
  - length of hospital stay
  - number of outpatient visits
  - medication use
  - number of emergency room visits.

The mean charge for initial hospitalization for myocardial infarction was higher for patients with diabetes than for those without the disease ($15,394 vs. $12,730). Patients with diabetes also incurred greater medical charges (including initial hospitalization) in the year following myocardial infarction ($26,414 vs. $18,577). Hospitalizations accounted for 88% of these charges. The authors concluded that patients with diabetes experience higher medical charges at the time of myocardial infarction as well as during the year following the event. This information may be helpful in conducting cost-effectiveness analyses for therapies designed to manage diabetic patients who experience myocardial infarction.

CASE STUDY 3

Direct medical charges associated with myocardial infarction in patients with and without diabetes

Cost analysis

Inner city patients with and without diabetes who experience myocardial infarction

293:87 with diabetes and 206 without diabetes

1 year

Direct medical charges for hospital stay, outpatient visits, drugs, and ER visits

Total differences in medical charges

Patients with diabetes experienced greater charges at the time of myocardial infarction as well as during the year following the event.

Smith et al.[26]

Case Study 4

Cost-utility analysis was used to evaluate second-line antibiotics for the treatment of acute otitis media in children.[27] Success rates and adverse events were compared among commonly used second-line agents (cefaclor, amoxicillin-clavulanate, and erythromycin-sulfisoxazole). This safety and efficacy information was used to assess the utilities (preferences) for treatment with various outcomes. The outcomes measured in this study included:

- treatment success and failure
- adverse events of treatment
- overall cost of treatment
- utility assessment for each health state
- quality-adjusted life day (QALD).

Using decision analytic modeling, cefaclor was the preferred treatment, given its lower overall cost ($108 for cefaclor vs. $119 and $120 for amoxicillin and erythromycin, respectively) and higher QALDs (28.15 for cefaclor vs. 27.98 and 28.03 for amoxicillin and erythromycin, respectively).

CASE STUDY 4

A cost-utility analysis (CUA) of second-line antibiotics in the treatment of acute otitis media in children

Children from 2 months to 18 years visiting family MD or clinic for acute otitis media

Decision analysis model used

30 days

Treatment success and failure, AEs, cost of treatment, utility, QALD

Cost differences, quality adjusted life days (QALDs), cost/cure, cost/QALD

Cefaclor had lower overall costs ($108 for cefaclor vs. $119 and $120 for amoxicillin and erythromycin, respectively). Cefaclor also had higher QALDs (28.15 for cefaclor vs. 27.98 and 28.03 for amoxicillin and erythromycin, respectively).

Oh et al.[27]

Case Study 5

A cost-effectiveness analysis was performed to compare two asthma treatments (formoterol vs. salmeterol).[28] Outcomes measured included:

- number of asthma episode-free days
- number of patients reaching a clinically relevant QoL improvement
- total treatment costs including:
  - medications
  - number of physician visits
  - length of hospital stay
  - number of emergency room visits
  - number of lung function tests and other tests
  - travel costs
  - work loss.

There were no differences in 6-month treatment costs between the groups ($828 with formoterol and $850 with salmeterol) or in QoL scores based on the St. Georges Respiratory Questionnaire. Additionally, with both treatments, about 60% of all days were episode-free. Average costs per episode-free day were approximately $9 in both groups. Costs per patient improving in QoL ranged from $1300 to $1400. The authors concluded that the drugs were equally cost-effective.

CASE STUDY 5

Cost-effectiveness analysis (CEA) of formoterol versus salmeterol in patients with asthma

Patients from randomized, open-label study in six European countries

482

6 months

Medical costs, number of episode-free days, number of patients with improved QoL

Cost per episode-free day, cost per patient improving in QoL

Formoterol and salmeterol had similar costs, QoL improvements, and episode-free days

Both treatments had average cost of $9 per episode-free day, and between $1300 and $1400 per patient improving in QoL.

Rutten-van Molken et al.[28]

Case Study 6

A study was conducted to assess whether QoL scores could be used as a predictor of mortality following coronary artery bypass graft (CABG) surgery.[29] Patients completed the Short-Form 36 (SF-36), a generic QoL questionnaire, prior to the CABG procedure. The outcomes measured included:

- all-cause mortality within 6 months following CABG
- QoL scores on Short-Form 36 (SF-36).

Within 6 months of the CABG surgery, 117 (4.7%) patients died. The physical component of the SF-36 was a statistically significant predictor of mortality (after adjusting for known risk factors for mortality post-CABG). Scoring 10 points lower on the SF-36 physical component corresponded with an odds ratio of 1.39 (95% confidence interval, 1.11–1.77; $p = 0.006$) for predicting mortality. The SF-36 mental component was not predictive of 6-month mortality in this patient population. The authors concluded that assessment of the SF-36 physical component prior to CABG surgery could be helpful for clinical decision making and patient management.

CASE STUDY 6

Health-related quality of life as a predictor of mortality following coronary artery bypass graft (CABG) surgery

QoL

Subset of patients from Veterans Affairs study assessing CABG surgery

2480

6 months

All-cause mortality 6 months after CABG surgery, SF-36 QoL scores

Odds ratio (QoL as predictor of mortality)

The physical component of the SF-36 was a predictor of 6-month mortality following CABG surgery. A 10 point lower score had an odds ratio of 1.39 (95% CI 1.11–1.77; $p = 0.006$). The SF-3 mental component was not a predictor of mortality following CABG surgery.

Rumsfeld et al.[29]

SUMMARY AND CONCLUSIONS

The interest in health outcomes and pharmacoeconomics has grown significantly in recent years. Health systems, such as managed care organizations and hospitals, are now frequently involved in collecting outcomes data in their own patient populations. There has been tremendous growth in research in these areas. It is very important to investigate variability in medical practice and determine the most cost-effective treatments. To accomplish this objective, it is critical to examine the range of outcomes including clinical, economic, and patient-centered outcomes. Important outcomes have been broadened beyond only clinical measures to include economic outcomes (e.g., encompassing resource utilization and cost of care) and patient-focused outcomes (e.g., quality of life, symptom control, functional status, activities of daily living, knowledge, behavior, and satisfaction). It is also essential to note that the interest in health outcomes analysis has emphasized the importance of effectiveness research in addition to efficacy data. Formulary committees in health systems now frequently want to know the likely implications on health outcomes when they assess new treatment options. Treatment guideline development and dissemination are natural results from outcomes analyses in health systems. In order to conduct these research projects, it will be important to have participation from a range of professional disciplines, improved data collection capabilities, and enhanced computer information systems. To make better decisions, these research projects will be data intensive and require expertise from a range of professionals. The ability to make improved decisions utilizing health outcomes data will continue to drive the demand for additional research on these topics.

REFERENCES

1. Relman AS: Assessment and accountability: the third revolution in medical care. *N Engl J Med* 1996;319:1220–1221.
2. Wennberg JE, Roos N, Sola L, Schori S, Jaffe R: Use of claims data systems to evaluate health care outcomes: mortality and reoperation following prostatectomy. *JAMA* 1987;257:933–936.
3. Basskin LE: *Practial Pharmacoeconomics: How to Design, Perform and Analyze Outcomes Research.* Cleveland: Advanstar Communications; 1998.
4. Kozma CM, Reeder CE, Schulz RM: Economic, clinical, and humanistic outcomes: a planning model for pharmacoeconomic research. *Clin Ther* 1993;15:1121–1132.
5. Lohr KN: Outcome measurement: Concepts and questions. *Inquiry* 1988;25:37–50.

6. Kleinman J: The physicians new agenda. In: Zander K, ed., *Managing Outcomes Through Collaborative Care*. Chicago, IL: AHA Press, 1995; p. 45.
7. Johnson NE, Nash DB (eds): *The Role of Pharmacoeconomics in Outcomes Management*. Chicago: All American Hospital Publishing, Inc.; 1996.
8. Cramer JA, Spilker B: *Quality of Life and Pharmacoeconomics: an Introduction*. Philadelphia: Lippincott-Raven; 1998.
9. World Health Organization. *Basic Documents: World Health Organization*. Geneva, Switzerland: World Health Organization; 1948.
10. Schron EB, Shumaker SA: The integration of health quality of life in clinical research: experience from cardiovascular clinical trials. *Prog Cardiovasc Nurs* 1992;7(2):21.
11. Spiker B (ed.): *Quality of Life and Pharmacoeconomics in Clinical Trials*, 2nd edn. Philadelphia: Lippincott-Raven; 1996.
12. McDowell I, Newell C: *Measuring Health: A Guide to Rating Scales and Questionnaires*, 2nd edn. Oxford, Oxford University Press; 1996.
13. Patrick DL, Erickson P: *Health Status and Health Policy: Allocating Resources to Health Care*. Oxford, Oxford University Press; 1993.
14. Bowling A: *Measuring Health: A Review of Quality of Life Measurement Scales*, 2nd edn. Philadelphia: Open University Press; 1997.
15. Bowling A: *Measuring Disease*. Philadelphia: Open University Press; 1995.
16. MacKeigan LD, Pathak DS: Overview of health-related quality-of-life measures. *Am J Hosp Pharm* 1992;49:2236–2245.
17. Patrick DL, Deyo RA: Generic and disease-specific measures in assessing health status and quality of life. *Med Care* 1989;27:S217–S232.
18. Coons SJ, Kaplan RM: Assessing health-related quality of life: application to drug therapy. *Clin Ther* 1992;14:850–858.
19. Coons, SJ: Health outcomes and quality of life. In: Dipiro JT, Talbert RL, Yee GC, et al., eds, *Pharmacotherapy: A Pathophysiologic Approach*, 3rd edn. Stamford: Appleton & Lange; 1997.
20. Drummond MF, Stoddart GL, Torrance GW: *Methods for the Economic Evaluation of Health Care Programmes*. New York: Oxford University Press; 1987.
21. Revicki DA: Relationships between health utility and psychometric health status measures. *Med Care* 1992;30:MS274–MS282.
22. Schulman KA, Johnson AE, Rathore SS: The use of satisfaction measures in oncology. In: Perry MC, ed., *Educational Book*. Denver: Americal Society of Clinical Oncology 1997;337–341.
23. Ellwood PM: Outcomes management: a technology of patient experiences. *N Engl J Med* 1988;319:1197–1202.

24. Bjornson DC, Hiner WO, Potyk RP, Nelson BA, et al.: Effect of pharmacists on health care outcomes in hospitalized patients. *Am J Hosp Pharm* 1993;50:1875–1884.
25. Jimenez FJ, Guallar-Castillon P, Terres CR, Guallar E: Cost-benefit analysis of *Haemophilus influenzae* type b vaccination in children in Spain. *Pharmacoeconomics* 1999;15(1):75–83.
26. Smith TL, Melfi CA, Kesterson JA, Sandmann BJ, Kotsanos JG: Direct medical charges associated with myocardial infarction in patients with and without diabetes. *Med Care* 1999;37:AS4–AS11.
27. Oh PI, Maerov P, Pritchard D, Knowles SR, Einarson TR, Shear NH: A cost-utility analysis of second-line antibiotics in the treatment of acute otitis media in children. *Clin Ther* 1996;18:160–182.
28. Rutten-van Molken M, van Doorslaer EKA, Till MD: Cost-effectiveness analysis of formoterol versus salmeterol in patients with asthma. *Pharmacoeconomics* 1998;14(6):671–684.
29. Rumsfeld JS, MaWhinney S, McCarthy M, Shroyer ALW, et al.: Health-related quality of life as a predictor of mortality following coronary artery bypass graft surgery. *JAMA* 1999;281:1298–1303.

C H A P T E R

4

Principles of Drug Literature Evaluation

William W. McCloskey

INTRODUCTION

With the increasing emphasis on cost in today's health care environment, pharmacists and other health care providers often find themselves needing to consult the medical and pharmacy literature for economic information related to drug therapies. This information may be used to make decisions concerning selecting of drugs for an organization's formulary, in developing disease state management programs, or in determining the most appropriate agent for a particular patient's medical condition. The pharmacoeconomic literature can also provide documentation as to how various pharmacy services compare in terms of costs and outcomes; therefore, it may be useful in making choices regarding what new programs to implement. Consequently, the ability to access pharmacoeconomic information is very important for a variety of clinical and administrative decision makers. However, one not only needs to have adequate drug information resources available to research information on pharmacoeconomics but one also must be able to appropriately evaluate the information after it has been retrieved. This chapter provides an overview of the types of sources most often used for obtaining economic information on drug therapies and discusses a systematic approach to evaluating the pharmacoeconomic literature.

INFORMATION RESOURCES

Drug information resources are organized into three classifications: tertiary, secondary, and primary. All three categories of resources may be helpful in researching information related to pharmacoeconomics, and for completeness, more than one may need to be consulted. The appropriate use of each of these resources requires an understanding of their relative advantages and disadvantages.

Tertiary Resources

Tertiary resources include textbooks, review articles, and computerized databases such as Micromedex® and Clinical Pharmacology®. These types of resources provide general overviews of a subject based on information that is compiled from previously published work. Consequently, tertiary literature does not provide new information on a subject. Because of their general availability, these are usually the references consulted initially in any drug information search.[1] The tertiary references, especially textbooks, also have advantages that include ease of use, compactness, and conciseness.[1] They are especially helpful in providing some general background on a subject that one may not be very familiar with. For example, if one is conducting a pharmacoeconomic analysis of drug therapy for a disease that may not be very common, one could consult an appropriate medical text to find more information about that particular condition.

Despite their advantages, tertiary information resources do have some significant limitations. Because of the publication cycle, the material may not be the most current. There may be a significant lag period, even years, between the time a textbook is written and when it is actually published.[1] Consequently, the publication date of a book may not accurately reflect how up to date the information is. In researching pharmacoeconomic issues, one is generally most interested in current information on new therapies, practice guidelines, and other areas where textbooks may not provide the latest information. To determine the timeliness of the material in a textbook, one should always evaluate the dates of the references used to compile the chapters. Although the textbook may be the most recent edition, if the chapter references are several years old, the material may be outdated.

Compared with hard copy, computerized full-text versions of textbooks are more frequently updated, and therefore are more likely to have the latest information on a topic. Computerized tertiary drug information databases such as Micromedex® are also regularly updated, and may provide more current information than that available in textbooks. In addition to the references cited, one should still check the most recent date that a particular section of the database was revised to determine if the information is current.

Another limitation of the tertiary literature is that the information presented is from the viewpoint of the author(s) of the chapter. Therefore, there is the potential that the author(s) could introduce a bias in the interpretation of the literature reviewed for the chapter. Individuals who reference their own published works too frequently may not be providing an objective perspective of the subject matter. In addition, the author(s) may have conducted an incomplete literature search in preparing the chapter or text, and therefore may not have included all the relevant information.[1] Therefore, in addition to assessing how current the information is, evaluation of the chapter references will give the reader an idea of the quality and nature of the material used to compile the chapter.

Since review articles are generally published in professional journals, they may not be initially considered as tertiary literature. One may think of journal articles as synonymous with primary literature. However, as are the chapters in any book, review articles are overviews and are subject to the same limitations as any tertiary reference. Since journals are published on a relatively frequent schedule (e.g., weekly or monthly), the information in a review article is likely to be more current than that in a textbook.

Many reviews are narrative in nature, and just provide an overview of subject, such as a review of a new drug or disease state. A more informative review is a *systematic* review, which focuses on answering a specific question. For example, is once a day dosing of a medication as effective for the treatment of a condition as multiple daily dosing? Systematic reviews employ a careful screening of the quality of the literature included in the review to provide the best evidence to answer the particular question that is addressed.[2] For instance, the review may only include well-controlled clinical trials to base a conclusion.

One type of systematic review is a meta-analysis. A meta-analysis is a *quantitative* systemic review that pools the data from previously conducted studies on a subject, that as a whole are inconclusive, and treats the pooled data as an independent study. By increasing the overall sample size through pooling, a meta-analysis may be able to detect statistically significant differences between treatment groups that were previously not reported. While some have questioned the merits of meta-analyses as a research tool,[3] they are considered a valuable source of evidence when clinical trials have been unable to provide a definitive answer to a question. Because they are "studies of studies," these quantitative reviews may be considered primary and not tertiary literature.

In summary, one often consults the tertiary literature for drug information because of its availability and ease of use. While tertiary references may provide valuable background information regarding matters related to pharmacoeconomics, this type of literature has limitations that generally require one to consult other types of drug information resources.

Secondary Resources

Secondary information systems include indexing and abstracting systems of the primary literature. When one is looking for the most current information on a specific topic, these systems provide an efficient means for searching the health care literature. Indexing systems provide only bibliographic information (e.g., title, journal, author), while abstracting services provide brief descriptions, or abstracts, of the information contained in a specific citation.[1] Ideally, one should access the primary reference itself, since abstracts alone may not provide adequate information. Certainly, one would never purchase a home based only on a brief description of the property in a real estate brochure! Similarly, one should not make a health care decision based only on an abstract from a secondary system. Since each secondary system differs in the nature and type of the journals indexed, it may be necessary to use more than one for an optimal literature search. Although it is beyond the scope of this chapter to describe the various secondary resources in detail, a brief review of those that may be especially helpful for researching pharmacoeconomic topics follows below.

MEDLINE

Perhaps the most recognized secondary system for researching the biomedical literature is MEDLINE. MEDLINE is produced by the National Library of Medicine and is one of the Medical Literature Analysis and Retrieval System (MEDLARS) collection of over 40 databases.[4] MEDLARS includes other databases such as AIDSLINE, CancerLit, and TOXLINE. MEDLINE is a computerized version of *Index Medicus* and includes nearly 10 million references to 3900 biomedical journals going back to 1966.[5] Approximately 75% of the references cited in MEDLINE include English abstracts.[5] MEDLINE is indexed using a controlled vocabulary called Medical Subject Headings (MeSH), and therefore requires some basic searching skills in order to use it most effectively.[6] Although it is available free of charge on the Internet (www.nlm.nih.gov), one may purchase MEDLINE interfaces from commercial vendors that help navigate individuals through the search process more easily.

Despite the large number of journals it indexes, MEDLINE includes relatively few pharmacy-oriented journals. Therefore, one may need to consult other secondary systems when researching certain subjects related to pharmacoeconomics.

Embase

Embase is a secondary system produced by Elsevier, Amsterdam, the Netherlands. It is similar to MEDLINE in scope and structure, but it is more international in nature. The database covers approximately 3500 journals from over 100 countries.[7] Consequently, if one is looking for published studies regarding a drug where most of the research has been conducted outside the United States, Embase may have citations on that particular agent that may not be in MEDLINE. However, Embase is considered relatively expensive, and therefore may not be readily available in many organizations.

International Pharmaceutical Abstracts (IPA)

IPA is produced by the American Society of Health-System Pharmacists (ASHP). Unlike MEDLINE and Embase, this secondary system focuses primarily on pharmacy literature, including international pharmacy journals. The database abstracts approximately 800 journals going back to 1970.[7] IPA also includes abstracts of presentations at ASHP and other major pharmacy meetings that may provide useful pharmacoeconomic information. While these meeting abstracts are not very comprehensive, they do provide author contact information, such as an e-mail address, that may be useful for follow-up and networking. Since it emphasizes the pharmacy literature, IPA would be the secondary resource of choice when researching information on pharmacy practice related topics (e.g., cost-benefit analysis of a pharmacist-coordinated anticoagulation clinic).

Iowa Drug Information Service (IDIS)

IDIS is produced by the Iowa Drug Information Service at the University of Iowa. It is specific for human drug therapy, and includes pharmacoeconomic subject matter. IDIS contains published information from over 180 biomedical journals.[1] One of the advantages of IDIS is that the user has access to the full text of the article. Although limited in scope compared with other secondary systems, IDIS would be a valuable resource if one did not have a large collection of health care journals readily available.

In addition to these secondary resources, there are a number of other indexing and abstracting systems that may be useful for obtaining drug information as well. Table 4-1 summarizes some of the most important aspects of some of these secondary information resources.

To summarize, given the tremendous volume of health care related journals, secondary indexing and abstracts resources are a very valuable tool in accessing this information. One needs to be familiar with their differences in order to use them most efficiently.

Primary Literature

The primary literature provides the most current resource for health care information. This literature includes the results of original studies or descriptive reports. Unlike the tertiary literature, the primary literature provides new information on a topic, and details the methodology which readers can personally evaluate. Since most economic studies are not conducted concurrently

TABLE 4-1.

Miscellaneous Secondary Literature Resources Useful for Drug Information

Current Contents	Published by the Institute for Scientific Information. Provides the table of contents of journals. Available in seven editions including *Life Sciences* and *Clinical Medicine*. Published weekly
Clin-Alert	Published by Technomic Publishing Company, Lancaster, PA. Provides abstracts from the primary literature focusing on adverse reactions and therapeutic misadventures related to drug therapy. Published semi-monthly
InPharma	Published by ADIS International, Langhorne, PA. Indexes and provides abstracts information from the literature focusing on pharmacotherapy. Also has mini-reviews on a topic of current interest and marketing information. Published weekly
Reactions	Published by ADIS International, Langhorne, PA. Indexes and provides abstracts on information from the literature focusing on adverse drug reactions, toxicology, and related topics. Also has a mini-review on ADR-related events. Published weekly

with clinical studies, information from the primary literature may be used to determine the data sources used in pharmacoeconomic analyses. For example, this literature could help establish what outcomes might be anticipated from a particular therapy (e.g., therapeutic benefit, adverse reaction) and what the likelihood of the outcome is (e.g., probability of treatment success or adverse event). Primary literature can appear in a number of different formats as described below.

Letters

Many health care journals have a "Letters to the Editor" section. These letters may be brief descriptions of pilot studies, first reports of a therapeutic use of a drug or an adverse reaction, as well as critiques of previously published works. Since they are only letters, the level of detail they provide is usually limited. In addition, depending on the journal's policy, letters may or may not receive external or peer review before publication. Consequently, while they may provide useful information on a drug-related subject, one needs to exercise caution when using information from letters in a decision-making process.

Abstracts

Journals associated with professional organizations often publish abstracts that provide brief summaries (approximately 200 words) of data presented at major medical or pharmacy meetings. For example, the journal *Pharmacotherapy* publishes abstracts of presentations at meetings of the American College of Clinical Pharmacy. Although most meeting abstracts undergo an external review process, it is not of the same rigor as that of a published manuscript. In addition, the study results presented as abstracts may never be published as a complete manuscript, which makes it difficult to accurately assess the quality of the data. However, as do letters, abstracts may be useful in providing some preliminary information on a subject when little or no other data exists.

Supplements

Supplements generally consist of a series of articles focused on a specific topic (e.g., a new drug) that are published in concert with a regular issue of the journal. Supplements may include some pharmacoeconomic information about a drug as compared with related agents. However, many supplements are sponsored by the pharmaceutical company marketing the drug being reviewed. Consequently, one must be aware that there may be some bias inherent in the information presented. While the data published in the supplement may be valid, it is unlikely that a paper that is unfavorable toward the manufacturer's drug would be included. Consequently, supplements tend to present a very positive perspective on a drug. In addition, not all supplements undergo peer review, and thus may be limited in the quality of the material they contain.

Results of studies or descriptive reports

The most important primary literature generally consists of descriptive reports or the results of original research, including both clinical and pharmacoeconomic studies. An understanding of the basic differences in these types of primary literature is important in order to interpret them properly.

Descriptive reports Descriptive reports include case reports or case series and *are not studies*. Unlike a study, the author does not establish a hypothesis and set out to test it. The author just describes the events that occurred in a patient (case report) or patients (case series or clinical series). For example, a case report describing an adverse reaction to a medication does not attempt to establish that the drug is associated with an increase risk of that complication. The report only suggests there may be a possibility that the drug could cause the reaction, and does not establish causality. While these reports often generate interest in conducting further clinical studies, they are typically not used to establish outcomes in pharmacoeconomic studies since they are not conclusive. Descriptive reports also include such topics as a discussion of implementation of a new program or service (e.g., pharmacy-based drug therapy compliance clinic, pharmacokinetic service). This may be useful for an organization contemplating establishing similar programs, and provides insight into what resources it would take to do so.

Clinical studies Clinical studies are usually classified as either *observational* or *experimental*. *Observational* studies include case-control studies, cohort (follow-up) studies, and cross-sectional (prevalence) studies. In these types of studies, the investigator does not intervene in the course of events, but rather tries to draw conclusions based on observing study subjects for some outcome that may happen in the future (prospective cohort studies), or reviewing events that have transpired in the past (retrospective cohort studies and case-control studies). In cross-sectional studies, an assessment is made of some outcome at a specific point in time, and is neither prospective nor retrospective. It provides a "snapshot" of an association between two variables only at the time the study was conducted (e.g., a survey of elderly hypertensive patients to determine how many are currently receiving nonsteroidal anti-inflammatory agents).

Observational studies can provide valuable information about risks associated with some exposure. For instance, the Framingham Heart Study is a large observational study that helped identify important risk factors for cardiovascular disease such as smoking, hypertension, and elevated serum cholesterol levels.[8] However, these studies do not establish cause and effect relationships; they only suggest an association between two variables (e.g., a drug and an adverse reaction). Only an experimental study, such as the randomized, controlled, clinical trial can determine such a relationship. In this type of study design, the investigator *intervenes* in the course of events and preassigns treatment groups by means of randomization. Randomly allocating subjects to various treatment arms of study attempts to reduce the potential for selection bias by limiting the control the investigator has in determining who gets what treatment. These studies also employ a control (e.g., placebo, active drug) to which the results of the experimental group can be compared and the treatment effect evaluated. Therefore, the randomized controlled clinical trial is the method by which drug efficacy is assessed.

Pharmacoeconomic studies There are some basic differences between pharmacoeconomic studies and the clinical trials described above. First, the clinical trial is targeted primarily at clinicians, while pharmacoeconomic studies generally have multiple audiences. Parties interested in pharmacoeconomic studies include not only clinicians but managed care organizations, insurance companies, and even patients. Another difference is that the results of a well-conducted clinical trial performed in one country can usually be extrapolated to other countries. However, the results of a pharmacoeconomic study may not be applicable outside the country where it was conducted due to differences in cultures and monetary exchange rates. Also, as noted above, clinical trials evaluate the *efficacy* of a treatment. However, clinical trials are conducted under very controlled conditions. The patient selection process for clinical trials often excludes patients who may benefit from the drug therapy, and very rigid treatment protocols are usually established for monitoring the patients. While these trials may establish whether a drug may be efficacious for an intended use, the *effectiveness* of a drug is based on its use in general practice, or the "real world." Pharmacoeconomic studies analyze the cost of a drug relative to its effectiveness; therefore, these studies aim at providing information on the *efficiency* of the drug in the health care system. Efficiency is a term economists use to describe the drug not only in relation to its indication but also taking into account a clinical management strategy as well as the local market. Basically, it defines the drug's value for money.[9] A fourth difference between pharmacoeconomic studies and clinical trials is that the latter are required by the Food and Drug Administration (FDA) for drug approval, and pharmacoeconomic studies currently are not.

There are four primary types of pharmacoeconomic study designs or methods reported in the literature. Although they are detailed in Chapter 2, these study designs will be briefly reviewed here as well. An understanding of these methodologies is important in order to most appropriately evaluate and interpret pharmacoeconomic literature.

Cost-minimization analysis (CMA) A CMA is the most basic of the pharmacoeconomic study designs. This study simply compares the cost of two or more alternatives, assuming equal outcomes of each alternative. In general, the least costly of the alternatives is selected. However, with this type of methodology, the investigators should provide evidence that the outcomes of the alternatives they are comparing are indeed equal in all respects. Although two agents of the same class may have the same efficacy in the treatment of a disease, they may differ significantly in the incidence of a serious side effect (e.g., nephrotoxicity). Therefore, a CMA would not be appropriate if there is a significant cost associated with managing that side effect (e.g., dialysis).

Cost-benefit analysis (CBA) In a CBA, the outcomes of the alternatives being studied are not considered equal. Both the costs and outcomes (benefits) of the alternatives are measured in monetary units. A cost-benefit ratio is then calculated to determine what alternative provides the greatest benefit relative to cost. A CBA is usually conducted when resources are limited and choices need to be made concerning the most appropriate alternative to select. One of the difficulties with this type of study is assessing a dollar value on clinical outcomes.[10] Therefore, this type of study design is more useful in conducting an economic analysis of health care services rather than therapies.

Cost-effectiveness analysis (CEA) In this type of analysis, the outcomes of the alternatives are not measured in monetary units, but rather in natural or physical units (e.g., years of life saved, complication avoided). Although a CEA does not assume equal outcomes, it should compare alternatives with similar objectives. For example, the objective of a treatment may be to reduce ulcer reoccurrence in patients with a history of duodenal ulcers. Various treatment modalities (e.g., antibiotics, antihistamines, proton pump inhibitors) could be compared, and a cost-effectiveness ratio for each alternative would then be established to compare the cost per ulcer prevented. This type of analysis does not necessarily mean the least costly or most effective alternative is selected, but different scenarios are possible. Perhaps the most expensive alternative may be considered cost-effective if it has an additional benefit worth the extra cost. On the other hand, a less expensive, yet less effective, alternative may be considered the most cost-effective if the extra benefit is not worth the additional cost.[11]

Cost-utility analysis (CUA) A CUA analysis is very similar to a CEA, but the measured outcomes take into account patient health preferences or utilities. Outcomes are measured as quality-adjusted life years (QALYs), which takes into consideration that not each year of life gained from a therapy is valued equally by a patient. A patient with a debilitating disease (e.g., amyotrophic lateral sclerosis) may not perceive a year of life saved the same as an otherwise relatively healthy patient with a very manageable condition such as asthma. While there are a number of methods available to measure utility values, the tools used in a particular CUA should be validated and specific.[10]

PHARMACOECONOMIC LITERATURE EVALUATION

Pharmacoeconomic studies are being published with increasing frequency in the medical and pharmacy literature. As noted previously, these studies are often used to assess the relative merits of treatment alternatives in making a variety of decisions, including formulary management or patient-specific treatment options. However, many of these studies are seriously limited in terms of their quality. Therefore, one should have a systematic approach for evaluating pharmacoeconomic literature in order to more effectively interpret the information and draw the most appropriate conclusions. A variety of different evaluation strategies have been described, most of which incorporate similar key components as outlined in Table 4-2. The following provides an overview of the pharmacoeconomic literature evaluation process, highlighting many of these major elements.

TABLE 4-2.

Steps to Pharmacoeconomic Literature Evaluation

1. Evaluate the quality of the journal
   a. Is it an "impact journal" or "throw away"?
2. Evaluate the qualifications of the authors
   a. Are the authors qualified to conduct pharmacoeconomic research?
3. Evaluate the title and abstract
   a. Are title and abstract unbiased?
4. Evaluate the study methodology
   a. What is the perspective of the study?
   b. What was the type of study design used?
   c. What are the outcomes or benefits of the therapies or alternatives studied?
   d. What are the alternatives studied and are they appropriate?
   e. What are the types of costs used or considered in analysis?
   f. If the study was conducted over time, was there a discounting of costs?
   g. Was a sensitivity analysis conducted?
   h. How was the data presented?
   i. What were the data sources used in the study?
5. Evaluate the results and conclusion
   a. Were results and conclusion consistent with the study that was conducted?
6. Evaluate sponsorship of the study
   a. If the study was sponsored by industry, was there a potential for bias?

Adapted from References 10–18.

Evaluation of the Quality of the Journal

The first step in evaluating any primary literature should be to assess the quality of the journal in which it was published. Is the journal a high impact journal or a "throw away"? Impact factors are calculated by *Journal Citations Reports*, a byproduct of *Science Citation Index,* a secondary literature resource.[12] The impact factors are based on how often material from various journals are cited in other works, and provide a quantitative assessment of what publications are used as important resources for medical and scientific information. High-impact or "power" medical journals include the *New*

England Journal of Medicine, the *Journal of the American Medical Association* (*JAMA*) and the *Annals of Internal Medicine*. These journals have a rigorous peer review process in which external reviewers carefully screen manuscripts for quality and appropriateness prior to publication.

Their reviewers are individuals who are demonstrated experts in a given area and who have a solid tract record in research and publishing. In general, high-impact journals usually provide the best evidence for making health care decisions.

The term "throw-away" refers to journals that are not usually archived, but are discarded after a period of time. These journals may be available through free subscriptions, and they are typically very strongly supported by pharmaceutical manufacturer advertising. Consequently, there may be potential bias in the nature of the material published in these journals. The articles in these journals tend to be very favorable towards those drugs that are reviewed or studied. In addition, the peer review process tends to be less rigorous than that of higher-quality journals. However, there still may be useful and relevant pharmacoeconomic information presented in these journals. One just needs to understand the limitations of the publication when evaluating the data.

Journals that are peer reviewed have their manuscripts externally reviewed by experts in the related field. These individuals, sometimes called referees, provide valuable input and make recommendations as to the suitability of the paper for publication. Many journals boldly state on the cover that they are "peer reviewed" in an attempt to increase their professional acceptance. While external peer review helps screen out poor-quality studies, one must remember that the peer review process is only as good as the individuals who are reviewing the manuscript. Peer reviewers for a pharmacoeconomic study may not necessarily be selected based on their knowledge of pharmacoeconomics, but rather their expertise on the drugs in question. Consequently, they may not be able to provide the most appropriate evaluation of the manuscript. Therefore, one should not assume that all peer-reviewed work is of equally high quality. In addition, not all information published in a peer-reviewed journal may be peer-reviewed. Depending on the journal's policy, letters to the editor or invited manuscripts may not undergo external review. The "information for authors" page that is published periodically in most journals is very helpful in determining the nature of the peer-review process for that particular publication.

Evaluation of the Qualifications of the Authors

The next step in the evaluation of any drug literature is to assess the qualifications of the authors. If it is a pharmacoeconomic study, is there evidence that the authors are qualified to conduct such a study? Although this may be sometimes difficult to ascertain, one can tell by the description of the authors and their affiliations whether they are in a position to participate in economic research. For example, an author who is identified as a member of a pharmacoeconomic research unit within their organization could be considered an appropriate individual to conduct an economic study. One would also have a higher comfort level with a paper if the authors had a history of publishing pharmacoeconomic studies. If the reader wanted to determine the publication record of the individuals performing the study, one could use a secondary information resource such as MEDLINE or IPA to search for information written by those individuals.

Evaluation of Title and Abstract

Both the title and abstract should accurately reflect the nature of the study. The title should not be biased and overstate the significance of any findings. For example, the reader should not be influenced by the title of a paper that a specific agent is the most effective of its class for treatment of a particular condition. The title should accurately describe the nature of the paper and not mislead the reader in terms of the study objectives or the methodology used.

While abstracts provide a useful summary of the study, including objectives, methodology, results, and conclusion, one should also not rely solely on the information from the abstract of the paper to base any opinion. Recent evidence indicates that the data in the abstract may be inconsistent with that in the body of the text, even in well-respected journals.[13] One must read the entire article to be able to accurately interpret the information presented.

Evaluation of the Study Methodology

There is ample evidence to indicate that there are problems with the methodology of published pharmacoeconomic studies. Lee and Sanchez evaluated cost-effectiveness and cost-benefit analyses published in the pharmacy literature.[14] They applied previously published criteria for evaluating pharmacoeconomic literature and reported that over 50% of the studies they reviewed failed to meet at least 7 of the 10 criteria established.

In another study, Udvarhelyi and colleagues attempted to determine whether or not published cost-benefit and cost-effectiveness literature adhered to basic analytic principles.[15] In their methodology, the authors outlined six basic principles that reporting of the results of cost-benefit and cost-effective studies should be expected to follow. However, of the 77 pharmacoeconomic studies published in general medical, general surgical, and medical subspecialty journals that they reviewed, only three articles met all six criteria.

More recently, Bradley and colleagues used a 13-item checklist to critique pharmacoeconomic studies published in pharmacy, medical, and health economic journals.[16] While they noted that the quality of these studies increased over time, there were still limitations to many published pharmacoeconomic analyses.

The following sections summarize the primary criteria that these researchers and others believe are important in evaluating the methodology of a pharmacoeconomic study.[10,11,14–18] The reader should carefully assess each of these points to determine if the study methodology described is sound.

Perspective of the study

As noted earlier, pharmacoeconomic studies may be conducted from the point of view of many different parties. Perspectives include those of the health care provider (e.g., physician, hospital), payer (insurers, managed care organization), patient, or the broader perspective of society in general. The specific perspective of the study will determine what will be measured, what the costs and benefits are, and how these will be valued.[18] Consequently, the perspective of the study guides and limits application of study results. For example, suppose the objective of a study is to assess the benefits of a drug in reducing length of hospital stay, and this study is conducted from the perspective of the hospital. The investigators may not address the matter of transferring health care costs to the outpatient sector once a patient is discharged, even though it may be significant. They would be concerned primarily with costs associated with hospitalization and not potential financial burdens in the ambulatory setting (e.g., cost of home care). This study would also not likely include indirect or intangible costs in their analysis since they would not be relevant to the costs borne by the hospital. On the other hand, a study conducted from a societal perspective would assess indirect costs associated with morbidity and mortality (e.g., loss of income due to illness), and perhaps cost associated with pain and suffering due to an illness. Therefore, pharmacoeconomic studies should clearly state from what perspective the analysis is being conducted. Unfortunately, this is often not stated clearly in many studies, and it is left up to the reader to assume the perspective.

Study design

As noted previously, there are several types of pharmacoeconomic studies. The reader needs to determine if the study design was appropriate to address the objective stated. For example, the authors of a CMA should provide evidence that the alternatives being evaluated are equal in all respects, including both positive (e.g., cure) and negative outcomes (e.g., adverse drug reactions). The premise of a CMA study is that cost is the only distinguishing feature of two or more alternatives. Consequently, if the alternatives are not equal in all respects, then a CMA is an inappropriate study design.

Sometimes a paper will misrepresent what type of study was actually conducted.[14] For example, the title of an article may describe the study as a "cost-benefit analysis," but the results are expressed in terms of cost-effectiveness (e.g., cost per years of life saved or complication prevented). Consequently, the reader should evaluate the methodology carefully to confirm that the study design described is actually what was performed.

Benefits of the therapies being studied

Pharmacoeconomic studies should clearly describe what the benefits (outcomes) of the specific therapies being evaluated are, and provide documentation of these benefits.[15] For example, a pharmacoeconomic study evaluating treatment strategies for lowering serum triglycerides may indicate that a benefit would be to reduce stroke. The authors should provide evidence that there is indeed a relationship between these two variables. In addition, if the benefits of a specific therapy have not been scientifically established, this should be stated as well. The reader needs to evaluate the references cited regarding the benefits of a therapy to determine the source of the information.

Alternatives studied

One should assess whether the alternatives being studied are relevant and appropriate, or are the investigators comparing apples and oranges. For example, if one is conducting a cost analysis comparing an oral antibiotic with a parenteral antibiotic, both should have similar therapeutic applications. Comparing a new "wonder drug" to a drug that is no longer considered a therapy of choice is also not appropriate. In addition, all relevant alternatives should be considered, even the "no treatment" option if reasonable. Not initiating antibiotic therapy in a patient with serous otitis media may be considered a possible treatment strategy, and it should be considered an option if evaluating various antibiotic regimens for this condition.

Practitioners also need to determine whether the alternatives evaluated in a study are relevant to their practice. A pharmacoeconomic study may conclude that a new drug is more cost-effective for treatment of a particular condition than an older drug from within the same therapeutic class (e.g., calcium channel blockers, nonsteroidal anti-inflammatory drugs). However, it would be difficult to extrapolate the results of this study to an organization where the older drug was not on the institution's formulary anyway.[18]

Types of costs used or considered in the analysis

Costs may include direct costs, indirect costs, and intangible costs. Direct costs are the costs to deliver services to the patient and include both medical and non-medical costs. Key direct costs for pharmacoeconomic studies include acquisition costs, preparation costs, administration costs, and monitoring costs.[15] The cost of toxicity or therapeutic failure or the negative consequence of treatment should also be measured. Failure to specify the appropriate direct costs may lead to erroneous conclusions. For example, when comparing the costs of an oral drug with an intravenous drug, one must take into account the preparation and administration costs of the parenteral medication to accurately compare the two therapies. Failure to do so would underestimate the cost of the parenteral product and would lead to an erroneous conclusion.

Indirect costs are primarily the cost of illness to the patient or to society and may be difficult to assess accurately. These costs typically include the loss of income due to an illness. Intangible costs are hard to assign a dollar value to and include the cost of pain and suffering. CUAs often incorporate tools to adjust these "costs" to QALYs.[11]

As stated previously, the study perspective will dictate what costs are being measured. A study conducted from a hospital perspective would not necessary be concerned with indirect or intangible costs, while a study with a societal perspective would be. However, studies should incorporate all relevant costs in their analysis.

One should also determine whether the costs used in the analysis are applicable in one's own practice setting. Many studies use average wholesale price (AWP) for acquisition cost. This is generally appropriate since it usually represents the most common denominator when comparing drug costs. However, if the acquisition cost for an organization significantly differs from the AWP because of a contract they may have with the pharmaceutical company or other agency, the study results may not be applicable. Similarly, if a study was done in another country, costs should be expressed in the equivalent US monetary units for a more valid comparison.

Discounting

Many economic studies evaluate costs and benefits over an extended period of time. For instance, a drug may be intended to prevent a long-term complication of a disease such as stroke, and the outcome may not be realized for several years after the therapy is started.[15] Consequently, all costs should be adjusted or discounted back to their present value. The rationale for discounting is that the value of a dollar today is worth more than its value would be in the future.[18] If values are not discounted, the benefit or cost in the first year will remain stable and may lead to a false conclusion about the value of the benefit. While there is no generally accepted consensus on how to discount or how much to discount, the discount rate used in studies is often between 5 and 10%.[18]

Sensitivity analysis

In many pharmacoeconomic studies, the researchers make certain assumptions regarding the costs or probabilities of important variables. For example, the cost of a drug regimen may be estimated based on an intermediate dosing regimen, or the probability of a certain event may be estimated to occur at the most frequently reported percent of the time. By using a variety of "what if" scenarios, a sensitivity analysis tests the validity of the results of a study by altering important variables and recalculating the study results. For instance, "what if" a different dosage regimen is used, or "what if" a higher or lower probability of an outcome is assumed, would the study results change? Therefore, a sensitivity analysis can determine whether the results of a study will hold up under a variety of situations, or whether they are only valid under the conditions of a specific premise.[15] Therefore, when evaluating the results of a pharmacoeconomic study that is based on certain assumptions or models, one should determine if a sensitivity analysis has been performed.

Data presentation

Data should be presented in a way that facilitates comparisons between alternatives.[15] For example, if it is a cost-benefit analysis, data should be presented as a benefit to cost (B/C) ratio. A B/C ratio >1 indicates the benefits exceed the costs, and that the strategy or therapy should be pursued. Conversely, a B/C ratio <1 indicates that the costs exceed the benefits and that the strategy or therapy should not be favorably received.

When two therapies are compared in a cost-effectiveness study, an incremental cost analysis (ICA) should be conducted. An ICA assesses what the added cost per net effect for the alternative therapy would be, and is the difference in *total costs* of two therapies divided by the difference in *effectiveness* of the two therapies. For example, if therapy A costs $3000 and saves 10 lives, it has an average cost-effectiveness (C/E) ratio of $300/life saved. If therapy B costs $6000 and saves 15 lives, it has an average C/E ratio of $400/life saved. However, the ICA for therapy B would be equal to ($6000 – $3000)/(15 – 10) or $600/life saved. Consequently, if one uses the average cost-effectiveness to evaluate therapy B against therapy A, one may actually underestimate the additional cost per life saved.[15]

Data sources

Since obtaining original data on the efficacy and toxicity of drug therapies is both time consuming and expensive, the authors of pharmacoeconomic studies often rely on previously published work to obtain outcome information for their analysis. Therefore, the reader should investigate references cited in the paper to ascertain the nature of this very important information. For instance, were the data sources obtained from information published in a reputable journal? Were they based on information published in an abstract, letter, or supplement, or were they based on a more scholarly work such as a clinical study? If this information in the analysis is based on studies conducted outside the United States, is it applicable in this country? If the data were from a clinical trial, does it represent the reality of clinical practice? For example, an adverse reaction rate reported in a clinical trial may be smaller than noted with general use due to the relatively small patient sample receiving the drug, and the strict controls incorporated in a clinical trial design. Since the results of a pharmacoeconomic study are only as good as the data it is based on, one needs to evaluate these issues critically when interpreting this literature.

One also needs to evaluate how current the data is: if a pharmacoeconomic analysis uses outcome data that is several years old, is it still valid? For example, would antibiotic resistance affect the response rate to an antimicrobial that has been on the market for several years? If so, then more recent efficacy data should be used in a cost analysis of this agent compared with alternatives. Also, the relative costs of therapies may change over time due to changes in patent rights or availability of new chemical entities.

Evaluation of Results and Conclusion

Two other key components of any pharmacoeconomic study are the results and conclusion. By systematically evaluating the methodology of the study, the reader will be able to make a more informed decision as to whether the results have merit. As noted above, failure to include appropriate costs, outcome measures and address all relevant alternatives will seriously limit the significance of the results. That is why it is essential that one carefully critiques the methods section of any pharmacoeconomic study and does not jump straight to the results and conclusion section in the interests of time.

The conclusion section should provide the reader with the significance of the findings, and this should be consistent with the study that was performed. The authors publishing a study conducted from a hospital perspective should not make assumptions that their results apply under all conditions. Consequently, the limitations of any pharmacoeconomic study should be the paper, so the readers can more accurately determine how applicable the results are to their practice setting.

The conclusion of the study should also not misinterpret the results. If a drug is found more cost-effective than the alternative, the authors should not conclude that it is either more effective or less expensive. In addition, "statistically significant" findings may not mean "clinically significant," and should not be presented as such.

Evaluation of Sponsorship

As with any published study, the reader needs to evaluate whether or not there may be potential bias due to pharmaceutical industry sponsorship. However, one should not assume just because a pharmaceutical manufacturer supported the study that there is inherent bias. While the pharmaceutical industry supports a number of well-designed studies, the quality of studies varies based on product, company, and type of study.[17] Variables such as the alternatives studied and outcomes measured may depend on who supports the analysis. A manufacturer may be trying to position their product more favorably against a specific competitor and limit the scope of the study to two agents, when analysis of multiple alternatives would be appropriate. One should also question if the study would have been published if the results were not favorable to the manufacturer's product. Negative results do not make the study less valid, and they should be shared in the interest of providing valuable information.

CONCLUSION

There is a variety of resources that practitioners have available to access information on pharmacoeconomic issues, and one needs to understand the benefits and limitations of these resources in order to utilize them more effectively. Most of the time, more than one type of resource needs to be consulted to research information on a topic. Organizations should develop a library of references that best meets their needs.

Also, given the deficiencies reported in published pharmacoeconomic studies, it is important that the practitioner critically evaluates these studies so that they are interpreted correctly. Using the systematic approach described in this chapter is one method that can assist with the evaluation process. While this process may seem time consuming, it is an effective means for using this information most appropriately to best service both patients and the organization.

REFERENCES

1. Mosdell KW, Malone PM: Drug information resources. In: Malone PM, Mosdell KW, Kier, KL, Stanovich JE, eds, *Drug Information—A Guide for Pharmacists.* Stamford, CT: Appleton & Lange, 1996;15–65.
2. Cook DJ, Mulrow CD, Haynes RB: Systematic reviews: synthesis of best evidence for clinical decisions. *Ann Intern Med* 1997;126:276–380.
3. Bailar JC III: The promise and problems of meta-analysis. *New Engl J Med* 1997;337:559–561.
4. Wood EH: MEDLINE: the options for health professionals. *J Am Inform Assoc* 1994;1:372–380.
5. National Library of Medicine Facts Sheet. www.nlm.nih.gov.
6. Lowe HJ, Barnett GO: Understanding and using the medical subject headings (MeSH) vocabulary to perform literature searches. *JAMA* 1994;271:1103–1108.
7. Ritchey DC: Medical and pharmaceutical databases. In: Millares M, ed., *Applied Drug Information. Strategies for Information Management.* Vancouver, WA: Applied Therapeutics, 1998;3.1–3.47.
8. Voelker R: A "family heirloom" turns 50. *JAMA* 1998;279:1241–1245.

9. Milne RJ: Evaluation of the pharmacoeconomic literature. *Pharmacoeconomics* 1994;6:337–345.
10. Sacristan JA, Soto J, Galende I: Evaluation of pharmacoeconomic studies: utilization of a checklist. *Ann Pharmacother* 1993;27:1126–1233.
11. Jolicoeur LM, Jones-Grizzle AJ, Boyer JG: Guidelines for performing a pharmacoeconomic analysis. *Am J Hosp Pharm* 1992;49:1741–1747.
12. Garfield E: How can impact factors be improved? *Br Med J* 1996;313: 411–413.
13. Pitkin RM, Branagan MA, Burmeister LF: Accuracy in data of abstracts of published research articles. *JAMA* 1999;281:1110–1111.
14. Lee JT, Sanchez LA: Interpretation of cost-effective and soundness of economic evaluations in the pharmacy literature. *Am J Hosp Pharm* 1991; 48:2622–2627.
15. Udvarhelyi IS, Colditz GA, Arti Ri AB, et al.: Cost-effectiveness and cost-benefit analyses in the medical literature. *Ann Int Med* 1992;116:238–244.
16. Bradley CA, Iskedjian M, Lanctot KL: Quality assessment of economic evaluations in selected pharmacy, medical, and health economic journals. *Ann Pharmacother* 1995;29:681–689.
17. Sanchez LA: Evaluating the quality of published pharmacoeconomic evaluations. *Hosp Pharm* 1995;30:146–152.
18. Johnson JA, Coons SJ: Evaluation of published pharmacoeconomic studies. *J Pharm Pract* 1995;8:156–166.

C H A P T E R

5

Use and Evaluation of Pharmacoeconomics from the Payers' Perspective

Patrick D. Meek
and
Amy Steinkellner

INTRODUCTION

Payers of Health Care

Health services in the United States are purchased and paid for by a variety of individuals or groups. The payer is the group or individual who pays the provider (hospitals, physicians, nursing homes, pharmacies) for the provision of health care services and is responsible for reimbursing all services provided to an individual or a population of beneficiaries.[1] Typical payers are individuals receiving care, third-party insurance companies, managed care organizations, and large self-funded employers who self-insure.[2–6] Health care services can be purchased by one group (the purchaser) and provided to insured individuals who pay premiums or other financial sources to insurance carriers or government agencies (e.g., Medicare). In this arrangement, health care services are purchased by one group and paid for by another: for example, self-insured employers who contract with health maintenance organizations and third-party insurance companies.

The major purchasers of health care in the public sector are Medicare for the elderly, Medicaid for the poor, and government organizations as group purchasers for veterans and government employees.[7] Purchasers in the private sector include self-funded employers, groups of employers (employer coalitions), groups of employees (unions), and patients who buy individual private insurance or pay for health care out of pocket.[8] When considering who the purchasers of health care are, it is also important to note that there are an increasing number of uninsured individuals, for example the working poor, whose employers do not provide health care benefits and who may not be eligible for public-sector programs.[2,8]

In general, payments for health care services are provided in various ways. The past 30 years has seen a transition from a fee-for-service model to a managed care model where payments to providers are capitated. The flow of resources for payment of prescription drugs and services in a managed care setting is illustrated in Figure 5-1. Pharmacy benefit managers (PBMs) play an important role in this process.[9] Pharmacy benefit management companies are corporate entities that control the utilization and concomitant cost of pharmacy products on behalf of private and public payers, most commonly managed care organizations, insurance companies, and self-insured employers. A PBM conducts activities such as formulary management, utilization review, and other programs to promote use of pharmaceuticals in accordance to clinical practice guidelines or formulary status. Pharmacy benefit managers provide a set of health care products or services for management of the pharmacy benefit. The services are available for reimbursement by a particular health insurance plan specific to a particular group of insured individuals, and to the financial and other terms of the coverage.

Health Care Investment

Purchasers make an investment in the health care system to improve the health of individuals in the population. Providers of health care are responsible for making appropriate health interventions by applying knowledge of existing preventative, diagnostic, therapeutic, or health promotional strategies. Interventions often require the use of drugs, devices, equipment, and other health supplies. The choice of whether to use a particular medical intervention over another alternative depends on multiple factors: comparative efficacy, effectiveness, toxicity, preferences, and cost. A determination of the relevant factors by clinicians at the level of the individual patient is inherent in the medical decision-making process and critical to obtaining the desired health outcomes.[10–17]

Health outcomes for a particular individual can be defined and monitored in terms of health status indicators. The health status of a population is often

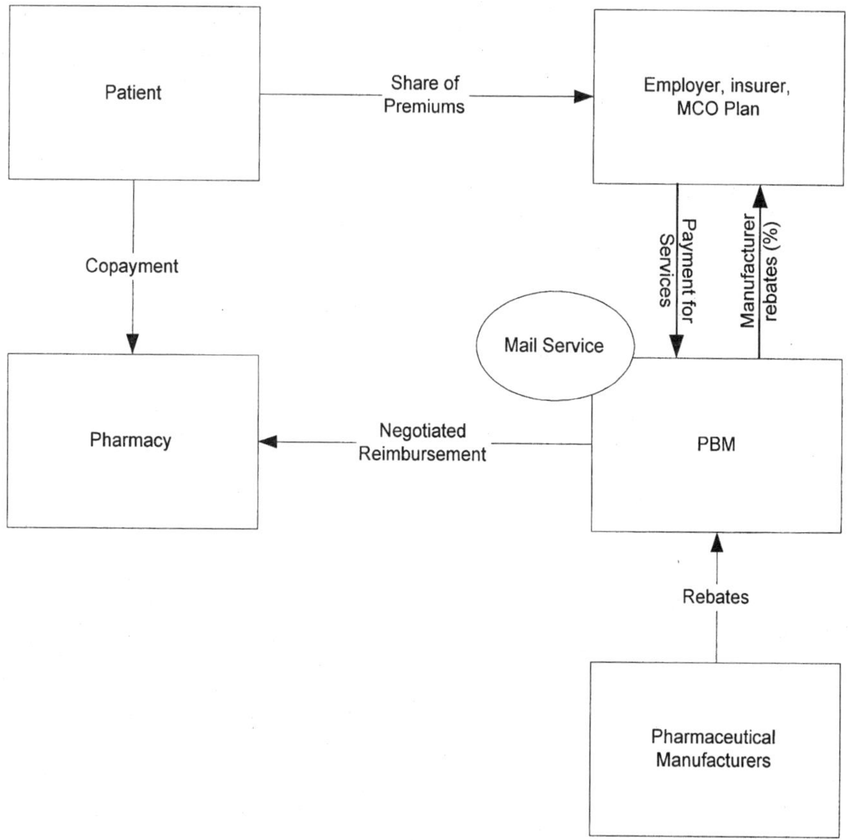

Figure 5-1. Flow of resources in purchase of prescription drugs and services. MCO = managed case organization; PBM = pharmacy benefit management company.

measured using birth and death rates, life expectancy, quality of life, morbidity from specific diseases, and presence of risk factors. The World Health Organization has adopted a measure of health-adjusted life expectancy, known as healthy year equivalents (HYE).[18] Other important determinants of health outcomes are those factors influencing the supply and demand for health services in the community, including use of ambulatory care and inpatient care, accessibility of health personnel and facilities, financing of health care, and health insurance coverage.[7]

THE VALUE OF PHARMACEUTICALS

Pharmaceuticals are an important component of the provision of health care in the United States.

In 1999, pharmaceutical and biotechnology companies added 40 new products to the market.[19] Many of these agents represent advances in the treatment of major diseases, including AIDS, infectious disease, cancer, cardiac arrhythmia, type 2 diabetes mellitus, osteoarthritis, and Parkinson's disease, and organ transplantation. The addition of new products to the existing mix of therapeutic alternatives offers decision makers the opportunity to evaluate the comparative value at several levels of the decision-making process (Figure 5-2).

Technology Advancement

The selection of pharmaceuticals is subject to a predictable life cycle, characterized in five distinct stages: investigation, promotion, acceptance and utilization, decline in utilization, and obsolescence. Technology assessments are generally considered to be most effective when made during the later stages of investigation, during the early stage of promotion, and during the phase of declining utilization. It is at these stages that determination of pharmacoeconomic outcomes may be evaluated with the goal of maximizing the value of the technology.

Expenditures for prescription drugs

Between 1970 and 1995, national prescription drug expenditures increased steadily, with a mean annual growth rate of 10%.[20] In 1997, prescription drugs accounted for $78.9 billion, or 7.2% of total health care expenditures (Figure 5-3).[1] In a second report from the National Institute for Health Care Management and Educational Foundation the rate of spending for prescription drugs was reported to have risen, between 1992 and 1997,[21] to a rate which is twice as fast as total national health spending (an average of 11% growth per year for prescription spending compared with 5.5% per year for total health spending).

Purchasers and policymakers are interested in identifying sources of cost without benefit in order to meet the challenge of providing high-quality health care at a manageable cost. Factors implicated in these trends include increases in the cost of drug therapy per day, the number of days of drug therapy per user, and the number of new drug users, each of which is fostered by recent increases in marketing efforts for pharmaceuticals.[20,21] Most purchasers look for programs that provide the highest value (highest health return for each dollar spent). Decision makers from the payers' perspective want to design health benefit programs, make formulary coverage decisions, design health

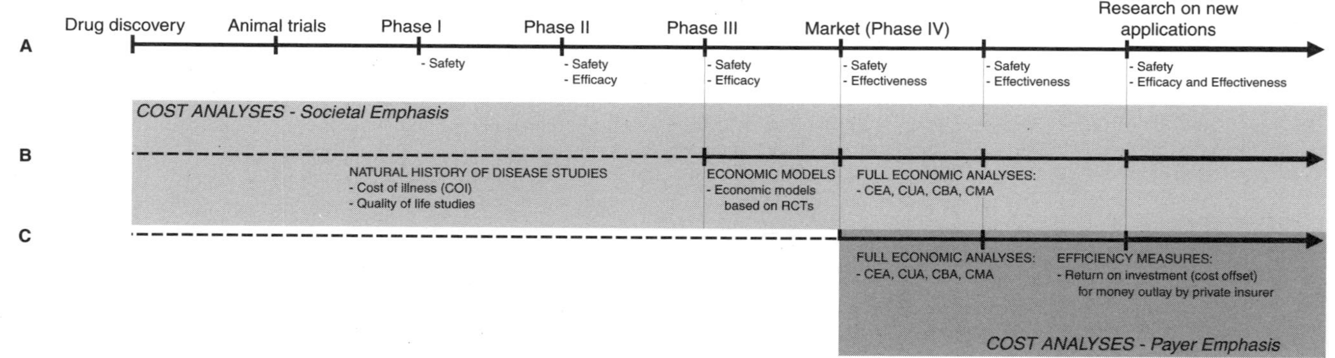

Figure 5-2. Drug discovery (from development to market). Information timelines for drug technology evaluation. Three discrete timelines are relevant for medical decision makers responsible for evaluating the value of competing drug technologies. Various types of information, and the timing of data collection, in relation to the FDA review cycle (line A), are illustrated in this figure. Line B represents evaluations performed from a societal perspective, and line C represents the perspective of the payer. The process of drug policy and development usually begins at the time of FDA approval and continues for the duration of time that the product remains on the market. Drug policy development activities may utilize any available information collected up to the time a decision is being made. CEA = cost-effectiveness analysis; CUA = cost-utility analysis; CBA = cost-benefit analysis; CMA = cost-minimization analysis.

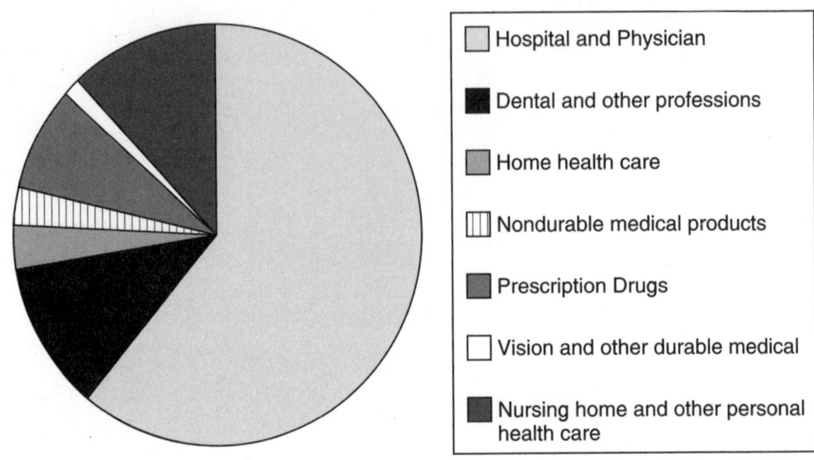

Figure 5-3. 1997 National health expenditures. Adapted from Iglehart.[1]

and wellness programs, and create a host of disease management programs that aim to improve the health of individuals in a population.

Measuring the value of drug therapy and other health care programs is an important component of quality improvement initiatives within the health care system. A range of definitions has been used to characterize the value of a pharmaceutical intervention. In its simplest form, value is defined as the lowest cost alternative among two or more alternatives of equal effectiveness. A more complex definition of "value" is the broad inclusion of the entire management of a particular disease with consideration of all relevant outcomes (costs and consequences) of therapy through rigorous clinical, epidemiological and economic analysis.

The disciplines of outcomes research[22] and pharmacoeconomics are evolving for this role and are being used by drug policy decision makers to evaluate the return benefit for an investment in drug therapy.[23] Drug policy decision makers in hospitals, clinics, managed care organizations [e.g., Pharmacy and Therapeutics (P&T) Committees], analysts within governmental payer institutions (Medicaid, Medicare), and researchers from pharmaceutical, and biotech manufacturers are active users of pharmacoeconomic information.

ROLE OF PHARMACOECONOMICS

The collection of economic information to evaluate a specific disease or treatment strategy occurs at a number of levels during the technology development and advancement process (see Figure 5-2). Information on the cost-effectiveness of treatment alternatives may be incorporated into the medical decision-making process at various levels, as illustrated in Figure 5-2.[24,25] Barriers to the use of the cost-effectiveness information in drug policy decision-making exist and have been described in the literature.[26–29]

Different Perspectives of Decision Makers

An important consideration in performing and evaluating the results of a pharmacoeconomic assessment is to note the evaluator's perspective.[30] Various purchasers of health care take different perspectives and have different expectations about the role of a medical technology or pharmaceutical agent. Depending on the perspective taken by the analyst, different conclusions might be drawn from the same set of pharmacoeconomic data.

Society

The societal perspective has been recommended by national health policy experts as the preferred perspective for cost-effectiveness evaluations of health technologies.[31] Adopting a societal perspective offers the broadest framework to evaluate the value of alternative therapies. The inclusion of a wide range of costs and outcomes provides information to make decisions that focus on the population as a whole, without exclusion. All purchasers of health care share a common interest in meeting the health needs of a population that is growing and aging. Developing and implementing policies and preventive interventions that effectively address the determinants of health can reduce the burden of illness, enhance quality of life, and increase longevity. The depth of topics covered by the objectives in Healthy People 2010 reflects the array of critical influences that determine the health of individuals and communities. For example, individual behaviors and environmental factors are responsible for about 70% of all premature deaths in the United States. Individual biology and behaviors influence health through their interaction with each other and with the individual's social and physical environments. Policies and interventions can improve health by targeting factors related to individuals and their environments, including access to quality health care. Pharmaceuticals play an important role in health care and are used widely in today's health care system.

Employers

Employers can provide health care benefits using a number of plan options including health maintenance organizations (HMOs); preferred provider organizations (PPOs); and traditional indemnity insurance. HMOs and PPOs may offer a discounted rate for a defined set of services or charge a fixed amount for each enrollee and provide for all the health care needs of each enrollee whether the costs are small or large (capitated). In either plan, the enrolled employee bears very little or no additional cost for services after the employer pays the initial enrollment fees. Frequently, HMOs assign a primary care physician to each employee to direct the provision of health care services and to arrange for any referrals to specialists that may be needed. PPOs generally limit their involvement in managing each employee's use of health care services to requiring that the employee use health care providers who are affiliated with the particular PPO. Traditional indemnity plans usually allow an enrolled employee to seek treatment from any legitimate health care provider of the employee's choice (fee-for-service plan). Unlike the other two plans, in an indemnity insurance plan, the employee is typically required to pay a percentage of the cost of services received up to a defined cost limit. Moderate-to-small employers tend to purchase health care insurance from a health care insurance company, which reduces the employer's exposure to significant financial loss if a number of their employees have catastrophic illnesses in a given year. Some large employers might contract with health insurance companies only to process health care claims and, in this case, such employers still assume the risk of covering all health care costs (self-funded employers). This approach may be more cost-efficient than purchasing health care insurance from a third-party insurance company.[32]

Employers are a major consumer of health care. From the perspective of an employer, decision makers responsible for managing coverage decisions, such as benefit design, generally do not want to be involved in formulary decisions. They want those decisions to be made by technical experts with knowledge of therapeutic alternatives, effectiveness, and cost. Employers are interested in the process of formulary decisions and consider the approach taken by policymakers to support formulary decisions when contracting for health care coverage.[33] Employers are interested in optimizing the quality of health care provided by managed care organizations. Some employers have strategically aligned to increase the purchasing power of a single employer within a coalition and monitor the quality improvement activities within health provider organizations.

Work productivity and performance In addition to providing high-quality health care at the highest value, employers also recognize that the health of the work force is a shared responsibility between employee and employer. Progressive companies may also support occupational health programs, wellness and disease management initiatives, which may be initiated through employer coalitions as a way to increase worker productivity, decrease worker absenteeism, and reduce the rate of disability.[34] There is increasing interest in measurements of productivity and performance as an additional measure of value.[35,36]

Medicare

The changing demographic profile of the United States is becoming more important in the cost of health care. The proportion of individuals over the age of 55 is expected to increase until the year 2040. These numbers are important because the elderly generally consume a disproportionate share of health care goods and services. In the United States this is especially true with pharmaceuticals, where 12% of the population over the age of 65 consumes 30% of the prescription drugs.

The Medicare program is the primary funding source for payment of health care of individuals over the age of 65 and covers 40% of health care expenditures for the elderly. In 1998, the annual average cost for drug therapy for an elderly person was $1100.[37] Approximately half of all Medicare beneficiaries have some level of prescription drug coverage through former employers. Without such coverage, elderly individuals would be expected to pay at least 75% of the cost of drug therapy out of pocket.[38] Medicare drug policy developers will likely continue to encourage employers through federal subsidies to offer such programs for retirees, thereby reducing the economic burden faced by the over-65 population.

Role of Pharmacy Benefits Managers

Pharmacy benefit management companies (PBMs) provide services that range from electronic and paper claims adjudication to sophisticated clinical management and decision-support technology. These services may be offered on a "carve-out" basis, meaning the pharmacy benefit management is separate from the health plan or health insurer. For employers, the most popular services offered by PBMs have been claims processing, generic substitution, pharmacy network development and management, mail service prescriptions, and formulary management. Currently, approximately 90% of US patients obtain their pharmacy benefits through a PBM.[39] Tracking the flow of money (Figure 5-2) for purchasing pharmaceuticals in the United States health care system is not easy since funds for personal health services come from multiple sources—employers, government, and individuals.

As part of the electronic claims processing function, many PBMs have developed databases of prescription drug claims information that is useful in pharmacoeconomic analysis. More sophisticated PBMs have integrated those drug claims with medical (inpatient and outpatient) claims as well as laboratory values when available to provide the foundation for powerful pharmacoeconomic and outcomes assessments. These studies can analyze the value demonstrated by a variety of drug therapies.

USE AND EVALUATION OF PHARMACOECONOMIC INFORMATION

Drug Policy Development Mechanisms

Formularies

The Academy of Managed Care Pharmacy defines a formulary as "a continually updated list of medications which represent the current clinical judgment of physicians and other experts in diagnosis and treatment of disease and preservation of health."[40] A minimal consideration in the formulary review process is a demonstrated safety and efficacy profile that meets the standards of the Food and Drug Administration (FDA). Comparative effectiveness in terms of clinical, economic, and quality of life outcomes is also important to consider when adding products to the formulary. According to the Academy of Managed Care Pharmacy position statement on formulary management,[40] P&T Committees should meet regularly to review medical and clinical literature, including clinical trials, relevant patient utilization, and experience; current therapeutic guidelines and the need for revised or new guidelines; economic data; provider recommendations; and the safest, most effective drugs that will produce the desired goals of therapy at the most reasonable cost to the health care system.

The National Committee for Quality Assurance (NCQA) requires managed care organizations to establish a policy for evaluation of new technology. The definition of new technology includes medical procedures, drugs, and devices. This policy must include a written description of the process used to determine whether medical technologies will be included in the benefit package. Technology assessment must include a thorough review of the clinical literature as well as a description of how this information will be used. Objective criteria may include demonstrable improvement in health outcome as well as favorable health risks and benefits compared with established procedures and products.

The concept of having a defined list of drugs serves a number of purposes; most importantly, it provides prescribers with a descriptive list of pharmaceutical and biotechnology products that have been evaluated and approved by physicians, pharmacists, nurses, and other health care professionals who serve on the P&T Committee that oversees the medication review process of the organization. Products selected for inclusion are agents that are considered highly efficacious and of sufficient safety profile for the treatment of conditions in the populations served. The use of pharmacoeconomic information is most evident when making decisions intended to preserve pharmacy budgets.[41] This does not mean, however, that pharmacoeconomic information should supersede efficacy and safety data. Instead, P&T Committees could use pharmacoeconomic and outcomes studies as additional tools to extend the formulary management process. Using these data helps expand the process beyond simply containing costs to optimizing drug therapy and controlling overall health care expenses.

Restricted access

Restriction may take various forms. A plan may control access to a specific class of drugs such as proton pump inhibitors by allowing only gastroenterologists to prescribe these agents or by mandating that other drug classes be used prior to the proton pump inhibitors.[33] An assessment of the impact of such strategies on the clinical and economic outcomes of patients affected by the approach should be determined. In a study conducted by Holzer and colleagues on the impact of proton pump inhibitor use on the cost of therapy over a 2-year period, the value of the use of proton pump inhibitors was a result of the superior efficacy over the alternatives, and reductions in the need for diagnostic testing and hospitalizations.[42]

Interchange programs

Interchange programs, such as generic substitution and therapeutic substitution, are examples of strategies that aim to optimize the value obtained from a particular drug therapy while optimizing beneficial outcomes. In either program, clinically equivalent but more cost-effective alternatives are suggested to prescribers as an opportunity to provide savings to the patient and/or the payer.

Clinical practice guidelines

Ideally, decision makers would have access to sufficient numbers of published pharmacoeconomic analyses performed in environments similar to their own.[43] Those analyses can be found in a comprehensive review of the clinical literature. Guidelines exist for evaluating the literature.[44] Managed care organizations, hospitals, and government-subsidized health care programs rely on economic analyses of health care technologies to help support formulary decisions. There are many costs to consider when a health plan creates a list of "approved" or "preferred" drugs as a way of controlling expenditures. The case of medications for gastroesophageal reflux disease is an example. The most effective class of drugs for treatment of gastroesophageal reflux disease may be the proton pump inhibitors. The cost of these medications is greater than alternative agents and often accounts for a large portion of an organization's drug budget. As a result, proton pump inhibitors are a common target of restrictive formulary policies.

EMPLOYERS' MECHANISMS FOR ENSURING QUALITY

Employer Coalitions

Large employers can benefit by contracting directly with components of the health care system, providers of health care services, physician groups, hospitals, or pharmacy benefits managers.[45] Corporations have been the driving force behind the move to compare health care providers and plans based on their performance. Most employers work directly or indirectly with health plans to produce information to support the assessment of quality of care. The Health Plan Employer Data and Information Set (HEDIS) makes available information to employers to rate plans based on their quality measurements. The HEDIS measures (Table 5-1) are performance measures used to generate report cards of plan performance that can be used to compare plans

TABLE 5-1.

HEDIS-2000 Measures Requiring Assessment of Drug Therapy[79]

Effectiveness of care measures	*Medicaid*	*Commercial*	*Medicare*
Childhood immunization	×	×	
Adolescent immunization status	×	×	
Chlamydia screening in women	×	×	
Controlling blood pressure	×	×	×
Beta-blocker treatment after a heart attack	×	×	×
Cholesterol management after acute cardiovascular events	×	×	×
Comprehensive diabetes care	×	×	×
Use of appropriate medications for people with asthma	×	×	
Follow-up after hospitalization for mental illness and antidepressant medication management	×	×	×
Advising smokers to quit	×	×	×
Flu shots for older adults			×
Use of services			
Outpatient drug utilization	×	×	×

which the employer contracts.[46–49] The HEDIS data are also used to identify specific medical interventions for which health plans should target continuous quality improvement initiatives.[45]

Accrediting Organizations

Purchasers of health care may rely on accrediting agencies, such as the Joint Commission on Accreditation of Healthcare Organizations (JCAHO) and the National Committee for Quality Assurance (NCQA), to evaluate the quality of health care services. These agencies are also involved in the collection of health outcomes, which are useful to the purchasers of health care—federal government, insurers, and employers.

National Committee for Quality Assurance

With accreditation organizations, such as NCQA—a not-for-profit organization committed to evaluating and publicly reporting on the quality of managed care plans—focusing their evaluation criteria on patient outcomes (e.g., HEDIS), it is likely that the measurement and management of improved patient outcomes will increase. As providers and purchasers of health care attempt to contain health care expenditures and maintain the desired quality of health care services, the importance of measuring effectiveness, costs, and outcomes of medical interventions has gained significance.

Measures of quality allow employers and consumers to negotiate contracts using performance-based indicators. Integrated into these measures are interventions considered to be of the highest value, based on studies of clinical effectiveness and cost. Pharmacoeconomic studies are useful in determining this value, and are used by NCQA to support the performance measures used in the HEDIS dataset.

HEDIS-2000® The purpose of the HEDIS initiative is to work in concert with providers to address the health care challenges of today and tomorrow. The HEDIS is a set of standardized performance measures designed to ensure that purchasers and consumers have the information they need to reliably compare the performance of managed health care plans.[46–48] The HEDIS initiative is sponsored, supported, and maintained by the NCQA. The HEDIS attempts to address a broad range of health care issues, from prevention and early detection to acute and chronic care for children, adolescents, adults, and seniors and for conditions of high prevalence such as AIDS, breast cancer, smoking addiction, heart disease and diabetes. The measurement standards are a combination of public and private sector measurement efforts—an equal set of measures are applied to both Medicaid beneficiaries, commercial enrollees, and Medicare risk populations. Examples of measurements having a component of drug therapy are provided in Table 5-1. This is important for comparing care across health plans. The HEDIS-2000 addresses information important to purchasers and consumers when choosing a health plan, including clinical results, access to needed services, satisfaction with care, and the cost of care.[50] The HEDIS was developed by representatives from both public (Medicaid and Medicare) and private purchasers: consumers, organized labor, medical providers, public health officials, and health plans. The committee that organizes HEDIS focuses on measures in eight areas: effectiveness of care, access/availability of care, satisfaction with care, cost of care, health plan stability, informed health care choices, use of services, and health plan descriptive information.[50]

HEDIS RECOGNIZES VALUE OF PHARMACEUTICALS

The use of pharmaceuticals as a means of eliciting favorable health outcomes is a component of the HEDIS-2000 "effectiveness of care" section. HEDIS topics where pharmaceuticals play an important role (see Table 5-1) include childhood immunizations, smoking cessation, use of antibiotics for preventing recurrent childhood ear infections, use of beta-blockers after a myocardial infarction, use of aspirin after a myocardial infarction, use of appropriate medications for individuals with asthma, prevention of stroke in individuals with atrial fibrillation, use of ACE inhibitors as outpatient care for individuals hospitalized for congestive heart failure, cholesterol management of individuals hospitalized for coronary artery disease, management of high blood pressure, use of antibiotics for the prevention of HIV-related pneumonia, use of medications for individuals with schizophrenia, and use of continued drug therapy for individuals with depression.[50]

PROGRAM DEVELOPMENT

To manage the health care needs of a group of individuals properly, a health care purchaser might incorporate a process of continuous quality improvement as an integral part of the health services it provides. Data must be translated into information useful to the design of health care benefit packages. Employers must be able to identify groups with special health and medical needs in order to deliver specialized services for such needs. Evaluations of programs, as well as the general health benefit program, before and after implementation of the program is essential. Regardless of plan type, large employers are at risk for health issues that impact the rest of the US general population. These include developing a chronic disease and the issues associated with its diagnosis and management. The top 10 leading causes of death in the United States in 1997 were heart disease (726,974), cancer (539,577), stroke (59,791), lung disease (109,029), accidents (95,644), pneumonia and flu (86,449), diabetes (62,636), errors in treatment (44,000), suicide (30,535), and kidney disease (25,331) (Sources: Centers for Disease Control; Institute of Medicine).[51]

Individuals in the population, are also susceptible to lifestyle factors associated with diminished health status. Purchasers of health care might develop programs that address the safety and wellness needs of the group. These include substance abuse (nicotine addiction); lack of physical activity or conditioning; and inappropriate diet. With steady employment comes opportunity for a wide variety of recreational activities and their associated injury risks. The employees are at risk, as everyone is, of the health consequences of negative social interactions such as being involved in an abusive domestic situation or simply being in the wrong place at the wrong time (car accidents or robbery).

Use of Clinical Practice Guidelines

The evaluation of available pharmacoeconomic data may allow policymakers to support various disease-specific initiatives. Several national consensus committees, representing a range of diseases have included pharmacoeconomic assessments in the decision process alongside the efficacy and effectiveness literature.[52–56] The foundation formed by the development of such national clinical practice guidelines contributes to the quality and cost-effectiveness of care, and supports the investment in disease management programs by the payers of health care.

Investment in Safety and Wellness Management Programs

Another important area for health care investment is in programs that promote safety and wellness and prevent illness. Companies realize that effective management of health care resources requires continuous improvement of the services for which the company contracts and in the manner in which these services are provided to employees. Evaluation and improvement of health care services at the level of an individual employee can provide useful information for future decisions. An example of such an evaluation is the use of employer data to identify and intervene with persons at elevated risk for cardiovascular disease.[32]

EXAMPLES OF SPECIFIC INITIATIVES

HEDIS Prevention Programs

Vaccination programs

A substantial proportion of vaccine-preventable diseases occur in adults of working age (15–65 years of age). These diseases include infections from influenza, pneumococcal, diphtheria, hepatitis B, tetanus, rubella, and measles. Most adults are not adequately immunized, despite vigorous efforts to implement strategies to reduce the incidence, morbidity, and death among adults. In the late 1980s, it was estimated that of the 40,000 deaths per pneumococcal epidemic, approximately 20,000 deaths and 80,000 hospitalizations per year could be avoided.[57] These findings prompted recommendations for immunization policies and vaccine coverage by insurance programs to enhance the delivery of vaccines to adults.

The cost-effectiveness of vaccination of healthy working adults was evaluated in 1994. The authors reported a 25% reduction in upper respiratory illness, 43% fewer days of missed work due to upper respiratory illness, and an estimated cost savings of $46.85 per person vaccinated, compared with a placebo control group.[58]

Estimates of the cost-effectiveness of vaccination programs from the perspective of a managed care organization have shown that annual influenza vaccinations for the elderly result in a net savings to the HMO per vaccination of $6.11 for high-risk elderly patients and $1.10 for all elderly individuals. Cost savings resulted from reductions in the rates of pneumonia- and influenza-related hospitalizations.[59] These findings were confirmed in a study of community dwelling elderly persons.[60] The authors of this study reported a lower rate of hospitalization for all types of illness in the vaccinated group and a cost savings of $117 per person per year and a 39–54% reduction in mortality during the three influenza seasons evaluated in the study.

Smoking cessation

Considerable benefit is obtainable with cessation of smoking and is expected to be one of the most cost-effective uses of health care resources.[61–65] The estimated lifetime economic consequences of smoking cessation, resulting from a reduced likelihood of developing smoking-related disease (lung cancer, coronary heart disease, and emphysema) ranged from $20,000 for a smoker of less than one pack per day to over $56,000 for a smoker of more than two packs per day.[61] Two studies have examined the cost-effectiveness of smoking interventions. One found that counseling smokers to quit would cost only $705–988 per year of life saved for males and $1204–2058 per year of life saved for females.[62] The second study found that prescribing nicotine replacement therapy as an adjunct to counseling would cost only $4113–6465 per year of life saved for males and $6880–9473 per year of life saved for females. These cost-effectiveness ratios are more favorable than those of most other current health care interventions.[66] Using a model to estimate the cost-effectiveness of smoking cessation, it is projected that a 50% reduction in the number of cigarettes consumed would result in an increase in the life-expectancy of 35-year-old males and females by 1.2 years and 1.5 years, respectively. Eliminating smoking entirely would yield a gain of 2.3 years for both 35-year-old males and females.[64]

Research has also shown smoking cessation in pregnant women who smoke would result in considerable benefit,[63,65] and would save $77,807,054, or $3.31 per each dollar spent on smoking cessation interventions. Savings result from reduced perinatal death and reduction of the risk of low birth weight infants resulting in neonatal intensive care unit admission. The ratio of savings to cost increases to more than $6 to $1 when costs of long-term care for infants with disabilities secondary to low birth weight were considered.[63]

Pediatric Infections

In the late 1980s, the estimated annual costs of otitis media in the United States were approximately $3.5 billion.[67] In 1994, due in part to this large expenditure in health resources and the availability of extensive medical literature on the topic,[68] the Agency for Health Care Policy and Research developed a clinical practice guideline to address the use of antibiotics for young children with otitis media with effusion.[69] A published review of the effectiveness and cost of alternative antibiotics recommends that physicians consider costs other than the direct cost of the antibiotic when making a treatment selection.[70] For example, working parents with a child in day care, are potentially at risk for added expense associated with missed work if antimicrobial therapy is not effective. Parents will likely miss part of or up to a full day of work in order to attend the physician's office with their sick child. Choice of a less expensive and less effective antibiotic, such as amoxicillin might result in added costs to the family if it results in unsuccessful eradication of the causative organism. These added costs might exceed any savings resulting from avoidance of a more effective antibiotic of higher cost.

Other Infections

Chlamydia trachomatis infections

In the United States the most common of all sexually transmitted diseases are those caused by *Chlamydia trachomatis*. Data obtained from the Center for Disease Control's (CDC) National Reporting System in 1987 revealed that *C. trachomatis* caused approximately 1.55 million cases of clinical illness in men, including episodes of urethritis and epididymitis, and 776,200 cases of clinical disease in women, including mucopurulent cervicitis, urethritis, and pelvic inflammatory disease.[71] An estimated combined total cost of $1.4 billion per year in direct health care costs and indirect costs of lost productivity are attributed to disease caused by this organism. The combined risk of morbidity and mortality of diseases caused by *C. trachomatis* and the significant economic burden of these disease states revealed the need for effective *C. trachomatis* control programs. In 1993 the CDC released recommendations for prevention and management of *C. trachomatis* infections.[72]

Cardiovascular Disease

Acute myocardial infarction

In 1992, the estimated number of myocardial infarctions in the United States was approximately 750,000 per year. The associated cost, in terms of morbidity and mortality, from such events are considerable. Analyses of treatment strategies for myocardial infarction have revealed favorable cost-effectiveness values for reperfusion strategies with a thrombolytic agent. Likewise, the use of beta-blockers and angiotensin-converting enzyme inhibitors post-myocardial infarction in appropriate patients has been shown to be cost-effective.[73] After myocardial infarction, beta-blocker therapy has been shown to reduce mortality (21%), cardiac death (24%), sudden cardiac death (30%), and reinfarction (25%). Beta-blocker therapy appears most efficacious among high-risk post-myocardial infarction patients (i.e., those with arrhythmias, left ventricular dysfunction, or inducible ischemia). Patients are recommended to receive beta-blocker therapy starting at 5 to 28 days postinfarction and continuing for at least 6 months.

Hypertension and hypercholesterolemia

Hypertension is a prevalent and costly problem. Like other preventive therapies for heart disease, such as smoking cessation, exercise, and weight loss, blood pressure control and lipid lowering have been the focus of cost-effectiveness analyses. Treatment of hypertension has been found to be cost-effective in virtually all populations and circumstances and for a wide variety of drugs. The presence of coexisting risk factors makes interventions to reduce blood pressure even more cost-effective. Factors limiting the potential for cost-effectiveness are issues of compliance and out-of-pocket drug costs. Studies evaluating the cost-effectiveness of antihyperlipidemia therapy for primary prevention of heart disease generally consider it to be expensive when compared with other risk-reducing interventions such as smoking cessation. Secondary prevention with cholesterol-lowering drugs is favorable.[74]

Respiratory Disease

Asthma

Asthma is associated with an increased risk of morbidity and mortality and was estimated to affect nearly 12 million individuals in the United States in the late 1980s. Direct expenditures for hospitalization, outpatient services, emergency room services, physician visits, and drug therapy were estimated to approach $4.5 billion in 1985.[75] Drug costs accounted for $712.7 million of total direct costs. Estimates of indirect costs associated with lost workdays and days spent away from school were estimated to add an additional $2.09 billion to annual asthma costs.

The cost-effectiveness of therapies, such as cromolyn sodium use on a regular schedule in combination with bronchodilators and corticosteroids can provide cost savings. Fewer emergency room visits were reported in this retrospective analysis of cromolyn therapy.[76] The estimated average costs of emergency room visits were $33 and $624, respectively, for cromolyn users versus an age, gender, asthma-severity matched comparison group. Hospital costs were also lower for the cromolyn group. Cromolyn therapy was considered cost-effective in patients with chronic mild to moderately severe asthma. An analysis of inhaled corticosteroids in children in Sri Lanka with asthma showed that therapy improved the ability of patients to attend school, and reduced hospitalization and wheezing symptoms. This study concluded that inhaled corticosteroids for prophylaxis of asthma were cost-effective.[77]

Diabetes Mellitus

Diabetic patients are at considerable risk for developing complications, including eye, kidney, neurologic, cardiovascular, cerebrovascular, and peripheral vascular disease. Estimates of the total per-capita expenditure associated with health care for diabetic patients found that patients with diabetes had more than three times greater associated health care costs than patients without the disease. In 1992, 4.5% of the population of the United States had diabetes, but accounted for a disproportionate degree of health care expenditures (11.9% of the total US health care expenditures). The total health care expenditure for patients with diabetes in 1992 was estimated to be $85 billion.[78] A greater proportion of health care expenditures for diabetes were paid for by Medicare (27% for diabetics compared with 13% for non-diabetics).

CONCLUSIONS

Given the increasing investment in research and development, significant technologic advances in drug therapy are anticipated. Likewise, the need for continued, critical evaluation of the value of such new drugs will continue. While some new drugs are unique additions to existing therapies, others may offer more modest improvements at higher cost. As suggested by the National Institute for Health Care Management and Educational Foundation researchers' recent report of factors affecting rising pharmaceutical costs,[21] more research is needed on several important questions, such as:

- How do we capitalize on the benefits of new therapies and assure that the right drugs get to the right people safely and at the right time, to deliver the highest value of care?
- Under what circumstances is each new drug the most appropriate treatment, compared to the available alternatives?
- What impact will increasing expenditures on prescription drugs have on overall health care spending?

Affordability of health care will increasingly be a concern. As the cost of covering prescription drugs continues to grow, health plans, purchasers, and consumers will face difficult choices among promoting access to drug therapies, maintaining health insurance premiums at an affordable level, and continuing to offer other needed benefits. The money to pay for more expensive new drugs will likely come from higher premiums, higher out-of-pocket costs, lower benefits, and/or more restricted access to drugs (e.g. formularies). In addition, the possible inclusion of a prescription drug benefit in the Medicare program makes understanding what is driving the increase in pharmaceutical expenditures all the more important. For private third-party payers, which covers a younger, healthier population, prescription drugs already represent about 13% of health benefit outlays. Some plans with many retirees report that drug costs are approaching 30% of total benefits. Pharmaceutical research focused on new drugs that will target the chronic and disabling diseases of the elderly may drive those costs even higher. The experience of private insurers, particularly those covering older populations, suggests that the cost of Medicare coverage of prescription drugs will likely be substantial from the outset and increase significantly over time.[21]

All these elements are of concern to employers, who remain the largest purchaser of health care services outside of the federal government. The application of pharmacoeconomic and outcomes research to include the employers' perspective will guide the ongoing outcome debate around optimal health care coverage.

REFERENCES

1. Iglehart JK: The American health care system—expenditures. *New Engl J Med* 1999;340(1):70–76.
2. Kuttner R: The American health care system—health insurance coverage. *New Engl J Med* 1999;340(2):163–168.
3. Iglehart JK: The American health care system. Managed care. *New Engl J Med* 1992;327(10):742–744.
4. Kuttner R: The American health care system—employer sponsored health coverage. Special report. *New Engl J Med* 1999;340(3):248–252.
5. Iglehart J: The American health care system—Medicare. Special report. *New Engl J Med* 1999;340(4):327–332.
6. Iglehart J: The American health care system—Medicaid. Special report. *New Engl J Med* 1999;340(5):403–408.
7. Kindig DA: *Purchasing Population Health: Paying for Results.* Ann Arbor: University of Michigan Press; 1997.
8. Rosenbaum DE: Health insurance provides buffer to rising drug prices for most Americans. *New York Times* Thu, 1 Jun 2000;24.
9. Lipton HL, Kreling DH, Collins T, Hertz KC: Pharmacy benefit management companies: dimensions of performance. *Ann Rev Publ Health* 1999;20:361–401.
10. Richardson WS, Detsky AS: Users' guide to the medical literature. VII. How to use a clinical decision analysis. B. What are the results and will they help me in caring for my patients? Evidence Based Medicine Working Group. *JAMA* 1995;273(20):1610–1613.
11. Wilson MC, Hayward RS, Tunis SR, Bass EB, Guyatt G: Users' guides to the medical literature. VIII. How to use clinical practice guidelines. B. What are the recommendations and will they help you in caring for your patients? The Evidence-Based Medicine Working Group. *JAMA* 1995;274(20):1630–1632.
12. Drummond MF, Richardson WS, O'Brien BJ, Levine M, Heyland D: Users' guides to the medical literature. XIII. How to use an article on economic analysis of clinical practice. A. Are the results of the study valid? Evidence-Based Medicine Working Group. *JAMA* 1997;277(19):1552–1557.
13. Guyatt GH, Naylor CD, Juniper E, Heyland DK, Jaeschke R, Cook DJ: Users' guides to the medical literature. XII. How to use articles about health-related quality of life. Evidence-Based Medicine Working Group. *JAMA* 1997;277(15):1232–1237.
14. Barratt A, Irwig L, Glasziou P, et al.: Users' guides to the medical literature. XVII. How to use guidelines and recommendations about screening. *JAMA* 1999;281(21):2029–2034.

15. Guyatt GH, Sinclair J, Cook DJ, Glasziou P: Users' guides to the medical literature. XVI. How to use a treatment recommendation. *JAMA* 1999;281(19):1836–1843.
16. Richardson WS, Wilson MC, Guyatt GH, Cook DJ, Nishikawa J: Users' guides to the medical literature. XV. How to use an article about disease probability for differential diagnosis. Evidence-Based Medicine Working Group. *JAMA* 1999;281(13):1214–1219.
17. McAlister FA, Straus SE, Guyatt GH, Haynes RB: Users' guides to the medical literature. XX. Integrating research evidence with the care of the individual patient. *JAMA* 2000;283(21):2829–2836.
18. US Department of Health and Human Services. *Healthy People 2010—Understanding and Improving Health,* Volume 1. Washington, DC; January 2000.
19. Holmer AF (Pharmaceutical Researchers and Manufacturers of America): *New Drug Approvals in 1999*. January 2000.
20. Suh DC, Lacy CR, Barone JA, Moylan D, Kostis JB: Factors contributing to trends in prescription drug expenditures. *Clin Therap* 1999;21(7):1241–1253.
21. Sherman D, Bradshaw A, Tanamor M, Topolski C, et al.: (The National Institute for Health Care Management and Educational Foundation). *Factors Affecting the Growth of Prescription Drug Expenditures*. July 9, 1999.
22. Clancy CM, Eisenberg JM: Health care policy—outcomes research: measuring the end results of health care. *Science* 1998;282(5387):245.
23. Graham JD, Corso PS, Morris JM, Seguigomez M, Weinstein MC: Evaluating the cost-effectiveness of clinical and public health measures. *Ann Rev Publ Health* 1998;19:125–152.
24. Evans R: Principles of economic analysis of health care technology. *Ann Intern Med* 1996;124(5):536.
25. Sacristan J, Javier S, Hernandez J: Principles of economic analysis of health care technology. *Ann Intern Med* 1996;124(5):535–536.
26. Gifford F: Outcomes research and practice guidelines. Upstream issues for downstream users. *Hastings Center Rep* 1996;26(2):38–44.
27. Neumann PJ, Sandberg EA, Bell CM, Stone PW, Chapman RH: Are pharmaceuticals cost-effective? A review of the evidence. *Health Affairs* 2000;19(2):92–109.
28. Prosser L, Koplan J, Neumann P, Weinstein M: Barriers to using cost-effectiveness in managed care decision making. *Am J Managed Care Pharm* 2000;6(2):173–179.
29. Litvak E, Long MC, Schwartz JS: Cost-effectiveness analysis under managed care: not yet ready for prime time? *Am J Managed Care* 2000;6(2):254–256.
30. Reinhardt UE: Making economic evaluations respectable. *Soc Sci Med* 1997;45(4):555–562.

31. Gold M. In: Gold M, Siegel J, Russell L, Weinstein M, eds, *Cost-Effectiveness in Health and Medicine*, 2nd edn. Oxford, UK: Oxford University Press; 1996.
32. Reeve GR, Pastula S, Rontal R: A major employer as a health care services laboratory. *Int J Qual Health Care* 1998;10(6):547–553.
33. McCaffrey E: The acid test for formulary policy. *Business & Health* 1999; special report (Dec):19–24.
34. Institute WLD: *Official Disability Guidelines*. Riverside, CT: Work Loss Data Institute; 1996.
35. Goetzel RZ, Ozminkowski RJ, Meneades L, Stewart M, Schutt DC: Pharmaceuticals—cost or investment? An employer's perspective. *J Occup Environ Med* 2000;42(4):338–351.
36. Koopmanschap MA, Rutten FFH: Indirect costs—the consequence of production loss or increased costs of production. *Med Care* 1996;34(12 Suppl S):DS59–DS68.
37. Christensen S, Wagner J: The costs of a Medicare prescription drug benefit. *Health Affairs* 2000;19:212–218.
38. Steinberg EP, Gutierrez B, Momani A, et al.: Beyond survey data: a claims-based analysis of drug use and spending by the elderly. *Health Affairs* 2000;19:198–211.
39. Navarro R, Blackburn S: Pharmacy benefit management companies. In: Werthheimer AI, Navarro R, eds, *Managed Care Pharmacy Practice*. Gaithersburg, MD: Aspen Publ; 1999:221–241.
40. Sax, M, Emigh R: Managed care formularies in the United States. *JMCP* 1999;54(4):289–295.
41. Hatoum H, Freeman R: Use of pharmacoeconomic data in formulary selection. *Top Hosp Pharm Management* 1994;13(4):47–53.
42. Holzer SS, Juday TR, Joelsson B, Crawley JA: Determining the cost of gastroesophageal reflux disease—a decision analytic model. *Am J Managed Care* 1998;4(10):1450–1460.
43. Schrogie J, Nash D. Relationship between practice guidelines, formulary management, and pharmacoeconomic studies. *Top Hosp Pharm Management* 1994;13(4):38–46.
44. Task Force on Principles for Economic Analysis of Health Care Technology. Economic analysis of health care technology. A report on principles. *Ann Intern Med* 1995;123(1):61–70.
45. Institute for Clinical Systems Improvement. Annual Report 1999. Available at http://www.icsi.org/annual.pdf.
46. Corrigan JM, Nielsen DM: Toward the development of uniform reporting standards for managed care organizations: the Health Plan Employer Data and Information Set (Version 2.0). *Joint Commission J Qual Improv* 1993;19(12):566–575.

47. Corrigan JM, Griffith H: NCQA external reporting and monitoring activities for health plans: preventive services programs. *Am J Prevent Med* 1995;11(6):393–396.
48. Corrigan JM: How do purchasers develop and use performance measures? *Med Care* 1995;33(1 Suppl):JS18–23; discussion JS23–24.
49. O'Leary DS: Performance measures. How are they developed, validated, and used? *Med Care* 1995;33(1 Suppl):JS13–17.
50. Member of the Committee on Performance Measurement at NCQA. *Book I: HEDIS 3.0: Understanding and Enhancing Performance Measurement*, Volume 2. Washington, DC: National Committee for Quality Assurance; 1997 NCQA Reference Set.
51. Freudenheim M: New technology helps health care avoid mistakes. *New York Times* Feb 3, 2000;1.
52. American Diabetes Association. Clinical practice recommendations 1997. *Diabetes Care* 1997;20(Suppl 1):S1–70.
53. Cromwell J, Bartosch WJ, Fiore MC, Hasselblad V, Baker T: Cost-effectiveness of the clinical practice recommendations in the AHCPR guideline for smoking cessation. Agency for Health Care Policy and Research. *JAMA* 1997;278(21):1759–1766.
54. National Heart, Lung, and Blood Institute: Clinical guidelines on the identification, evaluation, and treatment of overweight and obesity in adults—the evidence report. National Institutes of Health. *Obes Res* 1998;6(Suppl 2):51S–209S.
55. Sullivan S, Elixhauser A, Buist AS, Luce BR, Eisenberg J, Weiss KB: National Asthma Education and Prevention Program working group report on the cost effectiveness of asthma care. *Am J Resp Crit Care Med* 1996;154(3 Pt 2):S84–95.
56. National Osteoporosis Foundation: Osteoporosis: review of the evidence for prevention, diagnosis and treatment and cost-effectiveness analysis. Executive summary. *Osteoporosis Int* 1998;8(Suppl 4):S3–6.
57. Williams WW, Hickson MA, Kane MA, Kendal AP, Spika JS, Hinman AR: Immunization policies and vaccine coverage among adults. The risk for missed opportunities. *Ann Intern Med* 1988;108(4):616–625.
58. Nichol KL, Lind A, Margolis KL, et al.: The effectiveness of vaccination against influenza in healthy, working adults. *New Engl J Med* 1995; 333(14):889–893.
59. Mullooly JP, Bennett MD, Hornbrook MC, et al.: Influenza vaccination programs for elderly persons: cost-effectiveness in a health maintenance organization. *Ann Intern Med* 1994;121(12):947–952.
60. Nichol KL, Margolis KL, Wuorenma J, Von Sternberg T: The efficacy and cost effectiveness of vaccination against influenza among elderly persons living in the community. *New Engl J Med* 1994;331(12):778–784.

61. Oster G, Colditz GA, Kelly NL: The economic costs of smoking and benefits of quitting for individual smokers. *Prevent Med* 1984;13(4):377–389.
62. Cummings SR, Rubin SM, Oster G: The cost-effectiveness of counseling smokers to quit. *JAMA* 1989;261(1):75–79.
63. Marks JS, Koplan JP, Hogue CJ, Dalmat ME: A cost-benefit/cost-effectiveness analysis of smoking cessation for pregnant women. *Am J Prevent Med* 1990;6(5):282–289.
64. Tsevat J: Impact and cost-effectiveness of smoking interventions. *Am J Med* 1992;93(1A):43S–47S.
65. Windsor RA, Lowe JB, Perkins LL, et al.: Health education for pregnant smokers: its behavioral impact and cost benefit. *Am J Publ Health* 1993;83(2):201–206.
66. Oster G, Huse D, Delea T, Colditz G: Cost-effectiveness of nicotine gum as an adjunct to physician's advice against cigarette smoking. *JAMA* 1986;256:1315–1318.
67. Stool S, Field J: The impact of otitis media. *Pediatr Infect Dis J* 1989;8(Suppl 1):S11–S14.
68. Williams RL, Chalmers TC, Stange KC, Chalmers FT, Bowlin SJ: Use of antibiotics in preventing recurrent acute otitis media and in treating otitis media with effusion. A meta-analytic attempt to resolve the brouhaha. *JAMA* 1993;270(11):1344–1351.
69. Stool S: *Otitis Media with Effusion in Young Children: Clinical Practice Guideline No. 12*. Rockville, MD: Agency for Health Care Policy and Research, Public Health Service, US Department of Health and Human Services; 1994 AHCPR Publication No. 94-0622.
70. Pichichero ME: Assessing the treatment alternatives for acute otitis media. *Pediatr Infect Dis J* 1994;13(1 Suppl 1):S27–34; discussion S50–54.
71. Washington AE, Johnson RE, Sanders LL, Jr: *Chlamydia trachomatis* infections in the United States. What are they costing us? *JAMA* 1987;257(15):2070–2072.
72. Prevention CfDCa: Recommendations for the prevention and management of *Chlamydia trachomatis* infections, 1993. *MMWR—Morbidity & Mortality Weekly Report*. 1993;42(RR-12):1–39.
73. Kupersmith J, Holmes-Rovner M, Hogan A, Rovner D, Gardiner J: Cost-effectiveness analysis in heart disease. Part III: Ischemia, congestive heart failure, and arrhythmias. *Prog Cardiovas Dis* 1995;37(5):307–346.
74. Kupersmith J, Holmes-Rovner M, Hogan A, Rovner D, Gardiner J: Cost-effectiveness analysis in heart disease. Part II: Preventive therapies. *Prog Cardiovas Dis* 1995;37(4):243–271.
75. Weiss KB, Gergen PJ, Hodgson TA: An economic evaluation of asthma in the United States. *New Engl J Med* 1992;326(13):862–866.

76. Ross RN, Morris M, Sakowitz SR, Berman BA: Cost-effectiveness of including cromolyn sodium in the treatment program for asthma: a retrospective, record-based study. *Clin Therap* 1988;10(2):188–203.
77. Perera BJ: Efficacy and cost effectiveness of inhaled steroids in asthma in a developing country. *Arch Dis Childhood* 1995;72(4):312–315; discussion 315–316.
78. Rubin RJ, Altman WM, Mendelson DN: Health care expenditures for people with diabetes mellitus, 1992. *J Clin Endocrinol Metab* 1994;78(4):809A–809F

GLOSSARY*

Absenteeism—end result of missing a predetermined appointment or work agreement; often measured as days off work or school lost by a worker or student

Co-payment—a relatively small fixed dollar fee required by a health insurer (as an HMO) to be paid by the patient at the time of each office visit, outpatient service, or filling of a prescription

Coverage—provision of insurance by a payer; full or partial exemption from incurred health care expenses or liabilities

Disability—a restricted or worsened ability to perform activities of daily living or work activities due to limitations brought on by some physical, emotional, or cognitive hindrance

Drug policy—defined, in the context of pharmacoeconomics, as a strategy, clinical practice guideline, or coverage decision created for the purpose of guiding the selection of pharmacologic therapy, with the intent of delivering the highest-quality, lowest-cost drug therapy to the largest possible population

Formulary—a list of selected pharmaceuticals judged to be the most clinically and economically useful for a group of patients, from which physicians are expected to select—may be open, no denial of reimbursement for non-formulary products by the payer; closed, only formulary products will be reimbursed by the payer

Functional status—the capacity of an individual to perform normal or usual activities in the presence of disease at a given level of activity

Health—the state of physical, mental, and social well-being, not merely the absence of disease or disability. Defined by Healthy People 2010 further to encompass concepts of quality of life, functional status, and productivity

---

**Source*: Committee on Performance Measurement at NCQA. *Book II: HEDIS 3.0: Measurement Specifications*, Volume 2. Washington, DC: National Committee for Quality Assurance; 1997 NCQA Reference Set.

Health benefit programs—a set of health products or services and providers of care available for reimbursement by a health plan
Health outcome—the result of therapeutic interventions measured in terms of clinical (e.g., symptom, laboratory, diagnostic) or humanistic (e.g., quality of life, functional status) endpoints
Health status—a measurement of healthiness using a systematic scoring of different domains of health (e.g., physical and social function, vitality, mental and general health, role impairment)
Indemnity insurance—*protection against incurred health care expenses or liabilities; indemnity systems reimburse on a fee-for-service basis or full rate of charge for health care services*
Insurance—a contract made between a payer and a beneficiary for the purpose of providing security against hurt, loss, or damage
Medical decision-making—a systematic approach to gathering and applying relevant information to support the selection of a health intervention from among various alternatives to optimize the likelihood of obtaining the most satisfactory outcome
Outcomes research—the study of the end results of health services that takes patients' preference and experience into account; intended to provide scientific evidence relating to decisions made by all who participate in health care
Payer (of health care expenses)—the person, group, or institution by which a medical bill has been or should be paid
Policy decision makers—those responsible for defining a definite course (e.g., formulary status, therapeutic interchange, clinical practice guideline) or method (e.g., disease management or health promotion approach), or of action selected from among alternatives and in light of given conditions to guide and determine present and future clinical decisions
Precertification—a form of utilization management that aims to reduce the frequency of hospitalization by shortening the length of hospital stays or substituting other types of care
Preferred provider organizations (PPOs)—a managed care arrangement that creates a contractual arrangement between a restricted group of caregivers to deliver health services to health plan members
Premium—a sum of money paid at periodic intervals in advance of or in addition to the nominal value of a medical service or therapy
Private sector—the economic subdivision of the health care industry represented by non-government, non-federal purchasers (e.g., private insurance, out-of-pocket payers)
Productivity—1, the quality or state of being productive; 2, rate of production of work output
Provider—hospital, physician or other health personnel that make available services or products required to diagnose, treat, or prevent disease or injury
Public sector—the economic subdivision of the health care industry represented by government or federal purchasers

Purchaser—an individual or group obtaining health care services or therapy for one's self or on behalf of a population of beneficiaries by paying money or its equivalent to a provider of health care services or contracting with a third-party payer or health maintenance organization to do the same

Rebate—a sum paid by a manufacturer or wholesaler to a customer health plan based on a contractual arrangement specifying a negotiated percentage of return, and the number of units of product utilized by members of the health plan

Self-funded—refers to those employers that indemnify or guarantee an employee against loss by a specified health contingency or peril (provide health care insurance) by contract to employees through the company's own funds

Utilization review—an assessment of the need for health services or products based on a retrospective, concurrent, or prospective review of the medical necessity, efficiency, and/or appropriateness of such services or products

CHAPTER

6

Variables in Pharmacoeconomics

Patty J. Keys and Daniel Touchette

INTRODUCTION

There are many competing interests that foster the complexity of today's health care environment. Chronic diseases requiring lifelong investments of technology and resources dominate our health needs. Additionally, new technologies are being developed at an increasingly rapid rate. Finally, limited economic resources impose restraints on consumption of health care resources. In this light, health care decision makers are repeatedly faced with the challenge of providing care in a way that maximizes health outcomes while minimizing expenditures.

Pharmacoeconomic evaluations provide tools to assist decision makers in this challenge by providing a method to balance costs and consequences of health care interventions. These tools assess economic investments while considering clinical and humanistic outcomes.

In general, health care is employed to improve the health of a person. In so doing, three important components are required to fulfill this purpose. First, a commonly accepted definition of health should be considered. The World Health Organization (WHO) definition has established health as "a state of complete physical, mental and social well-being and not merely the absence of disease and infirmity."[1] Secondly, the development and application of technologies and interventions are considered. The evolution of technologies is prominent in our society. In fact, great emphasis is placed on the development and availability of drugs and diagnostic tools. In this light, the issue of whether the intervention works is explored exhaustively. This addresses, in part, the concept of efficacy, which asks the question, "Under ideal circumstances (all things being equal), does the technology or intervention work better than doing nothing?" In contrast, little attention is given to the impact of competing technologies. This begs the question of effectiveness, which asks, "Under everyday circumstances, does the technology or intervention work better than an active competing one?" In short, is the impact of the technology or intervention being compared with a placebo (do nothing) or is it being compared with, at least, a reasonable standard of care. In light of the rapid development of new health care technologies, it is important to consider the concept of "improvement" in health. This is the third and final component to consider in fulfilling the purpose of health care. Since health is a reflection of well-being (physical, mental, and social), improved health should reflect a desirable change in at least one of these dimensions of well-being. Consequently, a health care intervention or new technology would ideally be able to produce a measurable improvement in health. In concept, this is easy to understand. However, in practice, it meets with various levels of complexity. Consequently, a production in health improvement is predicated on the ability to measure improvement. Furthermore, the ability to measure improvement of health is additionally dependent on the ability to measure health status.

Measurement of health status is implicitly required as a part of providing health care. Various health status measurements are fundamentally important in pharmacoeconomic evaluations. Along with economic measures, they are used to evaluate the economic efficiency of interventions and new technologies in achieving the purpose of health care.

Pharmacoeconomic tools of assessment comprise a diversity of data, including economic, clinical, and humanistic variables. In this chapter we detail the relationship between pharmacoeconomic outcomes and variables and consider different approaches to organizing them. Lastly, the impact of changing variable values on outcome parameters is discussed.

RELATIONSHIP BETWEEN OUTCOMES AND VARIABLES

Pharmacoeconomic Outcomes

Before looking specifically at the types of variables used in pharmacoeconomic assessments, let us consider the question, " What do pharmacoeconomic variables represent?" In general, a variable is used as a proxy for a concept of interest to the researcher. Variables are not usually of ultimate interest. In the case of pharmacoeconomic evaluations, outcomes are the primary focus.

Pharmacoeconomic outcomes can be categorized as monetary and non-monetary outcomes. The Economic Clinical Humanistic Outcomes (ECHO) model provides a theoretical framework used in characterizing the types of pharmacoeconomic outcomes.[2] In this model, outcomes are described as the economic, clinical, or humanistic impact of the disease and treatment. Economic outcomes represent the concept of opportunity cost. Clinical outcomes reflect the concept of physiologic health status. Humanistic outcomes address the concept of psychosocial health status.

Outcomes are not directly measured: they are intangible concepts and, as such, are not measurable entities. For example, mortality is a clinical outcome that cannot be directly measured, yet mortality rates are commonly reported in the literature. To reconcile this, one must recognize that "mortality" is not the same as a "mortality rate." Mortality is a concept that represents "the state of being mortal, destined to die."[3] In contrast, mortality rates are measures of the frequency of death. Thus, mortality is an immeasurable concept (i.e., an outcome) and mortality rate is used to reflect a measure of mortality (i.e., a variable).

What Outcomes Should be Used?

Outcomes can be either terminal or intermediate in their description of health events. Terminal outcomes represent the medical event of primary interest when evaluating an intervention or technology. Mortality is the most frequently used and widely accepted terminal outcome in evaluation of health interventions. It is a physiologic (clinical) consequence used in health care to assess the impact of an intervention. Mortality has several attributes that make it an attractive terminal outcome. It is clearly defined and is easy to recognize and measure. However, measuring terminal outcomes, such as mortality, may be problematic in several respects. First, the length of time required to observe terminal outcome may be protracted, resulting in unreasonably lengthy and expensive studies. Secondly, the outcome event may be difficult to measure such as when subjects are lost to follow-up. Thirdly, the reliability of the outcome measure may impose limitations on interpreting or applying the measure in the context of the study. And finally, the relationship between the outcome event and the intervention may be poorly defined. These challenges do not preclude the assessment of outcomes in pharmacoeconomic evaluations, yet they do establish the need to broaden consideration for outcome measures beyond terminal outcomes.

In clinical medicine, years of research have gone into refining the association between intermediate outcomes and terminal outcomes. Every aspect of clinical medicine provides examples of this: established correlation between serum lipid levels and cardiovascular-related mortality; bone density and fracture outcomes in osteoporosis; obesity and adult onset diabetes in endocrinology; and viral load and mortality in HIV/AIDS all serve as examples for successfully substituting intermediate outcomes in place of terminal outcomes. In each case, the use of intermediate outcomes was dictated by specific limitations associated with following terminal outcomes on a routine basis. A common motivator for each example is the ability to obtain results, draw conclusions, and make recommendations more expediently than possible using measures of terminal outcomes. An additional common motivator is the ethical implications of waiting for terminal outcomes to occur. Since terminal outcomes are traditionally associated with a demise in health status, it is inherently unethical to routinely wait for these negative consequences to occur. It fundamentally goes against the purpose of health care.

Likewise, in pharmacoeconomic evaluations, intermediate outcomes are used to expedite the process of obtaining results, drawing conclusions, and making recommendations. Unfortunately, there is not as much historical research in place to consistently link intermediate and terminal outcomes in pharmacoeconomic evaluations.

There is another concern associated with reliance on traditional terminal outcomes such as survival and cure. Today's health care interventions predominately target chronic disease processes. Since chronic disease terminal outcomes are not usually characterized in terms of survivals or cures, their use as terminal outcomes will be unresponsive to intervention-related change.

These considerations highlight the need for continued research to identify causative associations between intermediate and terminal outcomes. The relationship of these issues to the selection and use of variables in pharmacoeconomic evaluations is further elucidated in this chapter.

Pharmacoeconomic Variables

In contrast to outcomes, variables are measurable events or entities. They are either a categorical status or numeric quantities that describe some aspect of the outcome. In our example, mortality rates are variables, since they are frequencies that present as numeric values. They are summarized representations of a categorical depiction of mortality, dead vs. alive.

Variables can take on many different values. They are defined as "that which is inconstant, which can or does change as contrasted with a constant."[3]

The method used for estimating the value of a variable warrants some discussion. A variable's value can be acquired through deterministic or probabilistic methods. A deterministic value for a variable is a reflection of one observation or an explicit assignment of value. This is best understood by considering the price of a prescription drug. The price of a prescription drug in one specific pharmacy provides a deterministic assignment for the monetary value associated with the drug.

In contrast, a probabilistic value for a variable is a reflection of multiple observations of the value. There is additional information contained in a probabilistic variable that conveys the accuracy and precision of the estimated value of the variable. For example, the probabilistic estimate of prescription price can be reflected by computing the mean price of the drug from different pharmacies. Additionally, an estimate of the variability in prescription price is reflected in the variance or standard deviation.

Variables used in pharmacoeconomic assessments are commonly a combination of deterministic and probabilistic valuation methods. Probabilistic estimates are preferred since they contain more information about the estimated value of the variable compared with deterministic estimates. Unfortunately, probabilistic estimates are not readily available for some pharmacoeconomic variables. Consequently, deterministic estimates are used. This is frequently the case with economic variables and, to a lesser extent, with clinical and humanistic variables.

TYPES OF PHARMACOECONOMIC VARIABLES

Consistent with the ECHO model, each type of outcome can be characterized by economic, clinical, or humanistic variables. Economic variables are the measurable entities that reflect economic outcomes. Likewise, clinical and humanistic variables are the measurable entities that reflect clinical and humanistic outcomes, respectively.

Economic Variables

Economic variables are measures of the economic cost of the disease and disease management process. These costs can be categorized in three ways. Direct medical costs are those costs that are incurred as a direct result of diagnosing, managing, and treating the disease. They include laboratory, hospital, X-rays, doctor's visits, medications, emergency room visits, surgeries, and special diagnostic procedures. Other costs reflected as economic variables are direct non-medical costs. These costs are incurred as a direct result of the illness, but are not expended within the health care sector (i.e., day care, housekeeping, special tutors, and transportation). They account for illness-related non-medical resource consumption. Lastly, indirect costs are the costs of disability that results in lost productivity.

Economic variables are implicitly composed of two components: resource utilization and monetary valuation. Resource utilization variables are frequencies or counts of the resources used in the disease management process. Monetary valuation variables represent the economic value of each unit of resource consumed (i.e., dollars per laboratory test, dollars per doctors visit, etc.).

Clinical Variables

Health care interventions are employed to effect a change in the clinical status of a patient. Clinical variables serve as the measuring stick against which health improvement is gauged. The measure of health improvement finds its origin in the quality improvement literature where Donabedian first proposed the theoretical framework for quality improvement.[4] This framework describes the relationship between structural and procedural elements of the health care system and observed changes in health care outcomes. In light of the different types of outcomes, specific attention must be given to the definition process for outcomes. In terms of patient improvement, health outcomes are defined as "a change in a patient's current and future health status that can be related to previous health care."[5] Likewise, it can be said that a clinical outcome is "a change in a patient's current and future clinical status that can be related to previous health care." To assess for a change in clinical status, selected clinical variables should be monitored and measured. The specifics of the disease process dictate the variables used for monitoring clinical outcomes. First, the relevant clinical outcomes need to be established. Consider, for example, an intervention or technology affecting hypertension. An appropriate terminal outcome to consider is cardiovascular-related mortality. Similarly, relevant intermediate outcomes may include:

- reduction in blood pressure;
- reduction in cardiovascular events such as stroke or myocardial infarction; and
- reductions in disease-related consumption of health care resources.

Each outcome has several corresponding clinical variables that can be measured. Table 6-1 shows examples of clinical variables as they relate to their corresponding clinical outcomes. Pre- and post-intervention measures of diastolic and systolic blood pressures produce four clinical variables for the blood pressure reduction outcome. Number of strokes, number of myocardial infarctions, and number of cardiovascular-related deaths produce three variables for the cardiovascular event outcome. Similarly, number of cardiovascular-related hospitalizations, number of emergency room visits, and number of angioplasties produce three variables for the disease-related resource consumption outcome.

Clinical variables are frequently used to measure both terminal and intermediate outcomes. However, they also serve other purposes. For example, clinical variables may help to identify a subset of patients or disease states.

Three types of clinical variables are useful in identifying a subset of patients: patient-specific variables, disease-specific variables, and risk modifier variables. Patient-specific variables are typically referred to as patient demographics and include age, gender, ethnicity, socioeconomic status, weight, and height. They

TABLE 6-1.

Outcomes and Variables

Outcomes	*Variables*
Blood pressure	Pre-treatment diastolic blood pressure Pre-treatment systolic blood pressure Post-treatment diastolic blood pressure Post-treatment systolic blood pressure
Cardiovascular events	Number of strokes Number of myocardial infarctions Number of cardiovascular-related deaths
Disease-related resource consumption	Number of cardiovascular-related hospitalizations Number of cardiovascular-related emergency room visits Number of angioplasties

are frequently obtained from sources such as medical charts, computerized medical records, administrative databases, and existing research databases.

Disease-specific variables are employed to characterize different aspects of a disease state. Disease classification variables are produced using established disease classification systems such as (1) the American Psychiatric Association: Diagnostic and Statistical Manual of Mental Disorders, 4th edn; (2) the TNM cancer staging system; and (3) the New York Heart Association classification for congestive heart failure. They contribute valuable information regarding both disease diagnosis and severity. Although primarily used as research tools, disease classification systems are commonly encountered in daily clinical practice to assist in prognosis and establishing severity of illness.

Risk modifier variables are not systematically identified as in established disease classification systems. Risk modifier variables are those clinical factors that impact the predisposition to disease sequelae, disease progression, or responsiveness to treatment. For example, the hypertension intervention data may need to be expanded to include information about diabetic comorbidity. By documenting the presence of diabetes in the hypertensive patient population, the outcomes common to both illnesses can be accounted for, thus reducing the risk of bias in the clinical variable measures.

Humanistic Variables

The use of humanistic variables is not new to the health care environment. Some of the oldest humanistic variables are pain, mobility, and other symptom-level characteristics of a disease process. However, there are increasing efforts to expand the descriptive nature of these variables to include quantitative attributes. Two types of humanistic variables have been commonly used in pharmacoeconomic evaluations: utilities and quality of life. Their common link is the use of patient perspective as the source of data. Measures of utilities are a way of expressing patients' preference for existing in a given state of health, while quality of life measures are a way of ranking their state of health and their level of functioning in that state. Humanistic variables can be used to represent terminal outcomes, and are used to estimate the psychological, emotional, and role functioning (social) impact of treatment interventions. They are particularly useful in characterizing chronic disease outcomes by reflecting the attributes affected by chronic disease treatments.

There are four ways to describe quality of life measures.[6] Indicator measures are a single number that represents the response value of one specific concept or domain: for example, "on a scale of 1 (none) to 5 (lots), rate the amount of pain you experience." Examples of indicator measures commonly used in health care include reports of symptoms such as pain, counts of disease occurrence, days lost from work, mortality rates, reports of disability such as mobility, flexibility, and reports of level of functioning in specific roles (i.e., employee, domestic, parenting).

Indicator measures are not capable of distinguishing contributing effects from different sources. They only reflect the overall concept targeted by the indicator measure. Consequently, they may be difficult to interpret in terms of the contributing effects for each value. For example, pain caused by two different sources could not be distinguished in a pain symptom report item. The response to the question would reflect pain from both sources with no information to determine the magnitude of pain from each source, separately.

A second way of reporting humanistic data is with index values. Indexes are a single number that is computed from multiple concepts or domains. Each input value represents a specific concept. It is an aggregate representation of many concepts, which reflect the net impact or summarization. An analogous example of a familiar index measure is mean values. The mean represents a summary of information that is obtained from multiple values. There is information contained in mean values that originates in each of the disaggregate values. In quality of life index measures, the disaggregate values represent the specific concept, while the index value represents a summarization of several concepts.

Index values used in assessing quality of life included quality-adjusted life years (QALYs) and healthy years equivalent (HYEs). Each of these measures is a way to simultaneously assess mortality and some aspect of morbidity and disability.

Indexes are very convenient in that they provide information in a single interpretable value. The information contained within the index is a global representation of the humanistic interest for a given person. However, indexes are disadvantageous in regards to their level of responsiveness to change. Changes that effect only one dimension of the input for the index may not be sufficient to register a significant change in the overall value of the index. This is most troublesome, since response to interventions targeted at chronic disease processes may only demonstrate change in one or two dimensions of the index dimensions. Furthermore, since effectiveness research commonly compares two active treatment interventions, the treatment effect is going to be substantially smaller than placebo versus active treatment interventions. These reductions in treatment effects further compromise the ability of indexes to register significant treatment differences.

Profile measures are much more complex in their interpretation. They are grouped by dimension of interest, and then each dimension is reported separately. There is no single value upon which to evaluate change, making comparative analysis more complicated. Alternatively, the responses are organized into relevant and related dimensions. Because of this, response due to treatment is more effectively represented. For example, the SF-36 has eight dimensions, which are reported separately. Thus, the results of the findings of the SF-36 will have eight distinct values: one value for each of the eight dimensions. In doing this, the treatment effects on the two dimensions, pain and physical functioning, is not diluted by the absence of treatment effect on the other six dimensions. Consequently, the response to treatment can be analyzed separately for each dimension. However, the complexity of the analysis needed for profile measures can be a formidable deterrent to their use.

There is a strong emphasis to enhance the ability of humanistic variables to provide objective analytic insight. The impetus for this is driven by the prominence of chronic disease processes wherein humanistic outcomes are more important. Consequently, humanistic variables are becoming increasingly important.

Perspective as a Cornerstone

Perspective is a concept frequently seen in pharmacoeconomic evaluations. It is the notion of "whose point of view is being considered in the study." It is not, *per se*, a variable, but it has important ramifications on the variable selection process. It determines many aspects of study design, including time horizon, which data elements to collect, and valuation procedures for resource consumption.[7] Consequently, it is an important consideration when developing the framework of a pharmacoeconomic evaluation.

There are four major types of perspectives:

- the provider perspective represents those who are responsible for the delivery of care;
- the payer perspective represents private and public third-party payers, such as insurance companies, Medicaid, etc.;
- the patient perspective represents the person who is receiving care; and
- the society perspective represents the community at large: this perspective represents every other type of perspective.

The concept of time horizon of the different perspectives is most apparent when comparing the perspective of the insurer with that of the provider. The provider perspective is interested in the episode of illness that effects their resource consumption and may be as short as the length of a hospital stay. In contrast, the insurers have a longer time horizon: consumption of their resources extends through the duration of time the patient is covered under their plan.

The impact of perspective on which data elements to collect is depicted by comparing a public insurer perspective like Medicare with that of a provider in the community setting. Data elements of interest to Medicare would include an inpatient resource utilization parameter. Yet, the provider in the community setting is most interested in ambulatory resource consumption.

Lastly, the impact of perspective on valuation procedures for resource consumption is best explained using costs and charges. Charges generated in a hospital are represented as costs to the insurer. Consequently, hospital charges do not sufficiently reflect their costs but do reflect the costs of an insurer.

USES FOR VARIABLES

In addition to describing pharmacoeconomic variables by the type of data they represent, they can be described by their use in the evaluation process. Three categories best describe them: input variables, composite variables, and outcome variables.

The pharmacoeconomic evaluation process follows a specific path. Like other evaluative processes, data collection is one of the first methodological steps involving the handling of data. The process of capturing or extracting the desired data elements from the designated sources is responsible for the generation of the input variables. Input variables can be categorized according to their ECHO model outcomes. Economic input variables may include costs or counts of resources used. Clinical input variables may include clinical parameters, such as serum cholesterol levels, serum blood sugars, or mineral bone density values. Additionally, patient parameters such as patient demographics are representative of clinical input variables. Humanistic input variables would include response to specific items on quality of life or another humanistic assessment tool.

The next step in the evaluative process is data analysis, which applies mathematical and statistical computations to the input variables. The purpose of data analysis is to transform the input variables to reflect additional information not contained in the native data element. The transformation process is responsible for generation of the composite variables. There are several types of composite variables commonly used in research. Means, medians, standard deviations, and variances are a few that should be familiar to the reader. Pharmacoeconomic-specific composite variables can be broken into their respective ECHO model categories. Economic composite variables may include mean cost, mean number of resource units used (i.e., mean number blood tests, X-rays, doctors visits), and total cost of care. Clinical composite variables are less obvious. Some examples include variables such as body surface area, lean body weight, or absolute neutrophil counts. Humanistic composite variables include computed values such as utilities, QALYs, and HYEs.

The data analysis process is also responsible for the generation of outcome variables. These variables are used to support the decision-making process. What distinguishes outcome variables from other variables generated in the data analysis process is the *a priori* specification of the primary study objectives. The variables that correspond with the study objectives become the outcome variables. For example, if a pharmacoeconomic evaluation was undertaken to determine the more cost-effective agent, then the cost-effectiveness ratio for each intervention and the incremental cost-effectiveness (CE) ratios serve as the corresponding outcome variable. The reader should note that the CE ratio is characterized as a variable and not a definitive absolute value. The reason for this becomes apparent in the following sections.

FACTORS AFFECTING PHARMACOECONOMIC MEASURES

Pharmacoeconomic analyses assess the "relative efficiency" of competing alternatives in terms of both economic and non-economic variables. This is accomplished through an index of efficiency, commonly a ratio of cost to outcome (i.e., CE ratio, cost-benefit ratio, and cost-utility ratio).

$$\text{Index of efficiency} = \frac{\text{Costs (\$)}}{\text{No. of outcomes}}$$

$$\begin{aligned}\text{CE ratio} &= \frac{\text{Costs (\$)}}{\text{No. of desired outcomes}}\\ &= \text{Cost per desired outcome achieved}\end{aligned}$$

Issues of precision and accuracy are important considerations. There are statistical implications associated with computed ratios such as the pharmacoeconomic ratios of efficiency (i.e., CE ratio). The CE ratio estimates are inherently variable because of variability associated with input variables used in computing CE ratios. These input variables comprise estimates for economic and clinical outcomes associated with the intervention.

Many factors influence the accuracy and precision of the estimates for economic inputs. The cost value used in computing the numerator of CE ratios consists of disease-related costs. They are commonly heterogeneous composites obtained from literature values, local databases, national normative values, or an expert panel. The cost of each health resource used (R_x) in providing care is tallied to compute the total cost of care. These costs include physician visits, laboratories, X-rays, special procedures, surgical procedures, medications, etc.

Computing Resource Costs

$$RCost(R_1) = Qty(R_1) \times Cost(R_1)$$
$$RCost(R_2) = Qty(R_2) \times Cost(R_2) \ldots$$
$$RCost(R_n) = Qty(R_n) \times Cost(R_n)$$

where R_x = type of resource; Rcost(R_x) = accumulated cost of resource (R_x); Qty(R_x) = quantity of resource (R_x); and Cost(R_x) = unit cost of resource (R_x).

Computing Total Costs

$$\text{Total cost of care} = \sum_{n=1}^{n} RCosts(R_x)$$

Consumption of health resources and their associated costs can vary by patient, physician, institution, and region. Consequently, the computed value of total cost can take on different values.

When estimating costs for a sample population, total costs provide acceptable estimates. However, total costs have inherent variability associated with them. By incorporating this value into the numerator of CE ratios, variability is introduced into the value of CE ratios.

Outcome measures also have inherent variability associated with them. Data sources for outcome measures include clinical trials, observational studies, and various databases. Data obtained in clinical trials have the potential to produce biased estimates of the outcome measure. First, the clinical trial population is specially selected to facilitate sufficient statistical power and maximize internal validity. Consequently, these populations are very homogeneous in their clinical status and often represent a specific subpopulation with the disease.

Women, minorities, extremely ill people, or those with major comorbidities are characteristically underrepresented in these trials. Furthermore, clinical trials are commonly designed to address efficacy of the intervention in terms of a limited range of disease severity. These selection criteria serve to increase the power and precision of the estimate. However, they have the potential to induce a bias on the value of the outcome measure.

For example, debilitated patients may not respond as readily to an intervention as those represented in the clinical trial sample. Consequently, clinical trial results may overestimate the number of favorable outcomes in the debilitated subpopulation receiving the intervention. Such a bias would reflect a CE ratio that overestimates efficiency of the intervention for debilitated patients. In this scenario, debilitated patients actually achieve fewer desirable outcomes than is reflected in the findings of clinical trials. Thus, the actual CE ratio for the debilitated population would be higher than the ratio computed for the clinical trials' population.

In contrast to clinical trials, data obtained from observational studies are more heterogeneous because the selection criteria are not as restricted. These measures are more likely to be reflective of the general population with the disease. However, randomization procedures are not required for such studies. Without randomization, it is difficult to ensure that treatment groups were comparable at the beginning. This fosters the possibility that a pre-treatment difference existed which may obscure or augment the treatment effect.

Let us consider an example comparing two treatment alternatives for hypertension. In the absence of randomization, there may be a selection bias that determines which of the two alternatives a physician chooses for each patient. Consider the therapeutic use of angiotensin-converting enzyme (ACE) inhibitors for hypertension. Captopril requires dosage reduction for patients with renal insufficiency while selected other ACE inhibitors do not (i.e., benazepril).[8] Thus, an observational trial comparing captopril and benazepril is likely to have a bias in operation where the captopril population has better renal function than the benazepril population. Such population differences may introduce confounding effects on response to treatment and effect patterns of resource consumption as well as clinical outcomes.

WHAT MAKES A VARIABLE USEFUL?

There are many types of variables, each having a specific purpose. In pharmacoeconomics, variables are used to represent variability in the value of the economic and outcome measures. As described above, the input variables for economic, clinical, and humanistic outcomes can be influenced and take on different values. Thus, CE ratios can have different values for the same model.

Consider cost inputs in a CE model. Assume a cost is assigned as a constant value, \$14,000 per patient, and desirable outcomes achieved in two of four treated patients. The total treatment cost equals \$56,000 (\$14,000 × 4). In this instance, the CE ratio would compute to a constant value, where CE ratio = cost/outcome = \$28,000 per outcome (\$56,000/2). This value for the CE ratio would be expected to reflect the level of efficiency for achieving desirable outcomes under all conditions specified in the model. The estimate can be highly accurate for the conditions in which it was computed. However, it can be extremely inaccurate for any conditions that did not match the conditions of the original computation.

For example, the \$28,000 per outcome may apply for patients who had adverse events associated with the intervention. In this instance, the estimate of \$28,000 per outcome would be highly accurate. However, for patients who did not experience as many adverse drug events, their associated costs would be lower. In this situation, the cost-effectiveness is expected to be lower than the computed \$28,000 per outcome. Thus, the model as originally composed would underestimate the level of efficiency for the intervention in the non-adverse drug event patients.

These variations in the value of the CE ratio serve to introduce unpredictability in this measure of relative efficiency. In doing so, the usefulness of this ratio in facilitating decision making is diminished; instead, it becomes another piece of information which further complicates the decision-making process.

Such concrete restraints on the value of input parameters limit the usefulness of CE ratios. However, by allowing and accounting for the inherent variability in the input parameters, a much more useful computation results.

Variables take into account the notion that an attribute may take on different values under different circumstances. Variability is an expected finding that can be measured and accounted for. It permits the analyst to plan for and assess the impact of the changing values of input variables on the research findings.

Two statistical parameters are used in this light: means or medians are commonly used measures of centrality, while standard deviations serve to estimate the measure of variability. Incorporating these two statistical estimates avails an entire venue for assessing the impact of different input variables can be explored and computed.

Let us first consider the cost as a variable. From the previous example, the constant cost of \$14,000 was assigned. This implies that every patient with the condition has a cost of \$14,000. However, this is not typically the case in health care. More commonly, different patients have different costs associated with their care. So to reflect this, let the \$14,000 cost represent the mean resulting from a sampling of patient costs for the intervention. The data inputs for the sample were: \$3,500; \$7,000; \$21,000; and \$24,500 = \$56,000. The mean cost, which represents the expected cost for each patient, is \$14,000. Likewise, the mean number of outcomes achieved per patient is 0.5 (desirable outcomes divided by the total number of patients treated = 2/4).

In this example, the computation for the CE ratio would still be $28,000 per outcome (using expected costs and outcomes values: $14,000 / 0.5 = $28,000; using total costs and outcomes values: $56,000/2 = $28,000). Additionally, the full range of CE ratios associated with the intervention can be computed using a modified box method.[9] We can compute a range for the CE ratios of $7000 per outcome to $49,000 per outcome. In this light, we could determine that, on average, the CE ratio for the intervention is approximated by $28,000 per outcome.

However, there may be selected circumstances that produce values as low as $7000 per outcome or values as high as $49,000 per outcome.

In this very simplistic approach, we have gained an additional level of understanding of the precision of the CE ratio. Our understanding has moved beyond one absolute value against which all other computations would be compared. In doing so, we have computed a central estimate for the value of the CE ratio, as well as established boundaries for extremes values.

In contrast to the non-variable example, we can now consider the full range of CE ratios for patients receiving intervention A (Table 6-2). By dividing each patient's cost by the expected number of outcomes, we are able to determine a CE range of $7000 to $49,000 per outcome achieved. Similarly, intervention B ($56,000 per outcome) has a CE range of $14,000–$98,000 per outcome achieved.

A more meaningful measure of the variability in CE ratios is confidence intervals. Computation for these 95% limits is more complex than computation of the ranges, but they add yet another level of information about the variability in CE ratio values. Confidence intervals provide additional insight into the probability of achieving CE ratios within the confidence interval based

TABLE 6-2.

Sample Cost-Effectiveness (CE) Ratio Calculations

	Intervention A	*Intervention B*	
Cost inputs by patient	$3500, $7000, $21,000; $24,500	$10,500; $21,000; $63,000; $73,500	
Total cost	$56,000	$168,000	
Outcomes achieved	2	3	
Expected number of outcomes per patient	0.5	0.75	
CE ratio ($ per outcome)	$28,000	$56,000	
CE ratio range	$7000–49,000	$14,000–98,000	
Incremental CE ratio ($ per outcome)			$112,000

on the probability distribution function of the variable. In this case, the cost variable is the value that was allowed to change, while the expected number of outcomes remained fixed. However, given sufficient input data about the variability of the number of outcomes achieved, it too, can be allowed to vary simultaneously with the cost variable.

The next step in assessing pharmacoeconomic variables is to determine which intervention is more efficient in achieving outcomes and by what magnitude it outperforms the alternative intervention. At first glance, intervention A appears to be more efficient in achieving outcomes. It only costs $28,000 per outcome compared with $56,000 per outcome for intervention B; yet, additional consideration should be given to intervention B since it produces more outcomes. The question then arises: "Is the additional benefit worth the additional investment?" Most certainly, given a choice, intervention B would be chosen as preferred, based on its ability to achieve more desirable outcomes in the target population. But does the additional outcome warrant the magnitude of the additional investment?

The answer comes in the form of an incremental CE ratio. By determining the difference in cost between the two interventions and comparing that to the difference in effect of the two interventions, it is possible to estimate how much the additional outcome is costing. In this case, the additional outcomes achieved using intervention B is costing $112,000. Relative to the cost per outcome in each of the interventions, it is apparent that the additional outcome comes at a premium. It is four times more expensive than the outcomes achieved using intervention A and twice as expensive as the outcomes achieved using intervention B.

Average and incremental CE ratios also have inherent variability. There are several techniques employed to measure and account for variability in the value of these outcome variables. Deterministic sensitivity analysis and probabilistic Monte Carlo simulations are commonly used. Sensitivity analysis employs deterministic techniques to set ranges for variables used to compute CE ratios. Then by changing the values of these variables, new CE ratios are computed. This method is used to assess if changing the values of the input variables can induce a decision change. Monte Carlo simulation requires information about the probability distribution function of the input variables. Using this information, random sampling for each of the distributions is undertaken. Using the values obtained in the random sampling procedure, new CE ratios are computed. The random sampling and recalculation is repeated to create a distribution of incremental CE ratios. If repeated enough times, it is possible to use this distribution to compute confidence intervals as well as estimate the decision frequency for the competing alternatives.

There are extensive research efforts to improve upon the methods, including both parametric and non-parametric methods to define the confidence limits for average and incremental CE ratios. The details of these discussions are beyond the scope of this chapter. However, it is important to acknowledge that variability in the form of input variables is the basis of uncertainty in estimating pharmacoeconomic ratios of efficiency.

CONCLUSION

Uncertainty in decision making is expected. In pharmacoeconomic evaluations, variables are the source of this uncertainty. Minimizing the magnitude of the uncertainty is the best approach to managing the variability associated with the input variables. These efforts should be employed throughout the evaluative process. Study design is the starting point where data source, variable selection, and valuation processes define the extent of inherent variability. Lastly, unrelenting diligence in data collection and analytic techniques is equally important.

REFERENCES

1. WHO: *The First Ten Years. The Health Organization.* Geneva: World Health Organization; 1958.
2. Kozma CM, Reeder CE, Schulz RM: Economic, clinical and humanistic outcomes: a planning model for pharmacoeconomic research. *Clin Therap* 1993;15(6):1121–1132.
3. Stedman TL: *Stedman's Medical Dictionary.* Baltimore, MD: Williams & Wilkins; 1995.
4. Donabedian A: The definition of quality and approached to its assessment. In: *Explorations in Quality Assessment and Monitoring I.* Ann Arbor, Michigan: Health Administration Press; 1980:1–31.
5. Donabedian A: Promoting quality through evaluating the process of patient care. *Med Care* 1968;6:181–202.
6. Patrick D, Erickson P: Health status and health policy: quality of life in health care evaluation and resource allocation. New York: Oxford University Press; 1993:113–142.
7. Davidoff AJ, Powe NR: The role of perspective in defining economic measures for the evaluation of medical technology. *Int J Technol Assess Health Care* 1996;12(1):9–21.
8. Weibert RT: Hypertension. In: Herfindal ET, Gourley DR, eds, *Textbook of Therapeutics: Drug and Disease Management*, 6th edn. Baltimore, MD: Williams & Wilkins; 1996.
9. Polsky D, Glick HA, Willke R, et al.: Confidence intervals for cost-effectiveness ratios: a comparison of four methods. *Health Econ* 1997;6:243–252.

C H A P T E R

7

Application of Pharmacoeconomics: Cost-Effectiveness Analysis in Behavioral Health

Linda Simoni-Wastila

INTRODUCTION

It is estimated that over 40 million, or 29.5%, of the US population aged 15–54 suffers from a mental illness at some point in their lives.[1,2] In addition, 22.9% of Americans will have a substance problem during their lifetime.[1] The costs of providing treatment for mental and substance abuse disorders is staggering—in 1990, the costs associated with these problems was estimated at $480.7 billion.[3] Of these costs, $105.8 billion can be attributed to medical and health care costs alone. Increasingly, concern about the treatment costs for schizophrenia, depression, alcoholism, and other behavioral health problems has led clinicians and other treatment decision makers to focus on the cost-effectiveness of new treatments.

Cost-effectiveness analysis (CEA) is a useful approach that can be utilized by clinicians, health care providers, and administrators of mental health services provided to patients with behavioral health conditions. This technique can be used as the basis for formulary decision making and allocation of resources, as well as for guiding treatment decision making for individual patients. CEA is also employed in the development of treatment protocols and guidelines.

CEA is increasingly important in the evaluation of new medications for treating mental health and substance abuse. In Australia, CEA studies are required for new drug approvals, and in Canada, pharmacoeconomic assessments are used in reimbursement decisions for newly approved medications. While not mandated in the United States, many managed care organizations, insurers, and other providers of health care are increasingly relying on cost-effectiveness studies in order to make formulary and reimbursement decisions about drugs used to treat behavioral health conditions.

In this chapter, we:

- review the prevalence of mental and substance abuse disorders;
- review treatment options for mental and substance abuse disorders;
- examine cost issues particular to behavioral health; and
- consider issues relevant to defining outcomes and measuring effectiveness in behavioral health.

This chapter also provides three examples in which cost-effectiveness analysis can play a role in treatment decision making and resource allocation situations. Each example presents the information critical to conducting or evaluating a CEA study.

MENTAL ILLNESS AND SUBSTANCE ABUSE: EXTENT OF THE PROBLEM

Behavioral health includes both mental illness and substance abuse disorders. The Diagnostic and Statistical Manual of Mental Disorder (DSM), the guideline used by psychiatrists and other clinicians in assigning mental disorder diagnoses, considers substance abuse disorders as one of a category of mental disorders. The five behavioral health domains defined in the DSM include:

1. affective disorders (major depressive disorder, manic episodes, dysthymia);
2. anxiety disorders (panic, agoraphobia without panic disorder, social phobia, simple phobia, generalized anxiety disorder);
3. substance use disorders (alcohol use with and without dependency, drug dependency, substance use);
4. antisocial behavior disorders; and
5. nonaffective psychoses (schizophrenia, delusional disorders, and atypical psychosis).

Based on findings from the National Comorbidity Study, it is estimated that the lifetime prevalence of any psychiatric disorders is as high as 48.0%.[1] Further, in any one year, 29.5% of the US population will have at least one psychiatric disorder.[1] As Table 7-1 illustrates, substance abuse disorders are the most prevalent of the behavioral health disorders, with more than one-quarter of the United States adult population having an abuse problem at least

TABLE 7-1.

Lifetime and 12-Month Prevalence of Most Common Psychiatric Disorders

Psychiatric condition	*Lifetime prevalence (%)*	*12-month prevalence (%)*
Anxiety disorders	24.9	17.2
Affective disorders	19.3	10.3
Substance abuse disorders	26.6	11.3
Non-affective disorders	0.7	0.5
Antisocial disorders	3.5	Data not available

Source: Kessler et al.[1]

once during their lifetimes. Nearly one-quarter of adults report having an anxiety disorder in their lifetimes. Finally, depression and other affective disorders affect nearly one in five adults.

Complicating both diagnosis and treatment of behavioral health problems is that some individuals suffer from more than one malady. Many individuals are "dually-diagnosed"; that is, they suffer from both a mental health and substance abuse disorder. It is estimated that 56% of the adults are dually-diagnosed.[1] Further, those individuals with at least one psychiatric disorder have, on average, 2.1 psychiatric problems.[3]

Mental illness and substance abuse disorders can strike anyone at any time in their lives. Some prevalence patterns, however, are notable. Considerable research has shown that men are more likely than women to have substance use and antisocial personality disorders.[3] Conversely, women are more likely to have affective disorders (with the exception of mania) and anxiety disorders. Psychiatric disorders tend to decline with advancing age and with higher socioeconomic status. Further, Whites tend to have greater susceptibility than Blacks for substance use and affective disorders.[2,3] There is considerable debate as to whether these patterns are due to true propensity for disease, or due to differences in symptom presentation and diagnosis.

Despite the high prevalence and costs of mental illness and substance abuse problems, little research has been conducted assessing the relative cost-effectiveness of treatments for these conditions. The remainder of this chapter focuses on three behavioral health disorders: depression, schizophrenia, and substance abuse. These three behavioral problems form our focus because:

1. they are among the most common psychiatric disorders;
2. they are costly conditions; and
3. the greatest amount of cost, effectiveness, and cost-effectiveness research have been conducted on these conditions.

Depression

Major depressive disorders affect 17.1% of individuals aged 15–54 at least once in their lifetime.[1] Major unipolar depression is one of the most common psychiatric conditions and is characterized by chronic, remitting episodes which may occur over an individual's lifetime. Depression, which may affect as many as 7% of all women and 2.6% of men during their lifetimes, is estimated to have direct costs of $12.4 billion in 1990 in the United States.[4] These direct costs include hospitalizations, physician charges, and drugs. Not included are the indirect costs related to lost productivity, comorbidity, and reductions in health status and well-being. Indirect costs associated with depression have been estimated to exceed $14 billion annually.[5]

Schizophrenia

While schizophrenia is a less common malady than depression, the costs of treating this condition are staggering. In 1991, the direct costs of schizophrenia in the United States exceeded $8.6 billion; the indirect costs are estimated at $46.5 billion.[6] This figure accounts for 22% of all mental illness costs and 2.5% of total health care costs.[7] The costs of schizophrenia are high, primarily due to the increased risk of hospitalization among this population as well as the prolonged length of stay experienced once hospitalized.[7] Comorbidity may also play a role in explaining high treatment costs. Among schizophrenic individuals, the most common comorbid disorder is substance abuse, especially alcohol abuse[8] and stimulant abuse.[9]

Substance Abuse

Substance abuse is also costly, to both society and to the health care system. The costs to society of substance abuse include lost productivity related to increased morbidity and mortality, as well as costs associated with criminal victimization. Societal costs of substance abuse are estimated at $276.3 billion.[3] The United States annually spends approximately $10.6 billion on treatment for alcohol dependency and $3.2 billion on other forms of substance disorders.[10]

TREATMENT

There are a multitude of treatments—both pharmaceutical and nonpharmaceutical—available to treat behavioral health conditions. Despite the availability of therapy, however, little has been done to examine the relative benefit or effectiveness of these treatments in treating mental and substance abuse disorders. There is a similar paucity of available comparative cost data for behavioral health conditions and therapies.

Pharmaceutical advances in the past decade have had a tremendous impact on patient outcomes. Pharmaceuticals have also had an influence on the costs associated with treatment. Improved availability of effective medications also has increased their share of treatment expenses. For example, some medications used to treat depression, notably the selective serotonin reuptake inhibitors (SSRIs), can exceed $2400 annually (see Table 7-2). Similarly, new treatments used in schizophrenia can approach $6300 annually. Finally, naltrexone, used to treat alcohol dependence, can cost $1660 per year. It is important to note that these costs, based on average wholesale prices in 1998, do not reflect markups (typically 15% or more) or patient out-of-pocket expenditures. Finally, because these conditions are often treated with more than one drug,

TABLE 7-2.

Selected Pharmaceutical Treatments for Schizophrenia and Depression

Medical condition and drug	*Common daily regimen (mg)*	*Daily cost ($)*	*Annual cost[a] ($)*
Schizophrenia—atypical antipsychotics			
Clozapine	400	14.09	5142.85
Risperidone	12	17.20	6278.85
Olanzapine	10	8.19	2989.35
Quetiapine	750	13.10	4782.96
Depression—SSRIs			
Fluoxetine	20	2.50	912.50
Paroxetine	40	2.33	851.67
Sertraline	150	6.63	2419.95
Fluvoxamine	200	4.56	1664.40
Nefazodone	400	4.04	1474.60
Venlafaxine (SNRI)	200	2.52	919.80
Alcohol abuse			
Naltrexone	50	4.55	1660.75

[a] Average wholsale price obtained from *Drug Topics Red Book*, March 1998 update, Montvale, NJ, 1998.

SSRIs, selective serotonin reuptake inhibitors; SNRI, selective norepinephrine receptor inhibitor.

and because patients are likely to have comorbid medical conditions, total medication costs for many patients can be extremely high.

CONSIDERATIONS IN CONDUCTING OR EVALUATING PHARMACOECONOMIC STUDIES IN BEHAVIORAL HEALTH

Pharmacoeconomic studies consist of a group of related methods for measuring and comparing the medical care costs and relevant health outcomes of different treatments.[11,12] Pharmacoeconomic studies examine the impact of various therapeutic interventions on patient psychopathology, daily functioning, quality of life, well-being, morbidity, and mortality, as well as costs. In medical and health care, CEA has become the primary pharmacoeconomic technique over other approaches, such as cost-benefit analysis (CBA) and cost-utility analysis (CUA). CEA's pre-eminence is due to a number of reasons, including the ethical difficulty in assigning a dollar value to morbidity, mortality, and quality of life.

Why use pharmacoeconomic techniques in assessing the benefits and costs of treatments used in behavioral health? One reason is that pharmacoeconomics can provide systematic methods for comparing different outcomes associated with competing treatment options. Using CEA, for example, may help an institution determine which antidepressants to include in its formulary. Pharmacoeconomic analyses can also provide a quantitative estimate for each outcome that is evaluated. This can be quite handy when dealing with psychiatric conditions, such as depression and anxiety, in which symptoms and treatment outcomes are subjectively reported. In mental illness and substance abuse disorders, most signs and symptoms of disease, as well as the effects of treatment, cannot be directly measured. Rather, measurement relies on patients' subjective reports of symptom changes. This is unlike symptom measurement seen with many somatic conditions, such as measuring blood sugar levels in diabetes or blood pressure in hypertension.

Pharmacoeconomic studies also provide a structure for comparing the outcomes of different studies. The use of standard rules and procedures in conducting pharmacoeconomic analyses allows comparison and pooling of studies that can provide better and more thorough information on the treatments under evaluation. For example, through the use of diagnostic and quality of life scales, such as the Hamilton Rating Scale for Depression (HAM-D) and the Medical Outcomes Study Short Form-36 (MOS SF-36), it becomes possible to compare the efficacy and treatment outcomes in similar populations.

Finally, pharmacoeconomic techniques can be used to identify the incremental impacts of clinical and demographic characteristics on treatment outcomes. For example, the use of sensitivity analyses can illuminate how treatment options differentially impact males and females, different doses of drugs, or different age groups.[13]

This can be extremely important in behavioral health, as drug dose titration and dose tapering has been shown to variably affect different patient subpopulations.

The Five Aspects of Conducting a Cost-Effectiveness Analysis

In conducting pharmacoeconomic analyses, it is important to consider five aspects: perspective; comparison of appropriate alternatives; outcomes; costs and cost savings; and the time horizon. Each of these aspects is discussed below and is illustrated in Case Studies 1–3.

CASE STUDY 1

Antidepressant Formulary Decisions in an HMO

Facing rapidly increasing pharmacy costs, a large staff-model health maintenance organization (HMO) in the New England region decides to examine its drug utilization by therapeutic category. The review finds that antidepressants are one of the most costly categories, and that the selective serotonin reuptake inhibitors (SSRIs) and selective norepinephrine receptor inhibitors (SNRIs) make up the majority of antidepressant budget outlays. The Pharmacy and Therapeutics (P&T) Committee decides to authorize a cost-effectiveness analysis of two of its more frequently used drugs: fluoxetine and venlafaxine. The average daily cost, based on the average wholesale price (AWP), of both drugs is comparable: venlafaxine is $2.52 per day, and fluoxetine is $2.50 per day. In preparing for the CEA study, the P&T Committee discuss the following parameters of the study:

Perspective
The perspective adopted for this analysis is that of an organization. This perspective is chosen because the research question is essentially a formulary and cost issue, and one that primarily affects the HMO rather than individuals or society at large.

Comparison of Alternatives
Venlafaxine is an SNRI and one of the latest introductions on the antidepressant market. Fluoxetine was the first SSRI and is considered the "gold standard" of depression treatment. Both drugs are approved for

the use of depression; in addition, fluoxetine is also indicated for bulimia nervosa and obsessive-compulsive disorder. Venlafaxine has the added advantage of dose flexibility: that is, increasing the venlafaxine dose may result in increased antidepressant efficacy and earlier therapeutic response than seen with other antidepressants.

Outcomes

Because the HMO is large and has a significant number of patients diagnosed with depression, outcomes and cost data can be collected prospectively as patients are newly diagnosed. For this study, the P&T decided to use a quality of life scale used in depression, the Global Clinical Impression scale, that is routinely administered to all HMO patients diagnosed with depression.

Costs and Cost Savings

Direct costs pertinent to this analysis include inpatient hospital (general and psychiatric) admissions, outpatient physician (general and psychiatric) visits, emergency department admissions, other psychiatric and psychology visits, fluoxetine and venlafaxine costs, and the costs of medications used to treat side effects of fluoxetine and venlafaxine. The data used for the study include service utilization data collected by the HMO, with associated billing data. Indirect costs were not assessed in this evaluation.

Time Horizon

Data for newly diagnosed patients started on either drug were collected for 12 months after the start of treatment. Only patients who stayed on the initial drug and were not switched during the 1 year were kept in the study.

Perspective

Perspective refers to the audience for which the CEA is intended. In both conducting and evaluating CEA studies, it is important to identify the perspective of the analysis *a priori* and to adjust the analytic plan to accommodate that perspective. Many analysts conduct pharmacoeconomic studies from a societal perspective. Such a perspective values all of the costs and benefits that affect the public, such as the costs associated with lost work productivity and criminal activity, as well as direct health and medical costs. Other perspectives are also possible, including the perspective of the patient, provider, or institution. Those who provide or manage behavioral health services may adopt the perspective of the provider or institution. For example, in the case of the health maintenance organization (HMO) deciding which antidepressants to include in its formulary, it is important to take the perspective of the institution. The HMO is interested in how the costs and benefits of its decisions will impact its budget.

CASE STUDY 2

Choice of Antipsychotic Treatment for Indigent Schizophrenic Patients

A large psychiatric group practice which treats a large number of schizophrenic patients in an outpatient setting is trying to determine whether olanzapine, a newly approved atypical antipsychotic, is a cost-effective alternative to clozapine, the first atypical antipsychotic approved to treat schizophrenia. The group practice intends to develop treatment protocols for its population, which is largely indigent. Although the state Medicaid program reimburses both drugs, it does have a total cap on the number of prescriptions it allows and has a significant patient copayment. Further, the state is currently focusing drug utilization efforts on antipsychotics, due to an unexpectedly large pharmacy outlay in this therapeutic category. The average daily costs of olanzapine and clozapine are $8.19 and $14.09, respectively.

Perspective
This study takes the perspective of the patient.

Comparison of Alternatives
Olanzapine has the advantage of once-daily dosing, which may improve drug compliance in a patient population noted for poor compliance. In addition, because clozapine has the rare but potentially fatal side effect of blood dyscrasias, use of the drug entails close blood monitoring, which can cost additional hundreds of dollars annually.

Outcomes
Data for this analysis are based on retrospective resource use and outcomes. Resource use is captured for all patients with a new diagnosis of schizophrenia 2 years prior. To assess quality of life, the research physicians used the Quality of Life scale and the Medical Outcomes Study Short Form-36, which are routinely administered to all patients at intake and quarterly thereafter. These instruments allow comparison of the acute effects of olanzapine and clozapine on the functioning, well-being, and quality of life of schizophrenic patients.

Costs and Cost Savings
Direct costs are collected and assigned for the following: inpatient hospital (general and psychiatric) admissions, outpatient physician (general and psychiatric) visits, emergency department admissions, other psychiatric and psychology visits, the costs of clozapine and olanzapine, the costs of medications used to treat side effects, and laboratory and monitoring

costs. Patients are briefly surveyed during each visit for their use of all medical and health-related services. Each patient is surveyed over a period of 4 months. Costs for all inpatient visits are estimated from diagnosis-related group (DRG) data available from public-use datasets; outpatient visits are approximated by using state-level Medicaid charge data available from the state's Medicaid bureau; drug costs are estimated using average wholesale prices (AWP), available from local pharmacy resources. Laboratory and monitoring costs are approximated by estimates provided by area laboratories. Indirect costs were not included in this study.

Time Horizon

Patients' service utilization is followed for 12 months, which is possible because the study is retrospective.

CASE STUDY 3

Cost-effectiveness of Two Treatments for Alcohol Dependence

The public health department of a large midwestern state would like to mandate the use of naltrexone, a newly-approved medication to treat alcohol dependence, in its public alcohol treatment programs. Currently, the only other medication available to treat alcoholism and alcohol dependence is disulfiram, which is infrequently used in treating alcohol dependence. Until the introduction of naltrexone, the treatment of alcoholism has been primarily based on psychosocial therapy and support. In bringing its request for funding before the state legislature, it is determined in committee that further study of naltrexone's cost-effectiveness is required. In particular, the state wishes to determine the impact of naltrexone compared to standard treatment for alcohol dependence on the state's drunk driving and alcohol-associated mortality. The state allocates sufficient funds to implement a one-year pilot project in which naltrexone is reimbursed for all public care recipients requiring treatment for alcohol dependence. The state also allocates money to conduct a cost-effectiveness study of the naltrexone compared to standard therapy with disulfiram in order to determine whether naltrexone should be reimbursed by the state.

Perspective

The perspective taken in this analysis is a societal one. The state is interested in the societal costs and outcomes of naltrexone.

Comparison of Alternatives

Disulfiram is rarely used, primarily because it has unpleasant side effects when taken with alcohol, therefore leading to poor compliance among individuals to whom it is prescribed. Naltrexone, originally used in the treatment of opiate dependence, is now approved for the treatment of alcohol dependence. It has few side effects and is therefore expected to result in higher patient compliance. The cost of naltrexone ($4.55 per day), however, is substantially higher than that of disulfiram, which is obtained for free from a generic manufacturer.

Outcomes

The state is most interested in how the use of naltrexone will affect the costs of alcohol treatment as a whole, as well as how it will impact the public's health. Because of this emphasis, outcomes considered for measurement include: changes in arrests for driving under the influence; changes in motor vehicle accidents in which alcohol use is implicated; and changes in admissions to inpatient and outpatient alcohol treatment centers.

Costs and Cost Savings

Both direct and indirect costs associated with naltrexone and disulfiram will be collected. Direct costs include: inpatient hospital (general and psychiatric) admissions, outpatient physician (general and psychiatric) visits, emergency department admissions, other psychiatric and psychology visits, admissions to inpatient, residential, and day treatment programs, disulfiram and naltrexone costs, and the costs of medications used to treat side effects. Direct costs associated with services utilization will be constrained to the public sector; thus, all data will be derived from state Medicaid claims data, as well as data available from the state public health department. Indirect costs include costs averted due to changes in the incidence of and morbidity associated with drunk driving. These data are procured from public health department sources and state and local police data.

Time Horizon

Data will be collected over two years. The first year will represent data collected before the introduction of naltrexone and will primarily be retrospectively captured. The second year of data will be prospectively collected as naltrexone use is implemented.

Comparison of appropriate alternatives

It is important that analysts select appropriate treatments for comparison; that is, analysts should select those treatments which have the most relevant clinical (or policy) significance. It does not make sense, for example, to compare the latest atypical antipsychotic to another that has been available for years and is rarely used in clinical practice. The comparative medications should be commonly used and clinically acceptable for the disease in question. Often the alternative medication is considered the "gold standard" prior to the introduction of the new therapy.

Outcomes

Outcomes measure the benefits, or "effectiveness", of the treatments in questions. Pharmacoeconomic analyses should identify the most relevant outcomes *and* be able to adequately define those outcomes. For some analyses, the avoidance of mortality is a desired (and easily measured) outcome. However, in most cases, and especially in behavioral health analyses, avoidance of particular morbidities, signs, and symptoms are desired outcomes. It is important for the analyst to determine which outcomes are pertinent to both the studied condition and the studied treatment, and to appropriately define the measurement of each outcome.

Costs and cost savings

Costs and cost savings must be as completely specified as possible. The costs and cost savings relevant to each analysis is, in part, dependent upon the perspective of the analysis. For example, costs and cost savings from a societal perspective may include the direct costs of the treatment, induced costs (such as the need to monitor the treatment for side effects), and indirect costs (such as administrative overhead costs). From a provider or management perspective, direct costs of the treatment, the costs of treating side effects, the costs of additional and/or substitute treatments, the savings from these treatments, and subsequent changes in morbidity are all costs to be included in the analysis.

Time horizon

Time horizon refers to the time period in which a treatment and its outcomes are considered. The time horizon may be short or long, but the analyst must specify the time period and justify its length in order to adequately interpret results. For example, a time period of 6 months to assess the cost-effectiveness of antidepressant medications may not be sufficient because most antidepressant treatment requires up to 2 months and longer to just determine the most effective dosage. Further, outcomes resultant from antidepressant therapy may not be measurable for 6–12 weeks, the length of time it takes most antidepressants to exert maximal benefit.[14] Although conducting analyses with relatively short time horizons may be more practical (and less expensive!), studies with longer time horizons provide a more realistic assessment of delayed side effects and drug tolerance problems. If a longer time horizon, on the order of more than 2 years, is used, then it is important to discount future costs and benefits.

Additional Issues in Behavioral Health CEA Studies

There are several issues unique to behavioral health CEA studies. One issue is that the diagnosis of a particular psychiatric disorder may be difficult to make. Unlike the assessment of many somatic conditions, the measurement of symptoms in patients with mental illness is more subjective and frequently less quantifiable than using a blood assay to determine whether an individual suffers from diabetes or hypercholesterolemia. For the same reason, it is often difficult to quantify changes in patient health due to the efficacy (or lack of efficacy) associated with behavioral health pharmacotherapies. One way to address these problems is to use standardized scales or indices developed to assess various psychiatric conditions. Some examples of such measures are included in Table 7-3.

When choosing a scale or index to diagnose or assess treatment progression, it is important to use measures validated in the study population of interest. In addition, consideration should be given to whether the scale requires professional administration or the patient self-administers the scale. While patient self-administration is usually less costly and time intensive, it may also result in less reliability and sensitivity. Finally, the length of time it takes to administer the scale is important, as longer scales may result in incomplete assessment due to patient frustration and boredom.

A second issue in conducting behavioral health CEA studies is reliability of diagnosis. Many mental health patients are misdiagnosed over a period of time. Such misdiagnoses are possible because patients may not initially present with a complete array of symptoms, may have symptoms that are indicative of several possible disorders, and/or because patients do not respond sufficiently to a course of therapy indicated for a possible condition. There is also growing evidence that some subpopulations present with different signs and symptoms for the same condition. For example, women with depression often present with symptoms of fatigue and sadness, whereas depressed men may complain of gastrointestinal and cardiovascular symptoms. Also, some screening instruments have not been validated in some patient groups. The use of screening instruments may have resulted in an overdiagnosis of schizophrenia and an underdiagnosis of bipolar disorder in African-American patients.[15]

Thirdly, effective treatment of both mental illness and substance abuse frequently consists of a combination of pharmaceutical and nonpharmaceutical approaches. Nonpharmaceutical approaches include 12-step/self-help recovery programs; cognitive behavioral therapy; individual and group counseling;

TABLE 7-3.

Selected Measures and Scales Used in Diagnosis and Quality-of-Life Assessment in Behavioral Health

Scale	*Description*	*Conditions used in*
CES-D	Center for Epidemiologic Studies Depression Scale. Requires trained interviewer.	Depression
DIS	Diagnostic Interview Schedule. Requires trained interviewer.	Affective disorders; anxiety; some psychoses; substance abuse
CIDI	Composite International Diagnostic Interview. Used in various cultures. Requires trained interviewer.	Affective disorders; anxiety; psychotic disorders
CAGE	Assesses lifetime problem drinking with four questions. Self-administered.	Alcohol dependence
ASI	Addiction Severity Index. Covers seven domains of substance abuse. Requires trained interviewer.	Substance abuse
MOS SF-36 (also SF-12)	Medical Outcome Study Short-Form 36. Assesses limitations in functioning, well-being, and quality of life. Can be self-administered or use trained interviewers.	General health
HAM-D	Hamilton Rating Scale for Depression. Requires trained interviewer.	Depression
Quality of Life Interview	Requires trained interviewer.	Schizophrenia
Wisconsin Quality of Life Index	Self-administered instrument with 103 items on symptom severity, functioning, and well-being.	Schizophrenia

motivational therapy; behavioral therapy; and electroconvulsive therapy (ECT). It is important to control for the effects of nonpharmaceutical therapies when evaluating treatment outcomes in behavioral health. In conducting CEA, it is important to include the costs and effects of such nonpharmaceutical treatments, especially if their use varies by different pharmacotherapies.

DETERMINING COSTS AND OUTCOMES

The primary components of CEA are (1) the measurement of health and medical costs and (2) the measurement of health outcomes associated with alternative treatments.

Determining Costs

When measuring costs, the pharmacoeconomic analyst must comprehensively capture information on all medical services used and their associated costs. Costs can be direct or indirect. Direct costs reflect the use and costs of medical services associated with alternative treatments. For most behavioral health conditions, direct costs include:

- inpatient hospital admissions
- emergency department visits
- day hospital or rehabilitation admissions
- laboratory and diagnostic services
- physician office visits
- outpatient psychiatric services
- outpatient substance abuse services
- residential treatment admissions
- other mental health provider services
- medications (including medications used to treat the side effects of treatment drugs).

It is often difficult to obtain the actual accounting costs of provided services. Instead, several sources of information are often used to obtain charge and price data to approximate costs. Sources of cost data frequently employed include billing information, administrative data, acquisition costs, average wholesale price data, and patient costs, such as copayments and other out-of-pocket costs. These data may be collected from public sources (e.g., Medicaid and Medicare claims data are available from some states and from the Health Care Financing Administration), private sources (e.g., billing and claims data from hospitals and managed care organizations), patient and provider surveys, and time-in-motion studies.

Indirect costs represent the monetary value placed on the lost or impaired ability to work or function due to illness. Indirect costs also include the loss of economic productivity due to mortality. As with most pharmacoeconomic studies, those examining pharmacotherapies for mental and substance abuse disorders usually do not include indirect costs, due to the difficulty and subjectivity involved in measuring such costs.

Determining Benefits and Effectiveness/Outcomes

In CEA, health outcomes are measured in natural units (such as years of life saved) rather than in dollar units. The selection of outcomes, or the measure of treatment benefits, to be used in a CEA is determined by the medical condition in question. In deciding which outcomes to measure, investigators should consider (1) the potential differences between groups with respect to the main effects of the intervention; (2) the potential side or adverse effects of the intervention; and (3) the outcomes of interest to those whose perspective is taken in the analysis.

Measures of treatment effectiveness can include clinical outcomes (e.g., number of alcohol-free days), quality of life outcomes (e.g., improvement on a quality of life scale), and quality-adjusted life years (QALYs). In behavioral health, treatment outcomes might be measures of psychopathology, functional status, and quality of life. A standard of many CEA studies in all fields is the QALY. QALYs are the years of survival modified by changes in the quality of life associated with the treatment (e.g., mood improvements; side effects) or disease progression (e.g., relapse; remission).

QALYs are constructed by developing utility scores, which measure tradeoffs and health state preferences among patients with the disease in question. Utilities are quantitative measures of the strength of a patient's preference for a particular health outcome. These utilities are measured on a continuous 0 to 1 scale, where 0 represents death and 1 represents complete and perfect health. Few behavioral pharmacoeconomic studies have utilized QALYs, in part because of the difficulty in obtaining health state preferences in patients with mental health and substance abuse disorders.

As a result, most CEA studies in the behavioral health field to date have utilized quality of life measures, such as those listed in Table 7-3. A problem with this approach, however, is that there are so many potential quality of life scales available that different researchers rarely use the same ones. Hence, it is often difficult to compare findings across studies. Recent recommendations for the increased use of QALYs and other measures by the Public Health Service and the Food and Drug Administration may lead to increased standardization in the field.

CONCLUSION

As drug and other health care costs continue to rise, pharmacoeconomic evaluations of new medications to treat depression, schizophrenia, alcoholism, and other mental and substance abuse disorders will increasingly be requested by government and other health care decision makers. Cost-effectiveness studies provide additional and comparative cost, safety, and efficacy data on these new medications. Pharmacoeconomic analyses also provide much needed comparative information on quality of life and economic outcomes.

Unfortunately, CEA and other similar techniques have only recently become understood and applied by behavioral health investigators and policymakers. As a result, the field is relatively new, but expanding. Increasing numbers of clinicians, researchers, and administrators are adopting CEA as a mechanism to help guide treatment and resource allocation decisions. As a result of increased demand for this information, pharmacoeconomic studies are likely to become more standardized and, hence, more comparable and generalizable. It is important that both the conductors and users of pharmacoeconomic studies keep abreast of advances in CEA and other pharmacoeconomic techniques.

REFERENCES

1. Kessler RC, McGonagle KA, Shanyang Z, et al.: Lifetime and 12-month prevalence of DSM-III-R psychiatric disorders in the United States. *Arch Gen Psychiatry* 1994; 51:8–19.
2. Rouse BA, ed.: *Substance Abuse and Mental Health Statistics Sourcebook*. Washington, DC: Superintendent of Documents, United States Government Printing Office; 1995.
3. Rouse BA, ed.: *Substance Abuse and Mental Health Statistics Sourcebook 1998*. Washington, DC: Superintendent of Documents, United States Government Printing Office; July 1998.
4. Priest RG: Cost-effectiveness of venlafaxine for the treatment of major depression in hospitalized patients. *Clin Therapeut* 1996; 18(2):347–358.
5. Stoudemire A, Frank R, Hedemark N, et al.: The economic burden of depression. *Gen Hosp Psychiatry* 1986; 8:367–394.
6. Wyatt RJ, Hunter I, Leary MC, et al.: An economic evaluation of schizophrenia. *Soc Psychiatry and Psychiatric Epidemiol* 1995; 30:196–205.
7. Glazer WM, Johnstone BM: Pharmacoeconomic evaluation of antipsychotic therapy for schizophrenia. *J Clin Psychiatry* 1997; 58 (Suppl. 10):50–54.

8. Drake RE, Osher FC, Wallach MA: Alcohol use and abuse in schizophrenia: a prospective community study. *J Nerv Mental Disorders* 1989; 177:408–414.
9. Brady K, Anton R, Ballenger JC, et al.: Cocaine abuse among schizophrenic patients. *Am J Psychiatry* 1990; 147:1164–1167.
10. Rice DP, Miller LS: Costs of mental illness. In: Teh-Wei H, Rupp A, eds., *Advances in Health Economics and Health Services Research: Research in the Economics of Mental Health*, Vol. 14, 1992.
11. Drummond MF, Stoddart G, Torrance GW: *Methods for the Evaluation of Health Care Programmes*. Oxford: Oxford University Press; 1987.
12. Revicki DA: Methods of pharmacoeconomic evaluation of psychopharmacologic therapies for patients with schizophrenia. *J Psychiatry Neurosci* 1997; 22(4):256–260.
13. Wolff N, Helminiak TW, Tebes JK: Getting the cost right in cost-effectiveness analysis. *Am J Psychiatry* 1997; 154(6):736–743.
14. Association for Health Care Policy and Research: *Depression in Primary Care*, Vol. 2: *Treatment of Major Depression*. Clinical Practice Guideline Number 5. AHCPR Publication No. 93-0551. Rockville, MD; April 1993.
15. Baker FM, Bell CC: Issues in the psychiatric treatment of African Americans. *Psychiatric Serv* 1999; 50(3):362–368.

C H A P T E R

8

Application of Pharmacoeconomics and Decision Analysis in Gastrointestinal Disorders in the Context of Disease Management

Susan K. Maue
and
Richard Segal

INTRODUCTION

Disease management programs are developed and implemented for the purpose of improving the quality of care and patient outcomes while attempting to reduce unnecessary resource utilization. These programs are most successful when they are (1) based on clinical evidence and (2) designed with not only the patient population in mind but also the health care organization's structure and systems. During the development of these multifaceted programs, several components, such as drug selection for clinical guidelines, may rely upon structured decision-making techniques. Pharmacoeconomic analyses are one such technique used to assist in making logical, evidence-based, reproducible decisions during conditions of uncertainty.

Pharmacoeconomics is a process used to identify, measure, and compare the costs and consequences of relevant medical interventions (e.g., drugs, services, diagnostic tests) and their impact on patients, health care systems, and society. A number of influential factors may be considered during these analyses, the importance and relevance of which varies according to the perspective of interest. These factors, and their associated outcomes, are typically categorized into one of the three following categories: clinical, economic, or humanistic. While a number of different pharmacoeconomic methods are available, such as cost-minimization, cost-benefit, cost-utility and cost-effectiveness analyses, this chapter will center on the selection of cost-effective therapy for the eradication of *Helicobacter pylori* (*H. pylori*) infection. As such, only those variables relevant to this perspective of interest will be incorporated into the case study presented.

This chapter is organized into three major sections. First, an overview of disease management and the clinical management of peptic ulcer disease is presented. This section is followed by a description of a framework for a disease management program that underlies a pharmacoeconomic case study. Lastly, the chapter concludes with a case study illustrating how one pharmacoeconomic method—cost-effectiveness analysis—is used in decision making concerning the treatment of *H. pylori* infection.

DISEASE STATE MANAGEMENT

Disease management, or more broadly *health management*, is a concept that is rapidly gaining widespread acceptance and creating significant enthusiasm.[1,2] It is commonly defined as:

> An approach to patient care that coordinates resources across the entire healthcare delivery system and throughout the life-cycle of a disease.

or

> A systematic, population-based approach to identify persons at risk, intervene with specific programs of care, and measure clinical and other outcomes.
>
> Epstein and Sherwood[3]

Disease management has been embraced by many health care organizations as a promising approach to improve quality and decrease costs for selected patient populations.[4] Disease management strategies commonly focus on chronic conditions that have a significant long-term clinical and economic impact. The critical distinction between the disease state management approach and traditional attempts to control costs and improve quality is a shift in focus from discrete episodes of care to the health care continuum. This approach, which is obviously an attractive concept in an era of managed-care full-risk contracting, places increased emphasis on continuity of care and prevention. Many "players" have emerged in this area including integrated delivery systems, health maintenance organizations (HMOs), pharmaceutical companies, information technology vendors and others.

Three essential elements of disease management are as follows:

- An integrated delivery system that is capable of coordinating care across multiple disciplines over time.
- A continuous quality-improvement process that utilizes process information, outcomes, and new scientific literature to drive change.
- A comprehensive knowledge base that includes information about the economic structure of a disease and patient segmentation, and which maps treatment flow and identifies critical junctures or interventions. In addition, this knowledge base must include state-of-the-art guidelines, pathways, and algorithms to optimize care for the given patient population.

Another important, but less-recognized element of disease management is the incorporation of *evidence-based medicine* (EBM). EBM involves the use of scientific information to drive the interventions used in disease state management (DSM), and is a field that is receiving growing attention, for several reasons. These include:[5]

- First, by encoding optimal practice from the medical literature, the individual practitioner or team is most likely to improve patient outcomes. Many groups employ clinical practice guidelines and pathways to reduce variation. However, reducing variation around usual practice may be useful, but is unlikely to improve patient care dramatically. Reducing variation around optimal practice derived from the most rigorous medical literature through an EBM approach is most likely to improve clinical and economic outcomes.
- Secondly, EBM empowers all members of the multidisciplinary team to shape care. When a multidisciplinary team consisting of providers from different facets of patient care (including primary care physicians, specialists, pharmacists, nurses, case managers, etc.) begins to redesign the system through the development and implementation of guidelines and pathways, they may face difficulty associated with conflicting opinions and competing objectives. It is not unusual for a single individual, one who appears to have the greatest experience or expertise, or who has the most inflexible ideas about "optimal care," to attempt to force his/her opinions on the remaining team members. Given such a scenario, where team members may be intimidated by one particular individual, it

becomes difficult to design an effective, unbiased system of care that is likely to significantly improve the existing method of health care delivery. Using an EBM approach, however, allows the team to use the clinical literature as a neutral arbiter of optimal practice and potentially avoid conflicts based upon ego rather than best science. This approach empowers all members of the health care team and places them on an equal footing in designing all aspects of the program.

- Finally, EBM may be used to assist the team in preventing the micromanagement of those aspects of care that are unlikely to affect patient outcomes. If the team is unable to find clinical literature to support a particular practice or evidence indicating that outcomes are improved, the members may avoid devoting scarce resources to tracking or attempting to change practice around this particular element of care that offers no value.

CLINICAL BACKGROUND: PEPTIC ULCER DISEASE AND *Helicobacter pylori*

Peptic ulcer disease is a chronic inflammatory condition of the stomach and duodenum that affects as many as 10% of people in the United States at some point during their lifetime.[6] Currently, about five million people in the United States have peptic ulcers,[7] with the prevalence for men and women roughly the same.[8] The disease has relatively low mortality, but often is responsible for symptoms that can be debilitating, resulting in poor quality of life and high economic costs.

In the early 20th century, the pathogenesis of the disorder was believed to be associated with stress and dietary factors. Later, clinicians began suggesting that peptic ulcer disease was caused by injurious effects of digestive secretions such as gastric acid. Consequently, antacids became the standard of therapy. In 1971, Sir James Black identified a subtype of the histamine receptor (the H_2 receptor) that appeared to be the principal mediator of gastric acid secretion. Antagonists of this receptor were shown to be safe and effective therapy for peptic ulcer disease.[6]

More recently, inhibitors of the proton pump (H^+,K^+-adenosine triphosphatase) in gastric parietal cells have been shown to be rapidly effective and extremely potent as antiulcerative drugs. Despite these sophisticated therapeutic agents, however, the disturbing problem of the high recurrence rate of peptic ulcer, even after complete healing, remained.[6] In 1982, Warren and Marshall provided the first insight into another important pathogenic factor in peptic ulcer disease.[9] They isolated an organism (later called *Helicobacter pylori*) whose presence was shown to be highly correlated with antral gastritis as well as with gastric and duodenal ulcers. They showed that by eradicating this organism they were able to effectively eliminate ulcer recurrences.[10,11] Such studies suggest that *H. pylori* is a major etiologic factor in peptic ulcer disease, and that diagnosis and eradication of the organism are necessary to prevent recurrence.

In order to ensure sufficient understanding of the clinical rationale behind the case study presented in this chapter, several questions concerning the role of *H. pylori* in peptic ulcer disease are addressed:

- *What is the strength of the causal relationship?* While the clinical meaningfulness of the causal relationship between *H. pylori* and peptic ulcer disease has been questioned by some clinicians, nearly all patients with a duodenal ulcer have *H. pylori* gastritis.[12] Thus, infection with the organism may be a prerequisite for the occurrence of almost all duodenal ulcers in the absence of other precipitating factors, such as the use of nonsteroidal anti-inflammatory drugs (NSAIDs) or Zollinger–Ellison syndrome. The association between *H. pylori* infection and gastric ulcer is only slightly less, in that 80% of patients with nonNSAID-induced gastric ulcers are infected. Nevertheless, it is important to note that the majority of *H. pylori*-infected individuals do not develop duodenal or gastric ulcers.[6] These facts imply that host characteristics, strain variability, or other factors play a role in the pathogenesis of peptic ulcer disease.[6]
- *Does eradication of* H. pylori *infection benefit the patient with peptic ulcer disease?* According to a National Institutes of Health (NIH) Consensus Development Panel,[6] numerous studies have clearly demonstrated the benefits of eradication in patients with peptic ulcers. Specifically, *H. pylori* eradication has lead to a substantial reduction in the risk of ulcer recurrence, estimated at less than 10% in a 1-year period. The evidence is more complete for patients with duodenal ulcers than for those with gastric ulcers, although the benefits to the two groups of patients appear comparable. The side effects of current regimens for eradication of *H. pylori* infection are generally minor and seem to be outweighed by the benefit of reduced ulcer recurrence. The benefits of eradicating *H. pylori* infection in patients with peptic ulcer disease may vary depending on a variety of factors including those related to the host, the organism, and the environment. Specific factors include patient demographics (age, socioeconomic status, concurrent illness, and behavioral factors), frequency of reinfection, mode of transmission, and strain variation.
- *Should every patient who presents with dyspepsia be tested for* H. pylori*?* Fundamental questions remain concerning whether all patients who present with dyspepsia should be tested for *H. pylori* infection. The answers to these questions depend in part on whether antimicrobial therapy relieves symptoms in some or all symptomatic patients with *H. pylori* infection and gastritis, but without ulcers. Thus, the question arises as to

whether it is necessary, appropriate, and cost-effective to perform endoscopy or noninvasive testing in dyspeptic patients at initial presentation.[6]

- *Should* H. pylori *infection be treated in patients with nonulcer dyspepsia?* Approximately one-third of people in the United States have recurrent dyspeptic symptoms, many of whom have no evidence of peptic ulcer disease.[13] The reported prevalence of *H. pylori* infection in patients with gastritis and nonulcer dyspepsia ranges from 30 to 70%.[14] Several pharmacoeconomic analyses have examined whether or not it is cost-effective to treat all patients who might have an ulcer to benefit only a few.[15–17] Findings of these trials generally support the cost-effectiveness of treating *H. pylori* infection without an established diagnosis of peptic ulcer disease if the probability of peptic ulcer disease is 10% or greater.

FACETS OF THE DISEASE STATE MANAGEMENT PROGRAM THAT UNDERLIE THE PHARMACOECONOMIC CASE STUDY

Below are six steps[18] included in the DSM program that serve as the framework within which the pharmacoeconomic applications to *H. pylori* infection will be examined (Figure 8-1). For the purpose of the case study, assume that the DSM program is conducted within a group-model HMO that cares for approximately 200,000 members. This organization delivers primary care in 10 health centers with in-house pharmacies.

Step A: Formulate teams and scope of project

The DSM program begins with the formulation of two teams: a steering committee and a disease management team. These teams have differing roles, but function with the same ultimate goal in mind: to design an evidence-based gastrointestinal DSM program that improves the quality of patient care while simultaneously reducing unnecessary resource utilization.

The steering committee oversees the entire project, including organizational structure, assurance of adequate resources, coordination of the project, and ultimate assessment of success or failure. For this particular DSM program, the committee membership includes the chief executive officer of the health plan, the medical director of the medical group practice, the pharmacy director, and a disease management consultant.

The disease management team actually develops and implements the DSM program. The members of this multidisciplinary team, chosen on the basis of their expertise in clinical medicine, EBM and quality management, include a primary care physician who serves as the committee chairperson, a gastroenterologist, a pharmacist, a nurse, a quality improvement coordinator, an infor-

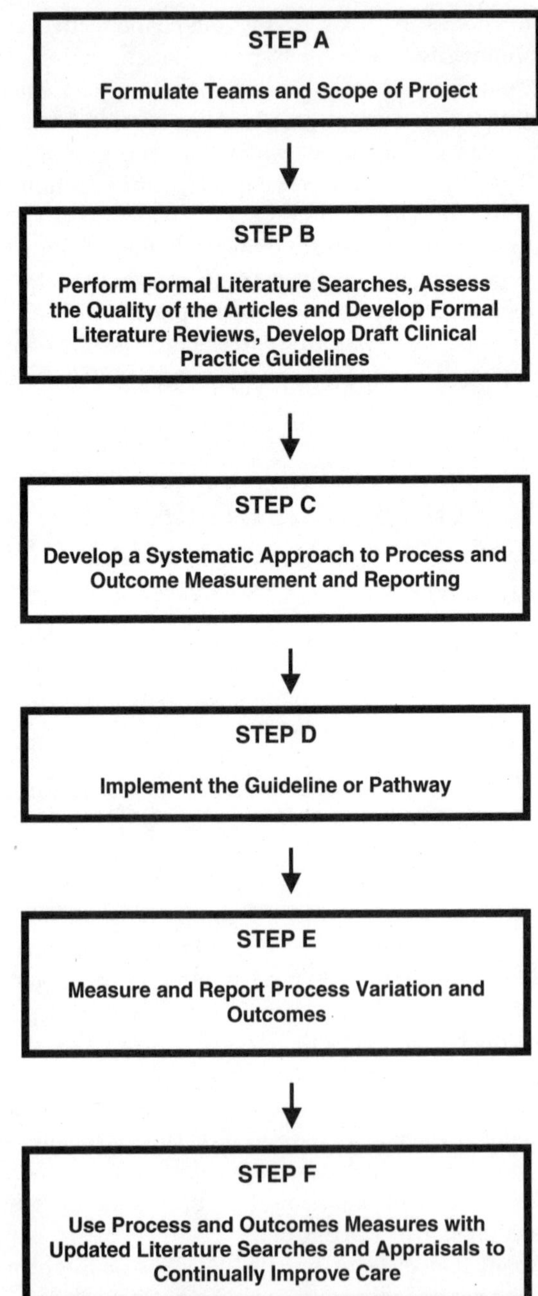

Figure 8-1. Disease state management framework.

mation technology/biostatistics representative, a consumer representative, and a disease management consultant.

With numerous questions raised in the literature concerning the potential gap between actual medical practices and recommended evidence-based practices for the appropriate management of *H. pylori* infection, the steering committee asked the disease management team to undertake an internal review of the management of acid peptic disorders in the plan's patient population. Results of their claims' database investigation and medical chart reviews revealed that over 3000 patients are receiving chronic histamine$_2$-receptor antagonists (H_2RA), 800 patients are receiving a prescription for an antisecretory agent along with an NSAID, and few patients, less than 1%, who presented with a history of dyspeptic symptoms, for more than 30 days, were tested for *H. pylori* infection. Based on these findings, the disease management team decided to focus their attention in five areas:

1. The initial diagnostic work-up for patients presenting with symptoms of dyspepsia.
2. The management of patients receiving concurrent prescriptions for an antisecretory agent along with an NSAID.
3. Testing for *H. pylori* infection.
4. Management of *H. pylori* infection.
5. Management of patients testing negative for *H. pylori* infection.

For the purpose of this case study, decisions about only the fourth area, "management of *H. pylori* infection," will be examined.

Step B: Perform formal literature searches, assess the quality of the articles and develop formal literature reviews, develop draft clinical practice guidelines

After formulating clear, pertinent clinical and economic questions about *H. pylori* infection eradication, formal literature searches are performed by trained practitioners (e.g., drug information pharmacists) with the assistance of a medical librarian, articles are reviewed, and formal literature reviews are prepared. These formal reviews are the scientific basis of the evidence-based practice guidelines that the disease management team will prepare and ultimately insert into clinical pathways and algorithms. They include descriptions of the relevant articles and are graded according to standardized evidence-based grading algorithms.[19]

The team decides to place the greatest weight on published articles in which randomized controlled trials were used to test the efficacy of *H. pylori* infection eradication treatments and on well-designed meta-analyses. Additionally, the team decides to focus only on the studies/articles that (1) discuss therapeutic regimens that include the use of antibiotic therapy, and (2) only those studies in which a follow-up assessment to test for successful eradication was performed 4 or more weeks after the completion of therapy. With these criteria, the team is able to focus the literature review on the studies with the greatest relevance.

During the review process, the trained practitioners (e.g., drug information pharmacists) gather, review, and develop concise appraisals of all relevant literature. These reviews are then provided to the multidisciplinary disease management team for further review and discussion. The team judges the information summarized in the clinical appraisals and weighs, for each recommendation, the expected benefits to the patient population against the anticipated harms and costs.

After the team undergoes a structured decision-making process that includes the use of the clinical literature, team member expertise, and understanding of the plan's operating structure, they develop the clinical practice guidelines that address the key clinical areas listed in step A (Figure 8-2 is an example of an excerpt of the clinical practice guideline developed by the disease management team—*note that this is an example guideline and is not intended to represent "best practices"*). It is within this decision-making process that the pharmacoeconomic example presented below is incorporated.

Step C: Develop a systematic approach to process and outcome measurement and reporting

Based on the proposed recommendations described in the clinical practice guidelines, the disease management team selects key process and outcome indicators to be used to demonstrate the impact of the program. The broad categories of outcome measures considered include (1) clinical quality; (2) patient satisfaction; (3) provider satisfaction; and (4) cost. To assess the degree of and value of the changes in care, the team first collects baseline measures for each of the identified indicators. Following the implementation of the program, the team then reassesses the same indicators to determine the influence of the program on the processes and outcomes of care.

The disease management team decides to focus on two primary outcomes related to the eradication of *H. pylori* infection: (1) reducing ulcer-related symptoms through the eradication of the infection, and (2) lowering total system costs from the perspective of the health plan. The team also decides to assess compliance with essential guideline recommendations that are believed to be associated with improved clinical and economic outcomes. Primary process measures that will be collected by the team include (1) the proportion of patients that meet inclusion criteria that are tested for *H. pylori* infection, (2) the proportion of *H. pylori*-positive patients for whom the recommended eradication treatment is prescribed, and (3) the proportion of patients failing on eradication treatment that are referred to a gastroenterologist (see Figure 8-2).

Data for the selected key process and outcome indicators are collected using methods specified by the disease management team (e.g., frequency of collection, retrieval methods). Most process and outcome measures are developed in

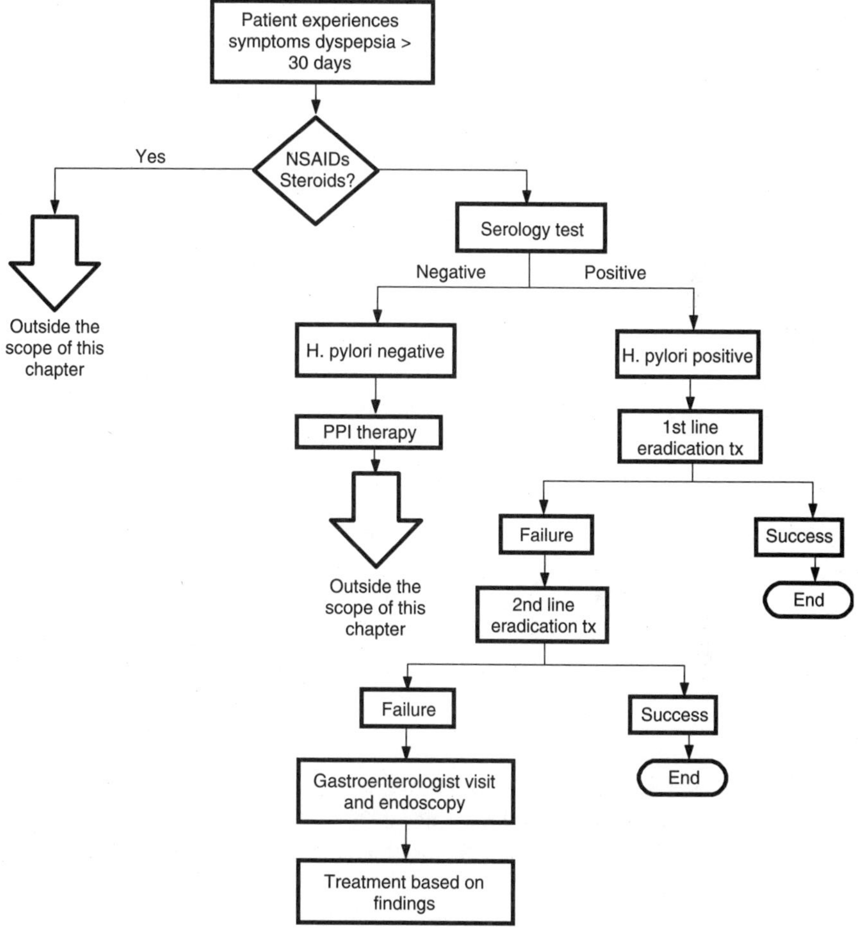

Figure 8-2. Excerpt of clinical practice guideline.

a way that allows for direct retrievability from the automated information system in a format suitable for analysis and reporting.

Step D: Implement the guideline or pathway

Once the team has developed evidence-based guidelines and pathways, and has a system in place to assess the process and outcomes indicators, the focus moves on to the challenge of implementation. This step represents one of the most challenging and difficult of all of the activities associated with DSM programs. Schwartz and Cohen[20] offer a useful framework for classifying strategies for changing physician behavior (Table 8-1). These researchers report that efforts to change behavior are likely to be most successful when several of these methods are combined and that most behavior is too resistant to change

TABLE 8-1.

Methods for Modifying Provider Behavior
Methods
Administrative structure/process
Education
Feedback
Incentives

to be altered consistently by any one method. Schwartz and Cohen argue that while education is often necessary, it is not usually sufficient to change behavior and that interventions that rely solely on education and do not address the complex behavioral, social, and organizational factors that influence behavior usually are not successful in changing behavior. Among the conclusions of Schwartz and Cohen's critical appraisal of the literature were the following:

1. The dissemination of printed educational materials had no detectable effect on prescribing patterns when used alone; however, these materials do lay a necessary foundation for more personalized educational efforts.
2. Merely distributing computerized listings of patient-specific medication profiles, without specific recommendations for change, is ineffective in reducing overall drug costs or use of inappropriate drugs. Their lack of effect may be due to the large quantity and clinical irrelevance of such data.
3. "Academic detailing" or face-to-face educational outreach visits, conducted by either specially trained clinical pharmacists or physician "counselors" and "opinion leaders," are effective in reducing prescribing of inefficient or contraindicated drugs in pediatric and adult primary care settings.

After considering the resources available to the disease management team and the culture of the provider groups, the disease management team selects several implementation strategies. These include:

- *Education*: Although traditional continuing medical education (CME) has not shown consistent effects, particularly when health outcomes have been measured, use of lectures and small group sessions to introduce general concepts and give overviews of specific guidelines and pathways may be useful. Thus, traditional CME may be considered necessary to achieve buy-in from practitioners, but insufficient to change behavior.

- *Academic detailing*: Personalized one-on-one sessions using pharmacists or physicians have been shown to be effective. This approach should be strongly considered, particularly in attempts to optimize drug prescribing and compliance. Some of the most important techniques of such "academic detailing" include: (1) conducting interviews to investigate baseline knowledge and motivations for current prescribing patterns; (2) focusing programs on specific categories of physicians as well as on their opinion leaders; (3) defining clear educational and behavioral objectives; (4) establishing credibility through a respected organizational identity, referencing authoritative and unbiased sources of information, and presenting both sides of controversial issues; (5) stimulating active physician participation in educational interactions; (6) using concise graphic educational materials; (7) highlighting and repeating the essential messages; and (8) providing positive reinforcement of improved practices in follow-up visits.
- *Opinion leaders*: Evidence also exists demonstrating that the early involvement of respected peers is effective in changing physician practice patterns. Involvement early in the guideline- and pathway-development process is important.
- *Remove disincentives*: A growing number of studies have revealed a number of internal and external barriers to implementing clinical practice guidelines. Asking providers to identify perceived barriers at the time of program rollout is an important step in uncovering challenges to implementing guidelines.
- *Use information technology*: The appropriate use of information technology can be critical in having guideline recommendations available to providers when they need it the most . . . during the clinician–patient encounter. Software and hardware solutions are used by the disease management team, allowing the primary care provider real-time access to clinical templates which incorporate guideline recommendations into the clinical work-up of patients.
- *Feedback*: Based upon the literature, the use of concurrent feedback by nurses, case managers, physicians, and pharmacists to assure the prompt compliance with guideline recommendations or delineate the reasons for lack of compliance is effective. Thus, the disease management team decided to incorporate physician profiling for the purpose of monitoring adherence to key recommendations included in the clinical practice guidelines.

Step E: Measure and report process variation and outcomes

Measurement, statistical analysis, summarization, and reporting of *both* process and outcomes measures provides the evidence of improvement. Although improved practitioner compliance with the evidence-based recommendations is likely to improve outcomes, it cannot be assumed. Improvement must be measured. As discussed in step C, the team first measures the indicators prior to implementing the new system of care. After the system has been in place for a specified amount of time, follow-up measures are taken and compared with the baseline measures to assess the impact. Following the assessment, further opportunities may be identified in an effort to continue improving the quality of care.

It is often possible that improvement is not shown. Potential explanations for failure to improve care despite apparent decreased variation and increased adherence to guidelines may include:

- Improper implementation, wherein patients are misclassified by the individuals applying the guideline. For example, patients not meeting the guideline inclusion criteria are managed according to the practice guideline.
- The practice guidelines do not reflect evidence-based best practices because of inadequate literature searches or poor assessments of the articles.
- Changes were made for one element of care on the pathway, which adversely impacted clinical outcomes downstream due to a failure to consider the entire system. For example, the test selected to diagnose *H. pylori* was not sensitive or specific, therefore patients who were candidates for antimicrobial therapy did not receive it and patients who were not candidates did.

Step F: Use process and outcomes measures with updated literature searches and appraisals to continually improve care

With the primary goal of the DSM program being to improve the quality of care provided to patients presenting with symptoms of dyspepsia, it is important for the program to run in a continuous cycle. Once the impact of the program is assessed, it is possible to further identify opportunities for improvement. In doing so, the team can then begin to repeat the cycle with the incorporation of the evidence generated from within the plan's own patient population. Incorporating the local data with updated literature appraisals will serve to strengthen the program, especially if the lessons learned are built into the program in a timely fashion.

PHARMACOECONOMIC APPLICATION

As part of the broad-based disease management program, the disease management team decided that the clinical practice guideline would include the use of *H. pylori* eradication therapy. The team's decision was supported by an accumulating body of evidence that has confirmed that patients with a diagnosis of *H. pylori* infection who undergo eradication therapy have better clinical outcomes and utilize fewer resources for the treatment of peptic ulcers.[21] In one particular study that assessed the effectiveness of *H. pylori* therapy, recurrence rates for duodenal ulcers were 95%, and 74% for gastric ulcers after acute therapy with H_2RAs. The recurrence rates in patients treated with a regimen containing antibiotics to eradicate *H. pylori* were only 12% and 13%, respectively.[10]

While antibiotics are effective, *H. pylori* eradication is difficult and requires the concurrent administration of two or more antimicrobial drugs.[22,23] Despite the difficulty, however, the acceptance of *H. pylori* eradication therapy has continued to grow over the past decade, and consequently, numerous regimens have been introduced as potential alternatives. For example, the Food and Drug Administration (FDA) has approved four regimens for the eradication of *H. pylori* infection and there are at least six other eradication treatments used in practice.[24] As such, the disease management team is faced with evaluating the effectiveness, safety, tolerability, and cost of these regimens as part of their decision-making process. Following the identification and structured evaluation of the various alternatives, the preferred regimen will be placed on the health plan's clinical practice guideline.

Applying a 14-Step Process to Assist in Decision-Making

Realizing the importance of using structured decision-making techniques to guide the team's decision, a 14-step process, adapted from earlier works,[25–27] is applied (Figure 8-3). Note that several of the steps may overlap due to the nature of the example and the context within which it is created (part of a broad-based DSM program).

Step 1: Define the pharmacoeconomic problem

The disease management team is charged with selecting the optimal regimen for the clinical practice guidelines. In view of the numerous alternatives available (Table 8-2), and the team's desire to select one preferred regimen, the team members must develop explicit, measurable criteria on which to base their decision. Developing these criteria will also help the team to better define the pharmacoeconomic problem at hand.

Rather than basing the decision on drug cost-savings alone, which is inappropriate for clinical practice and frequently may lead to excess costs in the long run, the team members determine that the two critical variables influencing the selection of the optimal regimen are (1) the effectiveness of the medication in successfully eradicating the *H. pylori* bacteria and (2) the cost of the regimen.

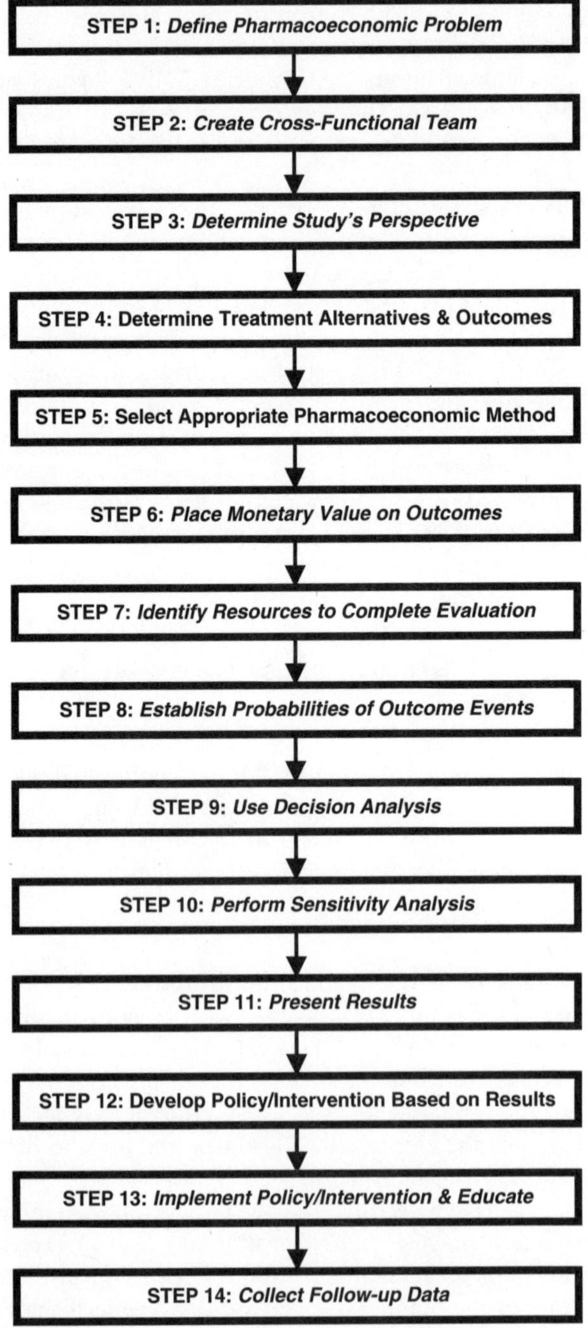

Figure 8-3. Fourteen-step pharmacoeconomic process.

TABLE 8-2.

Eradication Therapy

Regimen	*Duration (days)*	*Number of pills*	*Schedule*	*Eradication rate (%)*	*Cost ($)*	*Weighted average eradication*	*Eradication × compliance*
A	14	224	q.i.d.	91–96	136	0.92	0.79
B	10	180	q.i.d.	94–98	217	0.96	0.86
C	14	238	q.i.d.	87–92	192	0.91	0.78
D	10	60	b.i.d.	86–90	140	0.87	0.83
MX	14	70	b.i.d.	86–89	146	0.88	0.84

q.i.d., four times a day; b.i.d., twice a day.

The team phrases the pharmacoeconomic question as follows:

What is the most cost-effective regimen for *H. pylori* eradication given total health care costs associated with its management?

Step 2: Create a cross-functional project team

In order to ensure that all alternatives are appropriately considered and properly valued from the overall plan's perspective, a cross-functional team is assembled. The members of this team were previously identified in step A of the broad-based disease management program. This assemblage helps to ensure that all relevant viewpoints are considered and that specific expertise is at hand when particular issues are considered that may influence the final decision. As previously mentioned during the DSM discussion, the team members consist of a primary care physician, a gastroenterologist, a pharmacist, a nurse, a quality improvement coordinator, an information technology/biostatistics representative, a consumer representative, and a disease management consultant.

It is important to note that the number of individuals brought to the team should remain manageable. Given potential personality conflicts and competing objectives, along with questions regarding reliability of individuals and the difficulty of coordinating multiple schedules, the team members should be carefully selected. Additionally, a facilitator should be appointed to ensure that the team meetings are run efficiently and that team members are assigned reasonable tasks that help to drive the decision-making process. This team appoints the primary care physician as facilitator/committee chair.

Step 3: Determine the study's perspective

As this pharmacoeconomic analysis is a sub-component of a broad-based gastrointestinal DSM program, the study's perspective has been predetermined. The consequences and outcomes of interest should be based from the perspective of the health plan. Consequently, variables such as patient co-pay or time away from work due to side effects will not be considered in this example.

Step 4: Determine the treatment alternatives and outcomes

In order to select the optimal regimen, the team considers all reasonable alternatives. In doing so, they clearly specify each alternative and the associated costs and outcomes of each. For the purposes of this case illustration, only four of the more than nine commonly used eradication treatments will be considered in the analysis. As seen in Table 8-2, the expected clinical outcome associated with the use of specific regimens for the treatment of *H. pylori* infection is the eradication rate. Once again, only those regimens that included antibiotic agents that had been tested at 4 or more weeks following completion of therapy were considered.

Step 5: Select the appropriate pharmacoeconomic method

The next step is to choose the pharmacoeconomic method that is best suited for the pharmacoeconomic problem at hand. The team decided that the primary objective was to choose the regimen that was most cost-effective, thereby clarifying the method of choice. The team members must keep in mind that the treatment regimen that is cost-effective is not always less expensive than a comparator. An alternative regimen in this particular scenario may be considered cost-effective if it is (1) less expensive and at least as effective; (2) more expensive with an additional benefit worth the additional cost; or (3) less expensive and less effective in instances in which the extra benefit provided by the competing alternative is not worth the extra expense.[28]

Step 6: Place monetary values on outcomes

The next step requires placing a monetary value on the outcome(s) of interest. In this example, the outcome of interest is the successful eradication of *H. pylori* infection. It is important to consider the time value of money during this step, particularly if the data used for determining the monetary value either extends over a period greater than 1 year (not applicable for this example), or if values are extracted from different time periods, thereby preventing a simple justified comparison.

The costs in this particular scenario include (1) drug acquisition costs and other pharmacy costs, (2) the cost of office visits and cost of *H. pylori* serology test, and (3) cost of endoscopy and gastroenterologist visit (see Tables 8-2 and 8-3). The time period of interest for this program is the upcoming 12-month period and the costs associated with each alternative are taken from the most recently contracted prices for drugs, endoscopy, *H. pylori* serology tests, and physician visits (both primary care physicians and gastroenterologists).

The specific cost calculation for this example is found in step 9.

Step 7: Identify resources to complete evaluation

There are a number of different resources that a team may consider during a pharmacoeconomic evaluation. These may include claims data, medical literature, expert opinion, medical claims, or contracted pricing for pharmaceuticals. For the particular question at hand, the team members identify two sources

TABLE 8-3.

Additional Costs Associated with *H. pylori* Therapy

Variable	*Cost ($)*
Initial office visit and serology test	42
Subsequent office visits	35
Endoscopy and visit with gastroenterologist	440

they feel will be most useful in this analysis: (1) the medical literature and (2) the cost of each regimen based on contracted cost.

The medical literature will be used to estimate the range of effectiveness for each agent. Evidence-based clinical studies will be most strongly weighted, and those articles that emphasize expert opinion only will not be as highly regarded. For the cost of each regimen, the team considers the plan's contracted price, rather than the average wholesale price (AWP) (Table 8-2).

Step 8: Establish the probabilities of outcome events

Using the medical literature, the team identified the probability of successful eradication of each regimen previously selected for consideration. The findings are illustrated in Table 8-2 beneath the column labeled eradication rate. As the success of these particular regimens differed from study to study, the range of effectiveness is presented.

Step 9: Use decision analysis

Constructing the skeleton Once steps 7 and 8 are completed, the team members begin developing a decision tree that allows them to visually layout the alternatives and the associated outcomes. The skeleton of the decision tree, without probabilities or costs, is represented in Figures 8-4 through 8-6. Each therapeutic alternative listed in Table 8-2 is represented in the tree.

As displayed in Figure 8-4, the first step of building a decision tree is laying out the alternatives. In this tree, the four regimens for consideration are displayed, along with the possible outcomes of using each regimen: *success* or *failure* of eradicating the infection. These two options are listed at the "chance nodes," which are represented in the model by circles.

Following the top pathway in the tree, if regimen A is successful, the pathway ends. The end of the pathway is signified with a terminal node, which is represented by a triangle. However, per the clinical practice guideline, if initial therapy fails, a second course of eradication therapy is attempted. This is represented in Figure 8-5 by a square, a decision node.

For this example, the second therapeutic alternative is regimen MX, a regimen that does not contain metronidazole. The decision to use a therapy not including metronidazole was based on research showing that resistance to metronidazole is associated with impaired therapy. In one study of 933 patients who presented to a clinic between September 1988 and January 1997 with complaints of dyspepsia, abdominal pain, and peptic ulcer disease, the frequency of primary metronidazole resistance was 37.4%.[29] Assume for the purposes of this example that the decision to prescribe regimen MX was based on a previous pharmacoeconomic analysis performed by the team.

Regimen MX also has a chance of success or failure, as displayed in Figure 8-6. Once again, with successful eradication, the pathway ends. In the case of failure, the pathway also ends, but only after incorporating additional costs

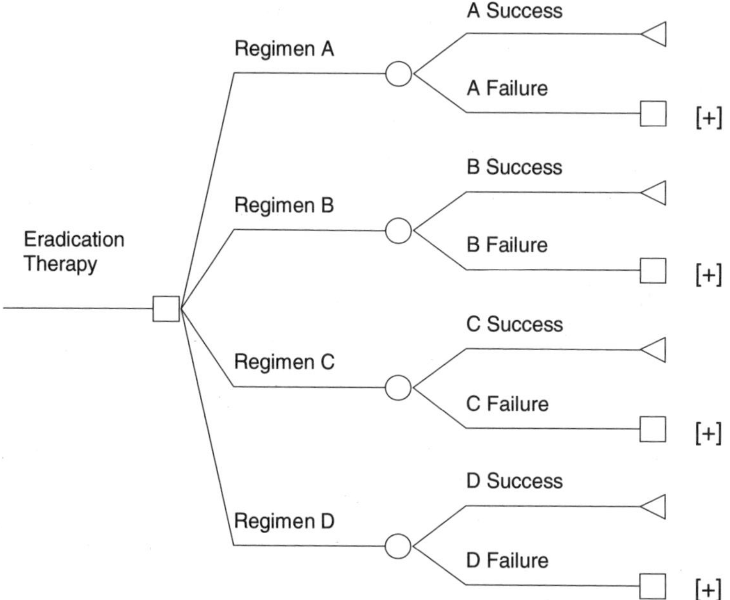

Figure 8-4. Skeleton of decision tree.

beyond those incurred at the point of the second therapeutic regimen. The incorporation of costs is addressed in the following section.

Inserting probabilities and costs Since each therapeutic alternative has a *range* of effectiveness (see Table 8-2), rather than a single probability of eradication, a weighted average is used in the model. The weighted average is based on the size of the population from each study considered in the decision-making

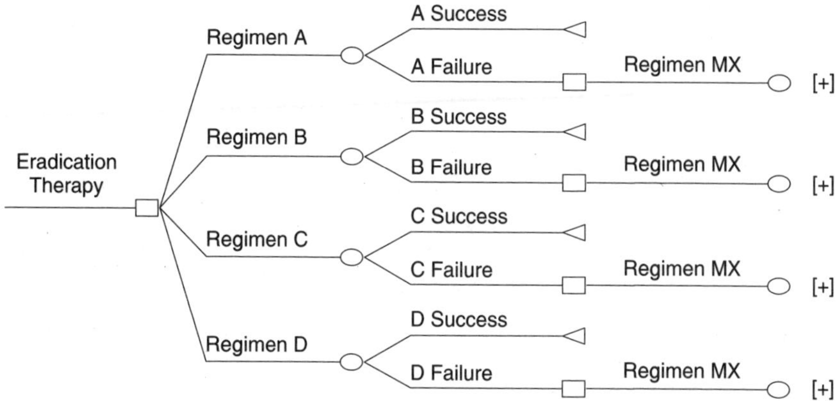

Figure 8-5. Expanded skeleton of decision tree.

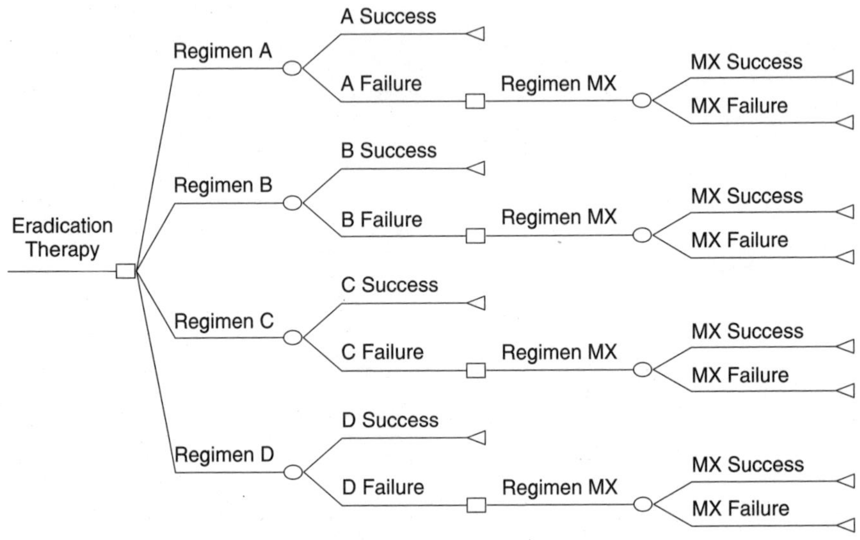

Figure 8-6. Completed skeleton of decision tree.

process. For instance, if the sample size and eradication rate for four published studies were as follows: 43 (95%), 125 (88%), 117 (92%), and 87 (89%), the rate used in the model would be 90%. For this example, the following probabilities of successful eradication were used for regimens A–D, respectively: 92%, 96%, 91%, and 89%, as listed in Table 8-2.

In cases where the therapeutic alternative is successful, the only costs incurred are the cost of the regimen and the cost of the initial office visit ($42), which includes the cost of the serology test ($7). In cases where the patient fails after initial therapy (meaning patient returns complaining of symptoms), the costs include the cost of the regimen, cost of the initial office visit, and serology test, cost of a second office visit, and the cost of the second regimen. If the patient fails after the second course of therapy, the cost of another physician visit is added, along with the cost for a gastroenterologist visit and endoscopy. For example, if a patient is given regimen B, fails therapy, is given regimen MX and has his/her *H. pylori* successfully eradicated, the costs are as follows: $42 + $217 + $35 + $146. If the patient fails on regimen MX, $35 for another primary care physician visit and $440 for a gastroenterologist visit and endoscopy are then included.

The costs and probabilities for each alternative in the model are displayed in Figure 8-7. The definitions for each variable included in the model are found in Table 8-4.

Determining the most cost-effective alternative Given the design of this model and the costs and probabilities associated with each alternative, regimen A is

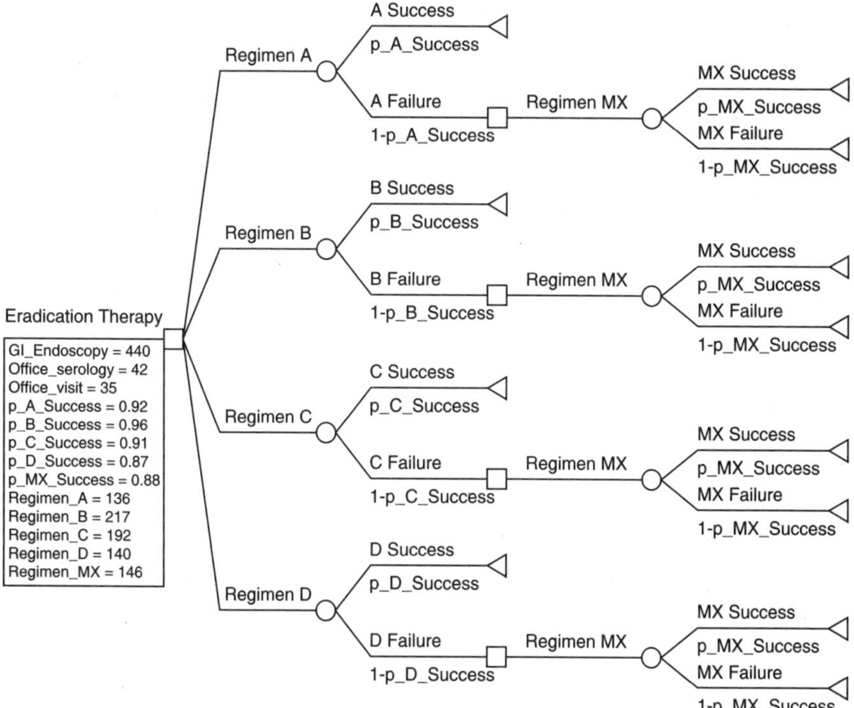

Figure 8-7. Decision tree with probabilities and costs displayed. Decision Analysis by *TreeAge*—Version 3.0 17/32-bit © 1988–1998 TreeAge Software, Inc.

determined to be the most cost-effective (Figure 8-8). The expected value, given the expected eradication rate of 0.92 and the associated costs of success and failure, is \$197. Note that this is a 14-day regimen that costs \$136.

Calculating the expected value of each alternative To illustrate how the decision tree calculations were made, let us examine how the expected cost of \$197 was calculated for regimen A (Figure 8-9). First, note the following:

There are three terminal nodes associated with regimen A. They correspond to following:

1. The probability of successful eradication using regimen A: This probability, as seen in Figure 8-9 and as noted in Table 8-2, is $P = 0.920$.
2. The probability of success with regimen MX, following regimen A: This probability, also seen in Figure 8-9, is $P = 0.070$, calculated by multiplying the probability of failure with regimen A (0.080) by the probability of success with regimen MX (0.880). [$0.080 * 0.880 = 0.0704$]

TABLE 8-4.

Definitions of Decision Tree Variables

Variable	*Definition*
Regimen A	1st *H. pylori* eradication therapy from Table 8-2
Regimen B	2nd *H. pylori* eradication therapy from Table 8-2
Regimen C	3rd *H. pylori* eradication therapy from Table 8-2
Regimen D	4th *H. pylori* eradication therapy from Table 8-2
Regimen MX	5th *H. pylori* eradication therapy from Table 8-2
"X" Success, where "X" corresponds to either regimen A, B, C, D, or MX	The probability of successfully eradicating *H. pylori* using regimen "X", where "X" corresponds to either regimen A, B, C, D, or MX
"X" Failure, where "X" corresponds to either regimen A, B, C, D, or MX	The probability of failing to eradicate *H. pylori* using regimen "X", where "X" corresponds to either regimen A, B, C, D, or MX
GI_endoscopy = 440	The cost of a visit with a gastroenterologist along with an endoscopy is $440
Office_serology = 42	The cost of the initial office visit and serology test is $42 ($35 for visit and $7 for test)
Office_visit = 35	All subsequent visits with the primary care physician are $35
P_A_Success	The probability of successfully eradicating *H. pylori* with regimen A is 0.92. Given this, the probability of failure (1 – p_A_success) is 0.08
P_B_Success	The probability of successfully eradicating *H. pylori* with regimen B is 0.96. Given this, the probability of failure (1 – p_A_success) is 0.04

(*continued*)

TABLE 8-4. *(continued)*

Definitions of Decision Tree Variables

Variable	*Definition*
P_C_Success	The probability of successfully eradicating *H. pylori* with regimen C is 0.91. Given this, the probability of failure (1 – p_A_success) is 0.09
P_D_Success	The probability of successfully eradicating *H. pylori* with regimen D is 0.87. Given this, the probability of failure (1 – p_A_success) is 0.13
P_MX_Success	The probability of successfully eradicating *H. pylori* with regimen MX is 0.88. Given this, the probability of failure (1 – p_A_success) is 0.12

3. The probability of failure after treatment with both regimens A and MX: This probability, also seen in Figure 8-9, is $P = 0.010$, calculated by multiplying the probability of failure with regimen A (0.08) by the probability of failure with regimen MX (0.120). [$0.080 * 0.120 = 0.0096$]

Note that these three probabilities sum to 1.0.

The expected value of regimen A can be calculated as follows. First, given the final probability of each alternative, as listed above, multiply each with the cost of the respective pathway, and then sum the values. This is demonstrated as follows:

4. 0.920 * $178 = $163.76, where $178 is the cost of success with regimen A: ($42 + $136, cost of office visit with serology plus the cost of regimen A)
5. 0.070 * $359 = $25.13, where $359 is the cost of success with regimen MX following failure with regimen A: ($42 + $136 + $35 + $146, cost of office visit with serology + the cost of regimen A + the cost of a follow-up primary care visit + the cost of regimen MX)
6. 0.010 * $834 = $8.34, where $834 is the cost of failure with both regimen MX and regimen A: ($42 + $136 + $35 + $146 + $440, cost of office visit with serology + the cost of regimen A + the cost of a follow-up primary care visit + the cost of regimen MX + the cost

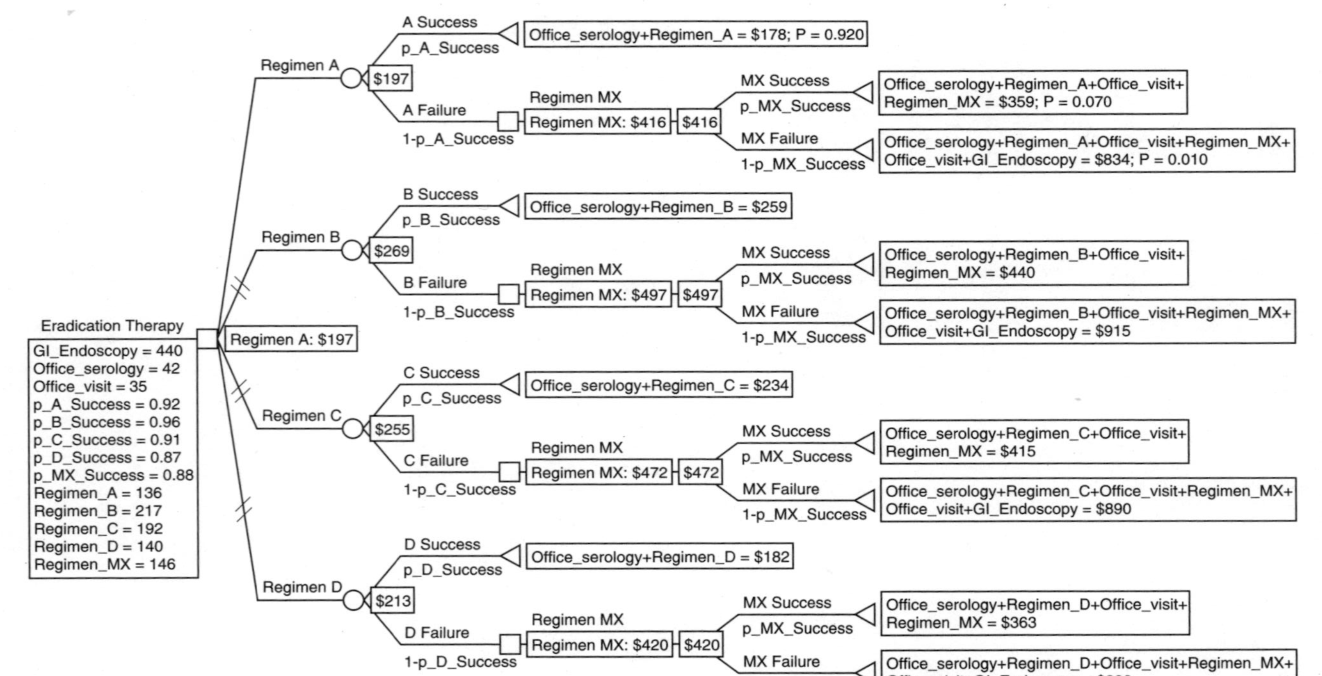

Figure 8-8. Final analyses. Decision Analysis by *TreeAge*—Version 3.0 17/32-bit © 1988–1998 TreeAge Software, Inc.

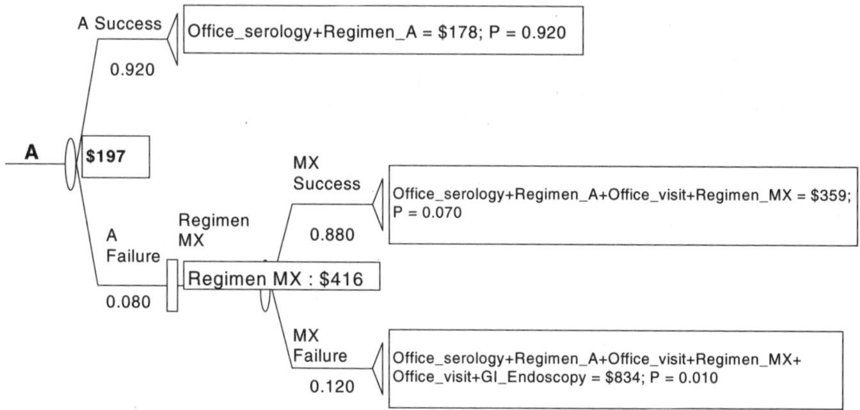

Figure 8-9. Calculating expected value of regimen A. Decision Analysis by *TreeAge*—Version 3.0 17/32-bit © 1988–1998 TreeAge Software, Inc.

of an additional primary care visit + the cost of a visit with a gastroenterologist and endoscopy)

7. $163.76 + $25.13 + $8.34 = $197.23: Considering each potential outcome associated with regimen A, and the corresponding probabilities, the expected value is $197.23.

A second method for calculating the expected value of regimen A, the rollback method, requires working backwards through the decision tree and considering the probabilities and costs simultaneously, rather than calculating the final probability of each alternative up front. During this process, it is helpful to consider entire sections of the tree one at a time. For this example, consider the cost of "regimen A success" as one section and consider the cost of "regimen A failure" as one section (i.e., split the tree in Figure 8-9 in half horizontally at the first chance node).

1. Identify the costs displayed at the three terminal nodes:
   Regimen A failure (2 terminal nodes)
   - $834 (failure with both regimen A and regimen MX)
   - $359 (success with regimen MX, following regimen A use)
     Regimen A success (1 terminal node)
   - $178 (success with regimen A)
2. Identify the probabilities associated with each branch emanating from the choice nodes:
   Regimen A failure (2 branches)
   - 0.12 (probability of regimen MX failure)
   - 0.88 (probability of regimen MX success)

A Regimen A success (1 branch)
   - 0.92 (probability of regimen A success)

3. Calculate the cost of regimen A failure, by considering the cost and probabilities associated with each alternative emanating from the regimen A failure node.
   Regimen A failure
   B • $834 ∗ 0.12 = $100.08
   • $359 ∗ 0.88 = $315.92
   Regimen A success
   • $178 ∗ 0.92 = $163.76
4. Add the values for each individual section
   Regimen A failure
   • 100.08 + $315.92 = $416
   Regimen A success
   • $163.76
5. Consider the probability of regimen A failure
   • 0.08
6. Multiply the cost and probability of regimen A failure
   • 0.08 ∗ $416 = $33.28
7. Add the value associated with cost and probability of regimen A success with the value associated with the cost and probability of regimen A failure
   • $163.76 + $33.28 = $197.04

Using this method, the same expected value of $197 for regimen A is calculated.

Step 10: Perform a sensitivity analysis

When dealing with uncertainty, as in this example where numerous variables have a range of values, such as costs and/or eradication rates, sensitivity analyses are conducted to test the robustness of the decision. In this example, several one-way sensitivity analyses were conducted.

Figure 8-10 shows the sensitivity of the decision analysis to the cost of the gastroenterologist visit and endoscopy. Consider the cost-effectiveness of these regimens if the cost was increased to $620. Regimen A remains the most cost-effective.

Figure 8-11 shows the sensitivity of the decision analysis to the eradication rate of regimen D. The sensitivity analysis uses 0.86–1.0 as the range of effectiveness for this alternative. As seen in Figure 8-11, in order for the cost-effectiveness of regimen D to exceed the cost-effectiveness of regimen A, the eradication rate must be greater than 0.937. However, as shown in Table 8-2, the highest reported rate in the published literature for regimen D was 0.90. Therefore, even when considering the maximum eradication rate possible for this alternative, regimen A remains most cost-effective. Likewise, when testing

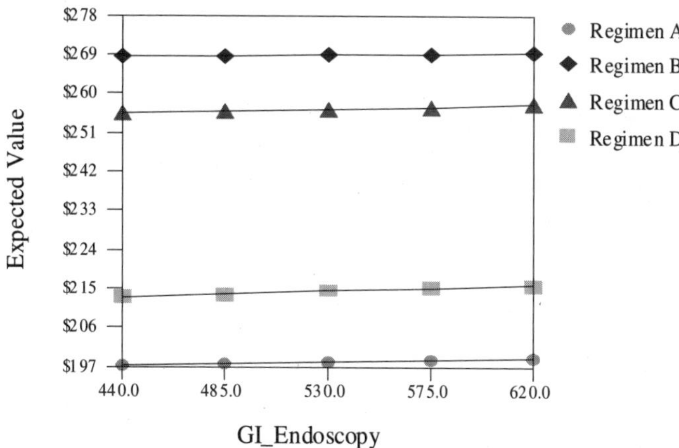

Figure 8-10. Sensitivity analysis using gastroenterology visit and endoscopy. Decision Analysis by *TreeAge*—Version 3.0 17/32-bit © 1988–1998 TreeAge Software, Inc.

the sensitivity of the decision to the eradication rates for regimens B and C, regimen A remained most cost-effective.

Figure 8-12 shows the sensitivity of the decision analysis to the cost of regimen D. The sensitivity analysis uses a range from $120 to $140 for this alternative. As seen in the figure, in order for regimen D to become more cost-effective than regimen A, the cost of this regimen would have to be less than

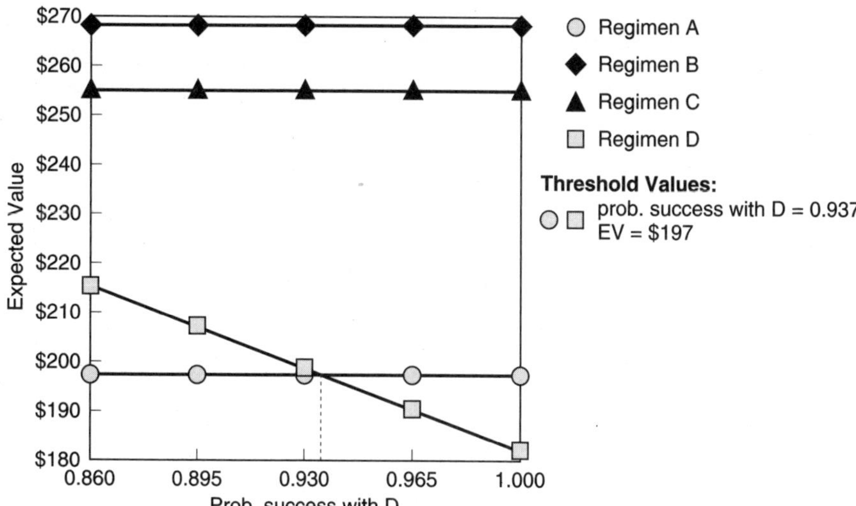

Figure 8-11. Sensitivity analysis using probability of success with regimen D. Decision Analysis by *TreeAge*—Version 3.0 17/32-bit © 1988–1998 TreeAge Software, Inc.

$124.10. However, given the contracted prices for each agent within this regimen, it is not possible to reduce the cost over $15 unless the price was lowered significantly by the pharmaceutical manufacturer to the health plan. Likewise, for regimens B and C, the costs would have to be below $145.50 and $133.60, respectively. These reductions are also unlikely.

Step 11: Present the results

The results of the decision analysis and sensitivity analysis are presented to the steering committee. Despite the overwhelming evidence from these analyses in favor of regimen A, the following question arises: Given the length of therapy (14 days), the number of pills (224) associated with regimen A, and the four times a day (*qid*) dosing, what is the expected rate of compliance and how will this affect the eradication rate? After much discussion, the disease management team agrees that the compliance rate will play a significant role in the success of the overall disease management program, and must be closely considered as a component of this decision. As a result, the team members develop a method that allows them to incorporate the impact of compliance into the decision.

As seen in Table 8-2, the team builds a compliance factor into the eradication rate. They assumed that for regimens with a b.i.d. (twice a day) dosing, the "real-world" eradication rate would drop by 5%, while the eradication rate for regimens with q.i.d. (four times a day) dosing would drop by 10%, due to

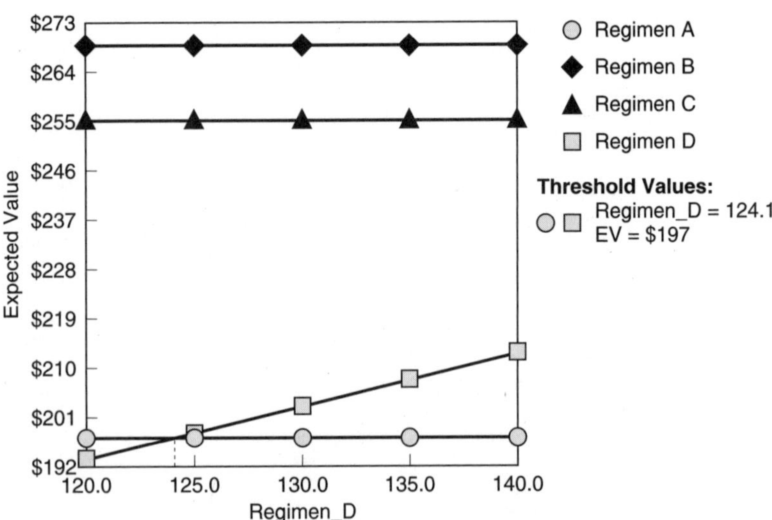

Figure 8-12. Sensitivity analysis using cost of regimen D. Decision Analysis by *TreeAge*—Version 3.0 17/32-bit © 1988–1998 TreeAge Software, Inc.

noncompliance. Additionally, for those regimens with duration of 14 days, the "real-world" eradication rate would be expected to drop by an additional 5% also due to noncompliance. Using these figures, the team calculated the "eradication × compliance rate", which is presented in the last column of Table 8-2. As an example, consider regimen A.

The weighted average eradication rate was 0.92. Considering the q.i.d.-dosing, this drops to just under 83% (0.92 * 0.90). Then, given that the patient must remain compliant for a full 2 weeks, the expected eradication rate drops another 5%, for a final rate of 0.79 (0.83 * 0.95).

These eradication rates were then substituted into the model developed in step 9. As seen in Figure 8-13, regimen D is the more cost-effective alternative when considering the compliance factor, with an expected cost of $226, versus $232 for regimen A.

When these results are presented, the team members provide mixed responses. Several members express great concern over the fact that the compliance issue raises the expected cost per patient by $29 ($226 – $197). This carries a great financial impact considering the size of the population of interest. After much discussion, the following proposal is placed on the table.

Realizing the value of increased compliance, the team members devise a plan that will allow the pharmacists within the plan's in-house pharmacies to receive compensation for the provision of pharmaceutical care. In this instance, the pharmacist would be charged with the responsibility of (1) thoroughly discussing the importance of medication compliance with the patient along with the associated consequences of noncompliance; (2) helping to select an appropriate reminder aid for the patient; and (3) monitoring the patient by contacting him/her during the course of therapy. The pharmacists will be compensated $15 for each patient.

The team members resort to the decision tree once again to determine the potential impact of this plan. They use the most conservative estimate by inputting the eradication rate of each regimen, without the compliance factor. The $15 charge per patient is then added only to the cost of regimen A. As seen in Figure 8-14, regimen A, despite the additional charge, once again becomes the most cost-effective therapy. The expected value is $212 for regimen A. The team makes the final decision: regimen A is the treatment of choice based on also implementing a pharmaceutical program intended to address patients' medication-taking practices.

Step 12: Develop a policy or intervention based on results (incorporate into guidelines)

As part of the disease management program, the selected regimen is built into the clinical guidelines, which are distributed to the entire provider population.

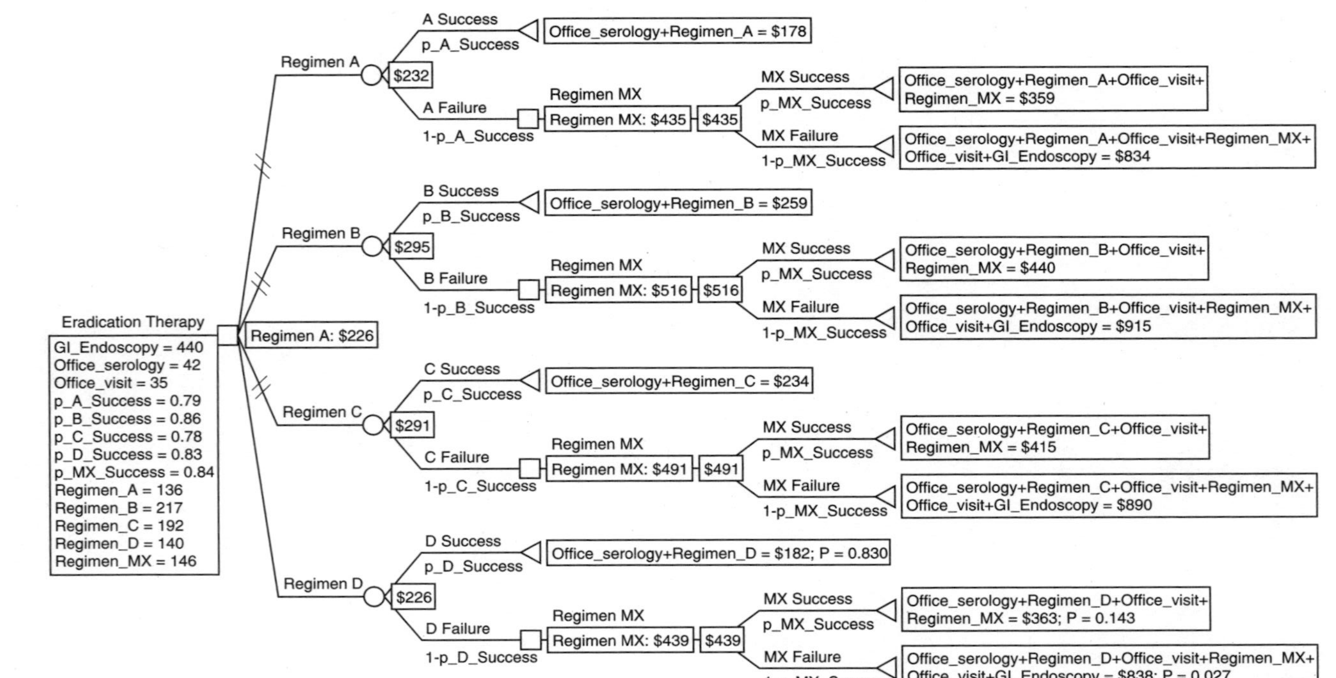

Figure 8-13. Cost-effectiveness using compliance factor. Decision Analysis by *TreeAge*—Version 3.0 17/32-bit © 1988–1998 TreeAge Software, Inc.

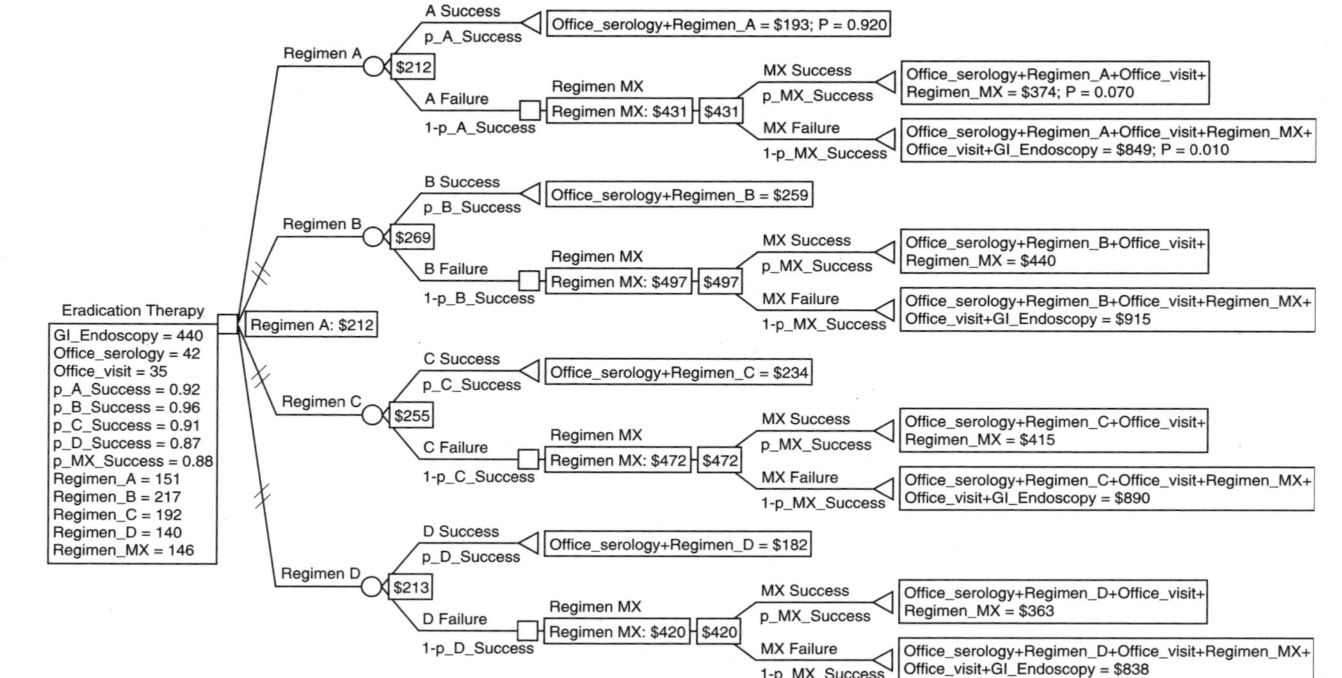

Figure 8-14. Cost-effectiveness when considering the cost of providing pharmaceutical care to increase compliance for regimen A. Decision Analysis by *TreeAge*—Version 3.0 17/32-bit © 1988–1998 TreeAge Software, Inc.

Step 13: Implement policy or intervention and educate

Additionally, as discussed previously, the team develops an implementation program to ensure provider buy-in and compliance with the recommendations.

Step 14: Collect follow-up data

Since the program is to ensure the delivery of the best care to patients, the team will collect follow-up data to assess the impact of program, staying alert to new developments in *H. pylori* therapy.

SUMMARY

The case study presented in this chapter was intended to show the role of pharmacoeconomics within the framework of disease management. The use of pharmacoeconomics and decision analyses is helpful for decision making under conditions of uncertainty, especially when clinical practice guidelines are under development. These structured decision-making techniques are particularly useful when there are numerous alternatives to consider that have a number of variable components, such as efficacy rates and cost. In the case study described within this chapter, the efficacy and cost were incorporated into a decision tree, which clearly demonstrated that the best alternative was regimen A. However, a significant issue was overlooked initially—that of compliance. As the effectiveness of medication use may differ significantly from the efficacy of the same agents in clinical trials, it is important to consider all factors that may influence the successful use of these agents. As demonstrated within this case, considering "real world" compliance significantly changed the findings of the analysis.

Conducting pharmacoeconomic analyses is not a simple task, as many factors must be addressed, proper evidence collected, and careful planning performed. Using the 14-step process outlined within this chapter will help to ensure that the analyses are properly conducted and that the decisions are based on evidence rather than opinions or cost alone.

REFERENCES

1. Todd WE, Nash D, eds: *Disease Management: A Systems Approach to Improving Patient Outcomes*. Chicago: American Hospital Association; 1997.
2. Bodenheimer T: Disease management—promises and pitfalls. *NEJM* 1999;340:1202–1205.
3. Epstein RS, Sherwood LM: From outcomes research to disease management: a guide for the perplexed. *Ann Intern Med* 1996;124:832–837.

4. Kibbe DC, Johnson K: Do-it-yourself disease management. *Family Practice Management* 1998;Nov–Dec: http://www.aafp.org/fpm/981100fm/disease.html.
5. Weingarten S: Zynx Health, personal communication; 1997.
6. NIH Consensus Development Panel of *Helicobacter pylori* in Peptic Ulcer Disease: *Helicobacter pylori* in peptic ulcer disease. *JAMA* 1994;272:65–69.
7. Sonnenberg A: Peptic ulcer. In: Everhart JE, ed., *Digestive Disease in the United States: Epidemiology and Impact*. Washington, DC: US Department of Health and Human Services, Public Health Service, National Institutes of Health (NIH), National Institute of Diabetes and Kidney Diseases; 1994. NIH publication 94-1447.
8. Berardi RR: Peptic ulcer disease. In: DiPiro JT, Talbert RL, Yee GC, et al., eds.: *Pharmacotherapy: A Pathophysiologic Approach*, 4th edn. Stamford, CT: Appleton & Lang; 1999;548–570.
9. Marshall BJ, Warren JR: Unidentified curved bacilli in the stomach of patients with gastritis and peptic ulceration. *Lancet* 1984;1:1311–1315.
10. Graham DY, Lew GM, Klein PD, et al.: Effect of treatment of *Helicobacter pylori* infection on the long-term recurrence of gastric or duodenal ulcer. *Ann Intern Med* 1992;116:705–708.
11. Guyton AC: Physiology of gastrointestinal disorders. In: *Textbook of Medical Physiology*, 8th edn. Philadelphia, PA: WB Saunders; 1991:736–742.
12. Cerda JJ, Fowler FC: Fighting the fire: managing and preventing peptic ulcer disease in the multi-risk patient. *Modern Med* 1994;62:40–49.
13. Jones R, Lydeard S: Prevalence of symptoms of dyspepsia in the community. *BMJ* 1989;298:30–32.
14. Armstrong D: *Helicobacter pylori* infection and dyspepsia. *Scand J Gastroenterol Suppl* 1996;215:38–47.
15. Fenfrick AM, Chernew ME, Hirth RA, Blom BS: Alternative management strategies for patients with suspected peptic ulcer disease. *Ann Intern Med* 1995;123:260–268.
16. Sonnenberg A: Cost-benefit analysis of testing for *Helicobacter pylori* in dyspeptic subjects. *Am J Gastroenterol* 1996;91:1773–1777.
17. Ofman JJ, Etchason JE, Fullerton S, Kahn KL, Soll AH: Management strategies for *Helicobacter pylori*-seropositive patients with dyspepsia: Clinical and economic consequences. *Ann Intern Med* 1997;126:280–291.
18. Modified from a 11-step framework described by S. Weingarten, Zynx Health, personal communication.
19. Guyatt GH, Sackett DL, Cook DJ: Users' guides to the medical literature. II. How to use an article about therapy or prevention. A. Are the results of the study valid? Evidence-Based Medicine Working Group. *JAMA* 1993 (Dec. 1); 270(21):2598–2601.

20. Schwartz JS, Cohen SJ: Changing physician behavior. In: Mayfield J and Grady M, eds, *Primary Care Research: An Agenda for the 90s*. Washington, DC: US Department of Health and Human Services Public Health Service/Agency for Health Care Policy and Research, 1990:45–54.
21. Soll AH: Medical treatment of peptic ulcer disease: practice guidelines. *JAMA* 1996;275:8.
22. Burette A, Glupczynski Y, Deprez C: Evaluation of various multidrug eradication regimens for *Helicobacter pylori*. *Eur J Gastroenterol Hepatol* 1992;4817–4823.
23. Chiba N, Rao BV, Rademaker JW, Hunt RH: Meta-analysis of the efficacy of antibiotic therapy in eradicating *Helicobacter pylori*. *Am J Gastroenterol* 1992;87:1716–1727.
24. Fennerty MB: Clinical issues and cost effectiveness of treating *H. pylori*. *Am J Managed Care* 1998;4(4):S2538.
25. Drummond MF, Stoddart GL, Torrance GW: Methods for the economic evaluation of health care programmes. Oxford, England: Oxford University Press; 1987.
26. Jolicoeur LM, Jones-Grizzle AJ, Boyer JG: Guidelines for performing a pharmacoeconomic analysis. *Am J Hosp Pharm* 1992;49:1741–1747.
27. Jones AJ, Sanchez LA: Pharmacoeconomic evaluation: applications in managed health care formulary decision-making. *Drug Benefit Trends* 1995;12, 15, 19–22, 32–34.
28. Doubilet P, Weinstein MC, McNeil BJ: Use and misuse of the term "cost effective" in medicine. *N Engl J Med* 1986;314:253–256.
29. Osato MS, Reddy R, Graham DY: Metronidazole and clarithromycin resistance amongst *Helicobacter pylori* isolates from a large metropolitan hospital in the United States. *Int J Antimicrob Agents* 1999 (Aug);12(4):314–347.

C H A P T E R

9

Application of Pharmacoeconomics in Cardiovascular Disease: Economic Evaluation of Lipid-Lowering Therapies

David Hawkins and Jay Jackson

INTRODUCTION

The leading cause of death in the United States is heart disease. More than 2600 Americans die each day of cardiovascular disease, an average of one death every 33 seconds.[1] This is more than the next seven leading causes of death combined. The morbidity associated with cardiovascular disorders is almost too much to fathom. According to the American Heart Association, more than 58 million Americans are afflicted with some type of cardiovascular disorder. The more prevalent conditions include hypertension, coronary heart disease (CHD; i.e., myocardial infarction and angina pectoris), stroke, and heart failure. Current estimates are:

- hypertension—50,000,000 Americans
- coronary heart disease—12,000,000 Americans
- myocardial infarction—7,000,000 Americans
- angina pectoris—6,200,000 Americans
- stroke—4,400,000 Americans
- congestive heart failure—4,600,000 Americans

The estimated cost of cardiovascular disease in the United States in 1999 was \$286.5 billion.[1] This estimate includes both direct costs and indirect costs.

Cardiovascular disease ranks first among all disease categories in numbers of hospital discharges. It accounts for more than 58 million physician office visits, 5 million hospital outpatient visits, and 4 million emergency room visits each year in the United States.[1] The Health Care Financing Administration in 1995 reported that \$24.6 billion in payments were made to Medicare beneficiaries for hospital expenses due to cardiovascular problems. That represented 32.9% of all hospital expenditures.

Because of the prevalence and economics of cardiovascular disease, millions of dollars are spent each year developing new cardiovascular therapies. The cost of synthesizing a new cardiovascular agent, testing it in human subjects, and eventually obtaining Food and Drug Administration (FDA) approval of the product exceeds \$20 million in most cases. Therefore, when the drug finally reaches the US market, it understandably carries with it a relatively high price tag. None of these therapies is curative. But there is evidence that new therapies reduce the incidence of morbid events and may prolong life. This then leads to the question: Is the extra benefit gained by a new cardiovascular intervention worth the extra cost? A careful economic evaluation is needed to answer that question.

Of all the cardiovascular therapies that have been subjected to economic analysis, lipid-lowering therapy has been the most extensively studied. This chapter will review the evidence that has been published in referred articles dealing with the cost-effectiveness of lipid-lowering agents, especially regarding the use of 3-hydroxy-3-methylglutaryl coenzyme A (HMG-CoA) reductase inhibitors (commonly referred to as the statins).

TYPES OF STUDY DESIGNS

Several different experimental and quasiexperimental designs have been used to estimate the costs and consequences of lipid-lowering therapy including the randomized controlled trial, the economic clinical trial, post-hoc analysis, and simulation designs. In the majority of published studies, the cost-effectiveness ratio is usually stated in terms of cost per life year saved (cost/LYS). The numerator usually includes the acquisition cost of the lipid-lowering agent (i.e., the average wholesale cost), the cost of monitoring therapy, and the cost of managing adverse drug effects minus the cost of treating coronary heart disease events avoided by the treatment. The denominator is the incremental change in survival achieved with lipid-lowering therapy. The alternative treatment in most studies has been no therapy, placebo, or a low-fat diet. Other outcome units which have been used to measure the cost-effectiveness of lipid-lowering therapies include cost per percentage of cholesterol reduction, cost to reach a specified target, cost per cardiovascular event avoided, and cost per quality-adjusted life year (QALY) gained.

PRIMARY VERSUS SECONDARY PREVENTION OF CORONARY HEART DISEASE

Before presenting the results of the economic evaluations of lipid-lowering agents, it is important to point out the clinical difference between primary and secondary prevention of coronary heart disease (CHD). Primary prevention applies to the patient who has no clinical or diagnostic evidence of CHD but is at risk of developing CHD. The intent is to prevent or delay the onset of disease. Since hypercholesterolemia is a powerful, independent risk factor of CHD, any strategy used to reduce serum cholesterol in patients without CHD is considered primary prevention.

Secondary prevention is designed to reduce the morbidity and mortality associated with CHD. The patient is known to have CHD as evidenced by a positive history of clinical coronary events or by a positive diagnostic work-up for atherosclerotic disease. The objective of secondary prevention is to prevent recurrence of clinical events and to increase survival.

Because patients with CHD are three to four times more likely to experience a coronary event (i.e., fatal or nonfatal myocardial infarction, angina, or unstable angina) than patients without CHD, it is easier to demonstrate the clinical effectiveness of a successful intervention in the setting of secondary prevention. It is also easier to demonstrate the cost-effectiveness of an intervention for secondary prevention than it is for primary prevention.

RESULTS OF ECONOMIC STUDIES IN PRIMARY PREVENTION

Many of the earlier pharmacoeconomic studies used a simulation design in which the benefits of cholesterol lowering were largely predicted from multivariate logistic risk equations derived from the Framingham Heart Study.[2,3] The necessary assumption in this approach is that the relationship between the relative risk of CHD and cholesterol levels derived from an epidemiological cohort can predict the CHD risk reduction in individuals given medication to lower their lipid levels. This type of design has been used particularly to evaluate the cost-effectiveness of lipid-lowering therapy in primary prevention.

Before the advent of the statins, the pharmacological agents used to lower cholesterol included the bile acid resins, fibrates, and niacin. These agents are not as effective as statins in lowering cholesterol nor are they as well tolerated.

Early clinical primary prevention trials with non-statin lipid-lowering agents showed a reduction in cardiovascular morbidity and mortality, but not total mortality. Economic evaluations of cholestyramine,[4,5] colestipol,[6] gemfibrozil,[7] and niacin[8] were principally based on simulation designs. For the most part, these studies found that only patients at an extremely high risk of CHD could be treated with lipid-lowering therapy in a cost-effective manner.

There are six statins currently available on the US market: lovastatin, fluvastatin, simvastatin, pravastatin, atorvastatin, and cerivastatin. These differ both in terms of cost and lipid-lowering potency. There may be other differences among the statins that impact their clinical effectiveness, such as decreasing fibrinogen levels, diminishing the uptake of oxidized low-density lipoprotein (LDL)-cholesterol by vascular smooth muscle cells, suppressing the release of tissue factor, and increasing endothelial-derived nitric oxide.[9] There are no head-to-head statin clinical trials, nor is it likely there ever will be. So the question of clinical superiority cannot be answered directly.

Economic evaluations of the statins have been carried out in the context of both primary and secondary prevention of CHD. For the most part, the statin has been pitted against no therapy in simulation designs and placebo when data from randomized controlled trials have been used. Very few economic studies have compared one statin against another: those that have are based on weak experimental designs and intermediate outcomes.

Lovastatin was the first available statin in the United States. The cost-effectiveness of lovastatin was initially investigated by Goldman and colleagues.[10] Their evaluation assumed a societal perspective and used a computer-simulation model based on data obtained from the Framingham Heart Study to predict outcomes. Only direct costs of CHD were included in the analysis. The investigators found that lovastatin was not cost-effective in any subgroup of women but was cost-effective in men who had other risk factors present (such as obesity, cigarette smoking, and hypertension).

Other investigators have found similar results in the evaluation of lovastatin for primary CHD prevention. Hay and his colleagues, using multivariate logistic risk equations derived from the Framingham Heart Study, found lovastatin to be cost-effective only in high-risk men (patients with cholesterol levels ≥260 mg/dl or patients with systolic hypertension).[11] In a study by Hamilton et al.[12] the lifetime cost-effectiveness of lovastatin for primary prevention of CHD was evaluated and also found to be cost-effective only in high-risk patients. When the theoretical benefit that statins have by increasing the high-density lipoprotein (HDL)-cholesterol was added to the model, the cost-effectiveness ratio was reduced by approximately 40%, and lovastatin was cost-effective even for low-risk middle-aged men and women.

In a Canadian study that compared the cost-effectiveness of fluvastatin with several other statins, Martens and Guibert[13] calculated the cost/LYS by estimating the CHD risk as a function of both LDL-cholesterol and HDL-cholesterol levels. A mathematical model for primary prevention was developed based on both the Canadian Heart Health Study and Framingham Heart Study. The model showed that in 45-year-old men who smoke and have pretreatment LDL-cholesterol levels in excess of 174 mg/dl, the cost/LYS ranged from $32,000 with fluvastatin to $46,000 with pravastatin (1993 US dollars).

Pharmacoeconomic evaluations of pravastatin have been performed using both a simulation design and randomized controlled trials. The results using the latter design will be discussed in the section on secondary prevention. Using a simulation design based upon Framingham risk equations, Johannesson et al.[14] projected the cost-effectiveness of pravastatin for primary prevention in a Swedish population. Costs were determined by subtracting the cost saved due to the reduction of cardiovascular morbidity from the cost of lipid-lowering medication and monitoring. The investigators found that pravastatin was not cost-effective even in relatively high-risk middle-aged men.

The cost-effectiveness of simvastatin has been assessed for both primary and secondary CHD prevention. More will be said about the studies in secondary prevention later. In the context of primary prevention, a study carried out in the Netherlands found simvastatin to be substantially more cost-effective than cholestyramine.[15] The study used a risk-reduction model based on multivariate logistic risk functions from the Framingham study. The superior cost-effectiveness ratio of simvastatin was limited to middle-aged men with an initial cholesterol level of 310 mg/dl and was sensitive to medication and treatment costs.

Huse et al.[16] conducted an incremental cost-effectiveness analysis of five statins (atorvastatin, fluvastatin, lovastatin, pravastatin, and simvastatin) at the recommended starting dose versus no therapy in primary and secondary prevention of CHD. The analysis was based on a mathematical model derived from Framingham Heart Study risk equations. Only estimates of direct medical costs were used in the analysis. The incremental cost/LYS was calculated according to the LDL-cholesterol concentration, age, and gender of the patient. The authors found that in primary prevention the statins were cost-effective only in women with the highest risk profiles and men at moderate to high risk.

Two recent large-scale primary prevention trials provide convincing evidence that statin therapy can reduce the morbidity and mortality associated with the development of CHD. The West of Scotland Coronary Prevention Study (WOSCOPS)[17] was a double-blind, randomized, placebo-controlled study that evaluated the effect of pravastatin on the incidence of CHD death and nonfatal myocardial infarction in more than 6500 predominantly asymptomatic men with elevated serum cholesterol levels. There was a 31% relative risk reduction in the combined endpoint of nonfatal myocardial infarction and CHD death in the pravastatin group. WOSCOPS also showed a 22% reduction in total mortality, which fell just short of reaching statistical significance ($P = 0.051$). The Air Force/Texas Coronary Atherosclerosis Prevention Study (AFCAPS/TexCAPS)[18] was a double-blind, placebo-controlled trial that evaluated the effect of lovastatin in over 6600 men and women who had hypercholesterolemia but were otherwise generally healthy. Compared with subjects in the placebo group, subjects in the lovastatin group had 37% fewer first acute coronary events (fatal or nonfatal myocardial infarction, unstable angina, or sudden cardiac death) and 33% fewer coronary revascularization procedures. There was no significant difference in mortality rates between the two groups.

In an economic study of simvastatin for primary and secondary prevention of CHD, Pharoah et al.[19] used a life table method to calculate the cost-effectiveness of simvastatin in people at various risk of fatal cardiovascular disease. Data from WOSCOPS was used in the primary prevention analysis. The secondary prevention arm was based on data from the 4S study; those results will be discussed later. The cost of primary prevention was estimated from the direct costs of treatment minus savings due to a reduction in coronary angiograms, nonfatal myocardial infarctions, and revascularization procedures. The authors found that the average cost/LYS in men without CHD was over $200,000.

Caro et al.[20] evaluated the cost-effectiveness of pravastatin for primary prevention based on the WOSCOPS clinical trial data and survival data obtained from the Scottish record linkage system. Costs estimates were based on the average direct 1996 cost of initial management of CHD events and the acquisition and monitoring costs of pravastatin. The major outcomes of the study included cost consequences, number of CHD events prevented, number needed to start treatment, and the cost per life year gained. The authors concluded that the use of pravastatin was cost-effective, especially in selected high-risk subgroups. These same authors performed a similar economic analysis on a more global basis and found that the cost-effectiveness ratios were less than $25,000 per life year gained for the UK, Canada, Sweden, Belgium, and South Africa.[21]

ECONOMIC STUDIES IN SECONDARY PREVENTION

In the study by Huse et al.[16] (already described under the section on primary prevention), all statins were found to be cost-effective in men and women with multiple risk factors for secondary prevention. Of the five statins included in this analysis, atorvastatin was the most cost-effective.

Ashraf et al.[22] calculated the cost-effectiveness of pravastatin in secondary prevention based on the pooled results of the pravastatin limitation of atherosclerosis in the coronary arteries (PLAC I)[23] and the pravastatin, lipids, and atherosclerosis in the carotid arteries (PLAC II)[24] regression trials. The Framingham Heart Study data were used to project the risk of mortality 10 years after a myocardial infarction. A Markov model was used to estimate the number of life years saved and a decision analysis was used to estimate cost.

The authors found that cost/LYS varied considerably with patient risk profile, ranging from $7124 to $12,665.

Pharoah et al.,[19] in a study previously described under primary prevention, found that treating hypercholesterolemia varies greatly according to patient risk factors. The average cost-effectiveness in secondary prevention was slightly more than $50,000/LYS. However, the cost-effectiveness ranged from just under $10,000/LYS in high-risk men to over $500,000/LYS in women with angina and a slightly elevated serum cholesterol. The authors concluded that a marginal cost-effectiveness analysis should be used in making clinical decisions regarding treatment.

Elliott and Weir[25] conducted an incremental cost-effectiveness analysis of the six currently available statins in a cohort of CHD patients between the ages of 60 and 85 years. The costs and effects of treatment were determined from a simulation model. The model takes an initial cohort of CHD patients and projects the number of survivors, the annual direct cost per survivor, and the annual indirect cost saving per survivor associated with a reduction in CHD events. The authors found that the cost/LYS ranged from $5421 with atorvastatin to $15,073 with lovastatin.

At least four economic evaluations of statin therapy in secondary prevention have been based on data obtained from a large randomized outcome trial—the Scandinavian Simvastatin Survival Study, or the 4S study. This study involved more than 4000 men and women with documented CHD and a total cholesterol level in the range of 213–309 mg/dl. During the 5.4 median years of follow-up, simvastatin therapy reduced all-cause mortality by 30%, CHD mortality by 42%, major coronary events by 34%, coronary revascularization procedures by 32%, and hospitalizations related to CHD by 26%.[26]

In a cost-minimization study that estimated the benefits of lowering cholesterol using data from the 4S study, simvastatin therapy produced a 10% decrease in length of hospital stay, a 26% reduction in the number of hospitalizations, a 31% reduction in hospital costs, and a 34% reduction in total hospital days.[27] As a result of these substantial cost savings, the cost of simvastatin was reduced from $2.29 per day to only $0.28 per day. In this study, the average wholesale price was used in calculating the cost of simvastatin therapy. In managed care organizations that negotiate contract prices, the cost associated with simvastatin would be even lower or might even be associated with cost savings.

Johannesson et al.[28] estimated the cost/LYS of simvastatin therapy based on the 4S study using a modified Markov model. Both direct and indirect costs were included in the analysis. Separate estimates of cost-effectiveness were prepared for men and women at different ages and pretreatment cholesterol levels. The authors found that simvastatin was cost-effective in both men and women of all ages and cholesterol levels studied. The cost-effectiveness ratios ranged from $27,400/LYS (based on direct cost only) in 35-year-old women with baseline cholesterol of 213 mg/dl to a cost savings (based on both direct and indirect costs) in 35-year-old men and women with baseline cholesterol levels of 213–309 mg/dl.

To forecast the long-term benefits and cost-effectiveness of simvastatin in the secondary prevention of cardiovascular disease, Grover et al.[29] developed a life-expectancy model based on the Lipid Research Clinics Program prevalence and follow-up data and the results of the 4S study. The economic perspective was that of a third party providing comprehensive coverage of all health care services. All costs were expressed in 1996 US dollars. The authors concluded that long-term treatment of hyperlipidemia in secondary prevention was cost-effective across a broad range of patients. The cost/LYS ranged from $4487 to $9548 for men and from $5138 to $13,747 for women, depending on other risk factors.

ECONOMIC STUDIES BASED ON INTERMEDIATE OUTCOMES

Fluvastatin is the least-expensive statin in the US market. It is also the least potent in terms of cholesterol reduction. In two separate economic studies that compared several statins in terms of the cost per percent reduction in LDL-cholesterol, the investigators concluded that fluvastatin was the most cost-effective lipid-lowering agent.[30,31] Such a conclusion, however, is tenuous since it is based entirely on a surrogate endpoint and the average wholesale price (AWP) of the statins, which no one actually pays. As a matter of contrast, Table 9-1 presents the cost per percent LDL-cholesterol reduction for each statin based on the AWP and the average negotiated contract price. The more important outcome of interest is the reduction in CHD events and mortality. It is certainly conceivable that a reduction in CHD events may substantially offset the cost of statin therapy. Projecting cost-effectiveness solely on drug costs and cholesterol reduction may underestimate the cost of other statins and overestimate the cost-effectiveness of fluvastatin.[32]

Atorvastatin is the most potent statin currently on the US market. In two separate economic studies, atorvastatin was found to be more cost-effective than other statins, but this was due strictly to its greater potency. The first study was based on a randomized economic trial design; the second study was a nonrandomized treat-to-target analysis carried out in patients attending a university-based lipid clinic.

In a randomized, 54-week, multicenter trial involving 662 patients, the mean total cost of care to reach National Cholesterol Education Program (NCEP) goals was determined.[33] Hypercholesterolemic patients were randomized to atorvastatin, simvastatin, lovastatin, or fluvastatin. Statin therapy was initiated at recommended starting doses and increased according to NCEP guidelines and package insert information. Colestipol was added to the regimen if the

TABLE 9-1.

HMG-CoA Reductase Inhibitors (Statins) with Average LDL-C Reduction and Cost

Drug/dose (mg/day)	*Average LDL-C reduction (%)*	*Annual cost—AWP ($/year)*	*AWP cost/%LDL-C reduction ($)*	*Average contract price/year[a] ($)*	*Contract cost/%LDL-C reduction ($)*
Atorvastatin					
10	39	685.84	17.59	514.38	13.19
20	43	1060.33	24.66	795.25	18.49
40	50	1276.77	25.54	957.58	19.15
80[b]	60	2553.54	42.56	1915.16	31.92
Cerivastatin					
0.2	25	517.94	20.72	388.46	15.54
0.3	31	517.94	16.71	388.46	12.53
0.4	34	517.94	15.23	388.46	11.43
Fluvastatin					
20	22	457.89	20.81	343.42	15.61
40	25	457.89	18.32	343.42	13.74
80[c]	36	915.78	25.44	686.84	19.08
Lovastatin					
10	21	482.17	22.96	361.63	17.22
20	27	849.72	31.47	637.29	23.60
40	31	1529.72	49.35	1147.29	37.01
80[d]	40	3059.44	76.49	2294.58	57.36
Pravastatin					
10	22	770.52	35.02	577.89	26.27
20	32	829.65	25.93	622.24	19.44
40	34	1364.01	40.12	1023.01	30.09
Simvastatin					
5	26	650.07	25.00	487.55	18.75
10	30	796.43	26.55	597.32	19.91
20	38	1389.19	36.56	1041.89	27.42
40	41	1389.19	33.88	1041.89	25.41
80	47	1389.19	29.56	1041.89	22.17

LDL-C = Low-density lipoprotein cholestrol; AWP = average wholesale price.
[a]Average contract price = AWP × 0.75
[b]80 mg atorvastatin = 2 × 40 mg tablet
[c]80 mg fluvastatin = 2 × 40 mg capsule
[d]80 mg lovastatin = 2 × 40 mg tablet
AWP obtained from *The 2000 Red Book*.
Average LDL-C reduction obtained from *1999 Physicians Desk Reference*.

goal was not reached at the highest recommended dose of statin therapy. Patients randomized to atorvastatin were more likely to reach the goal without the addition of colestipol. Consequently, atorvastatin was found to be associated with the least mean total cost of care.

In a population-based treat-to-target pharmacoeconomic analysis of various statins, atorvastatin was found to be the most cost-effective in high-risk patients (CHD present) and fluvastatin in low-risk (less than two risk factors for CHD) and moderate-risk (two or more risk factors for CHD) patients.[34]

At least two studies have examined the cost-effectiveness of low-dose combination lipid-lowering therapy compared with escalating the dose of statin monotherapy based on intermediate outcomes. In the study by Ito and Shabetai,[35] a randomized, open-label study was used to compare the combination of pravastatin 10 mg daily and cholestyramine 5 g twice daily with pravastatin 20 mg once daily monotherapy. After 6 weeks of therapy, pravastatin was increased to 20 mg in the combination group and 40 mg in the monotherapy group if the LDL-cholesterol remained above 100 mg/dl. The study was carried out in 59 men with moderate hypercholesterolemia and CHD. The outcome measured was the cost of treatment (AWP) per percent reduction in LDL-cholesterol. The authors found that significantly more patients reached the target LDL-cholesterol goal (≤100 mg/dl) with combination therapy and at a lower cost than pravastatin monotherapy.

In another study involving 96 patients with moderate hypercholesterolemia, a combination of low-dose colestipol and low-dose lovastatin reduced LDL-cholesterol levels significantly more than doubling the dose of lovastatin. The combination regimen was also found to be 25% more cost-effective than high-dose lovastatin monotherapy.[36]

LIMITATIONS OF ECONOMIC STUDIES

Conclusions drawn from economic studies based on intermediate outcomes, such as percent LDL-cholesterol reduction or extent to which LDL-cholesterol goals are achieved, may be misleading or incorrect, since important health outcomes do not necessarily correlate with surrogate endpoints. A proper cost-effectiveness study measures costs and relevant outcomes, and not surrogate or intermediate endpoints. Economic studies that employ simulation designs and various modeling techniques are also fraught with error. Some of the pitfalls associated with modeling include the difficulty of obtaining accurate data, the multiple assumptions that must be made regarding the clinical effectiveness of the intervention, and the fact that CHD risk equations underestimate the actual risks of nonfatal CHD events.[37,38]

A potential improvement on these designs is the pharmacoeconomic evaluation that is based on large-scale, prospective outcome studies that document the effectiveness of lipid-lowering therapy in reducing cardiovascular morbidity and mortality. However, even these studies have limitations that make it difficult to interpret the results. A fairly detailed discussion on the limitations of basing economic models on randomized clinical trials is provided by Schwartz[39] and Hlatky[40]and includes:

1. Lack of generalizability, since randomized controlled trials are usually restricted to specific patient populations
2. Results extrapolated beyond the study period
3. Post-hoc analysis performed on patients grouped according to risk factor status
4. Use of either a placebo or no treatment as the only comparator
5. Failure to include indirect costs
6. Failure to include quality of life assessments
7. Failure to consider all relevant CHD-related outcomes
8. Failure to measure the use of all relevant health care resources
9. Failure to measure the effect reduced patient compliance has on the cost and benefits of therapy
10. Failure to account for the impact different practice patterns and health care plans have on resource use and costs.

ACHIEVING COST-EFFECTIVENESS WITH LIPID-LOWERING THERAPY

Based on the evidence obtained from the economic studies that have been presented, one may conclude that the treatment for secondary prevention of CHD is cost-effective but the treatment for primary prevention is cost-effective only in high-risk patients. The issue in primary prevention then is to determine what patients are at high risk. An excellent discussion on CHD risk assessment is provided by Jacobson et al.[41] Basically, if a person's 10-year risk of experiencing a CHD event is 20% or higher, the patient can be considered CHD-equivalent and would benefit from aggressive lipid-lowering therapy. Whether this cut-off point is also cost-effective remains to be seen.

It is reasonable to postulate that if the optimal economic study could be performed, lipid-lowering therapy might prove more cost-effective for primary prevention than has been demonstrated with less rigorous designs. It might even prove cost saving in certain subgroups. A proper study has not been done that would allow one to conclude that one statin is more cost-effective than the others. Low-dose combination therapy appears to be a practical way of maximizing the cost-effectiveness of lipid-lowering therapy in patients who fail to achieve NCEP goals on the initial dose of the statin du jour.

A PROPOSED ECONOMIC STUDY DESIGN FOR PRIMARY PREVENTION

The economic randomized trial is perhaps the most rigorous design for conducting a cost-effectiveness analysis. It allows the researcher to collect clinical, economic, and humanistic data prospectively at predetermined time points from patients in different practice settings. It also provides both external validity and internal validity. Nevertheless, it is not without limitations. The economic clinical trial is extremely costly and requires an enormous study population to provide sufficient statistical power. Additionally, it is measured longitudinally, which often requires years to perform.

In the proposed study, three different practice settings will be utilized: managed care, academic medical center, and private practice. By including multiple practice settings, differences in cost factors can be accounted for in the analysis and generalizability of the results can be assessed.

Relevant cost factors and terminal endpoints will be collected for each practice setting. An example of these is listed in Table 9-2. Humanistic outcomes will also be collected prospectively using an appropriate general health survey. An analysis will be conducted to ascertain which therapy is cost-effective in each group of patients under different perspectives. Once the ratio is obtained, a sensitivity analysis will be run on drug costs and treatment costs. A sensitivity analysis will not be required for events because the actual events will be recorded. A diagram of the proposed study design is shown in Figure 9-1. The primary prevention study design examines patients with hypercholesterolemia and without coronary heart disease. Patients are stratified based on two criteria (CHD risk ≥20% and event risk <20%). The CHD risk of ≥20% is for a 10-year interval (2% per year based on weighted risk factors for CHD). The event risk of <20% is also based on a 10-year interval. After patients are stratified, they are randomized into one of three groups: (1) no drug therapy; (2) statin monotherapy; and (3) low-dose combination therapy. All patients will receive a step I/II diet. Patients randomized to statin monotherapy will begin treatment at the recommended starting dose and the dose will be increased until the NCEP goal is reached or the maximum dose has been given. Low-dose combination therapy consists of the starting dose of a statin plus resin, niacin, or a fibrate given in low doses. Patients will be followed for 5–10 years and all relevant costs and outcomes will be measured. To extrapolate results beyond the study period would require some type of modeling technique.

TABLE 9-2.

Cost and Outcome Variables

Costs	*Outcomes*
Direct costs	
1. Drug costs	
• Statin therapy (acquisition + dispensing + medical management)	1. Non-fatal acute MI 2. Fatal acute MI 3. Angina (includes unstable angina/coronary insufficiency)
• Related medication (acquisition + dispensing + medical management)	4. Sudden coronary death
2. Physician costs	5. Stroke/TIA
• Outpatient visits	6. CHF
• Inpatient care	7. Arrhythmias
• Monitoring	8. Stent
• Lab tests (lipid profiles, blood test)	9. CABG 10. PTCA (angioplasty)
3. Health care professional expenses	11. Heart transplantation
• Pharmacist	12. Pacemaker insertion and replacement
• Dietitian	
• Home health/nursing	
4. Hospital costs	
• Diagnostic procedures	
• Surgery	
• Hospital stay	
• ICU	
• CCU	
• Emergency room	
• Transportation to hospital	
5. Events costs	
• Nonfatal acute MI	
• Fatal acute MI	
• Angina (includes unstable angina/coronary insufficiency)	
• Sudden coronary death	
• Stroke/TIA	
• CHF	
• Arrhythmias	

(*continued*)

TABLE 9-2 *(continued)*

Costs	*Outcomes*
6. Procedure costs • Stent • CABG • PTCA (angioplasty) • Heart transplantation • Pacemaker insertion and replacement	
Indirect costs 1. Decrease in labor production • From morbidity • From mortality 2. Missed work days	

ICU = intensive care unit; CCU = critical care unit; MI = myocardial infarction; TIA = transient ischemic attack; CHF = congestive heart failure; CABG = coronary artery bypass graft; PTCA = percutaneous transluminal coronary angioplasty.

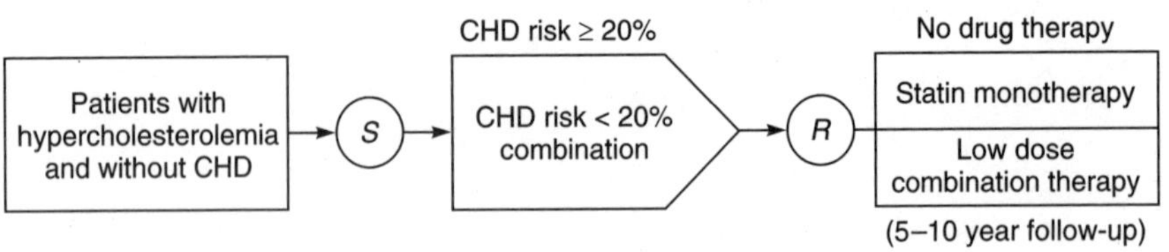

Figure 9-1. Proposed study design. S = stratification of patients; R = randomization of patients.

SUMMARY

The field of cardiovascular pharmacoeconomics relates to an important cause of morbidity, mortality, and impact on the health care delivery system. Although this chapter focused on lipid-lowering studies, the full range of pharmacoeconomic methods may be employed in this category. Differentiating primary versus secondary prevention of coronary heart disease is as important as essential versus primary hypertension as diagnosis.

Although there are numerous examples of pharmacoeconomic studies in the literature for the effect of lipid-lowering agents, researchers and users of this information must remain cautious. Study methods, parameters used or identified, and conclusions must be consistent in order to reach an appropriate evaluation of the study and its conclusion.

Finally, a proposed approach to study primary prevention effects was presented to illustrate ways to overcome common study limitations as well as to provide practical insights into the value of select cardiovascular drug therapies.

REFERENCES

1. American Heart Association: *1999 Heart and Stroke Statistical Update*. Dallas, TX: American Heart Association; 1999.
2. Castelli WP, Anderson KM, Wilson PW, et al.: Lipids and risk of coronary heart disease. The Framingham Study. *Ann Epidemiol* 1992; 2:23–28.
3. Levy D, Wilson WF, Anderson KM, et al.: Stratifying the patient at risk from coronary heart disease: new insights from the Framingham heart study. *Am Heart J* 1990;119:712–717.
4. Weinstein MC, Stason WB: Cost-effectiveness of interventions to prevent or treat coronary heart disease. *Ann Rev Public Health* 1985;6: 41–63.
5. Oster G, Epstein AM: Cost-effectiveness of antihyperlipidemic therapy in the prevention of coronary heart disease: the case of cholestyramine. *JAMA* 1987;258:2381–2387.
6. Kinosian BP, Eisenberg JM: Cutting into cholesterol: cost-effectiveness alternatives for treating hypercholesterolemia. *JAMA* 1988;259: 2249–2254.
7. Schulman KA, Kinosian B, Jacobson TA, et al.: Reducing high blood cholesterol level with drugs: cost-effectiveness of pharmacologic management. *JAMA* 1990;264:3025–3033.
8. Kelley MD: Hypercholesterolemia: the cost of treatment in perspective. *South Med J* 1990;83:142–145.
9. Knopp RH: Drug treatment of lipid disorders. *N Engl J Med* 1999; 498–511.
10. Goldman P, Lee TH, Weinstein MC, et al.: Cost-effectiveness of HMG-CoA reductase inhibition for primary and secondary prevention of coronary heart disease. *JAMA* 1991;265:1145–1151.
11. Hay JW, Wittels EH, Gotto AM: An economic evaluation of lovastatin for cholesterol lowering and coronary artery disease reduction. *Am J Cardiol* 1991;67:789–796.

12. Hamilton VH, Racicot FE, Zowall H, et al.: The cost-effectiveness of HMG-CoA reductase inhibitors to prevent coronary heart disease. *JAMA* 1995;273:1032–1038.
13. Martens LL, Guibert R: Cost-effectiveness analysis of lipid-modifying therapy in Canada: comparison of HMG-CoA reductase inhibitors in the primary prevention of coronary heart disease. *Clin Ther* 1995;16:1052–1062.
14. Johannesson M, Borgquist L, Jonsson L, et al.: The cost-effectiveness of lipid-lowering in Swedish primary health care. *J Intern Med* 1996;240:23–29.
15. Martens LL, Rutten FF, Erkelens DW, Ascoop CA: Clinical benefits and cost-effectiveness of lowering serum cholesterol levels: the case of simvastatin and cholestyramine in the Netherlands. *Am J Cardiol* 1990;65:27F–32F.
16. Huse DM, Russell MW, Miller JD, et al.: Cost-effectiveness of statins. *Am J Cardiol* 1998;82:1357–1363.
17. Shepherd J, Cobbe SM, Ford I, et al.: Prevention of coronary heart disease with pravastatin in men with hypercholesterolemia. *N Engl J Med* 1995;333:1301–1307.
18. Downs JR, Clearfield M, Weis S, et al.: For the AFCAPS/TexCAPS Research Group. Primary prevention of acute coronary events with lovastatin in men and women with average cholesterol levels: results of AFCAPS/TexCAPS. *JAMA* 1998;279:1615–1622.
19. Pharoah PD, Hollingworth W: Cost effectiveness of lowering cholesterol concentration with statins in patients with and without pre-existing coronary heart disease: life table method applied to health authority population. *Br Med J* 1996;312:1443–1448.
20. Caro J, Klittich W, McGuire A, et al.: The West of Scotland coronary prevention study: economic benefit analysis of primary prevention with pravastatin. *Br Med J* 1997;315:1577–1582.
21. Caro J, Klittich W, McGuire A, et al.: International economic analysis of primary prevention of cardiovascular disease with pravastatin in WOSCOPS. *Eur Heart J* 1999;20:263–268.
22. Ashraf T, Hay JW, Pitt B, et al.: Cost-effectiveness of pravastatin in secondary prevention of coronary artery disease. *Am J Cardiol* 1996;78:409–414.
23. Pitt B, Mancini GB, Ellis SG, et al.: Pravastatin limitation of atherosclerosis in the coronary arteries (PLAC I): reduction in atherosclerosis progression and clinical events. PLAC I investigation. *J Am Coll Cardiol* 1995;26:1133–1139.
24. Byington RP, Furberg CD, Crouse JR III, et al.: Pravastatin, lipids, and atherosclerosis in the carotid arteries (PLAC II). *Am J Cardiol* 1995;76:54C–59C.

25. Elliott W, Weir DR: Comparative cost-effectiveness of HMG-CoA reductase inhibitors in secondary prevention of acute myocardial infarction. *Am J Health-Syst Pharm* 1999;56:1726–1732.
26. Scandinavian Simvastatin Survival Study Group. Randomized trial of cholesterol lowering in 4444 patients with coronary heart disease: the Scandinavian Simvastatin Survival Study (4S). *Lancet* 1994;344: 1383–1389.
27. Pederson TR, Kjekshus J, Berg K, et al.: Cholesterol-lowering and the use of health care resources: results of the the Scandinavian Simvastatin Survival Study. *Circulation* 1996;93:1796–1802.
28. Johannesson M, Jonsson B, Kjekshus J, et al.: Cost-effectiveness of simvastatin treatment to lower cholesterol levels in patients with coronary heart disease. *N Engl J Med* 1997;336:332–336.
29. Grover SA, Coupal L, Paquet S, Hanna Z: Cost-effectiveness of 3-hydroxy-3-methylglutaryl-coenzyme A reductase inhibitors in the secondary prevention of cardiovascular disease: forecasting the incremental benefits of preventing coronary and cerebrovascular events. *Arch Intern Med* 1999;159:593–600.
30. Blum CB: Comparison of properties of four inhibitors of 3-hydroxy-3-methylglutaryl-coenzyme A reductase. *Am J Cardiol* 1994;73:3D–11D.
31. Spearman ME, Summers K, Moore V, et al.: Cost-effectiveness of initial therapy with 3-hydroxy-3-methylglutaryl coenzyme A reductase inhibitors to treat hypercholesterolemia in a primary care setting of a managed-care organization. *Clin Ther* 1997;19:582–602.
32. Hay JW, Yu WM, Ashraf T: Pharmacoeconomics of lipid-lowering agents for primary and secondary prevention of coronary artery disease. *Pharmacoeconomics* 1999;15:47–74.
33. Koren MJ, Smith DG, Hunninghake DB, et al.: The cost of reaching National Cholesterol Education Program (NCEP) goals in hypercholesterolemic patients: a comparison of atorvastatin, simvastatin, lovastatin, and fluvastatin. *Pharmacoeconomics* 1998;14:59–70.
34. Hilleman DE, Phillips JO, Mohiuddin SM, et al.: A population-based treat-to-target pharmacoeconomic analysis of HMG-CoA reductase inhibitors in hypercholesterolemia. *Clin Ther* 1999;21:536–562.
35. Ito MK, Shabetai R: Pravastatin alone and in combination with low-dose cholestyramine in patients with primary hypercholesterolemia and coronary heart disease. *Am J Cardiol* 1997;80:799–802.
36. Schrott HG, Stein EA, Dujovne CA: Enhanced low-density lipoprotein cholesterol reduction and cost-effectiveness by low-dose colestipol plus lovastatin combination therapy. *Am J Cardiol* 1995;75:34–39.
37. Szucs TD: Pharmaco-economic aspects of lipid-lowering therapy: is it worth the price? *Eur Heart J* 1998;19(suppl M):M22–M28.

38. Morris S: A comparison of economic modelling and clinical trials in the economic evaluation of cholesterol-modifying pharmacotherapy. *Health Econ* 1997;6:589–601.
39. Schwartz JS: Comparative economic data regarding lipid-lowering drugs. *Am Heart J* 1999;137:S97–S104.
40. Hlatky MA: Role of economic models in randomized controlled trials. *Am Heart J* 1999;137:S41–S46.
41. Jacobson TA, Schein JR, Williamson A, Ballantyne CM: Maximizing the cost-effectiveness of lipid-lowering therapy. *Arch Intern Med* 1998; 158:1977–1989.

C H A P T E R

10

Application of Pharmacoeconomics: Respiratory Diseases

Gireesh V. Gupchup,
E. Paul Larrat
and
Patricia Marshik

INTRODUCTION

The high human and economic costs of certain respiratory diseases present a unique opportunity for pharmacoeconomic evaluation and intervention. In 1992, International Classification of Diseases, 9th Revision, Clinical Modification (ICD-9-CM) codes related to chronic obstructive pulmonary disease (COPD) and pneumonia were ranked 4th and 6th as causes of death in the United States. The age-adjusted death rate for COPD and pneumonia increased by 36.3% and 13.4%, respectively, for the period 1979–1992.[1] Asthma prevalence and mortality has continued to increase in the 1990s despite dramatic advances in the diagnosis and treatment of the disease.[2] Morbidity and mortality associated with lung cancer is significant in that it is the leading cancer killer of both men and women.[3] The high economic burden of respiratory disease is a function of its high prevalence in our society, the chronic nature of these ailments, and the need for expensive hospitalization when therapeutic failure occurs.

Health providers and managers view respiratory disease as a ripe area for pharmacoeconomic evaluation for several reasons. First, and most obvious, is that the high cost and prevalence of the disease invites economic scrutiny. Secondly, ambulatory pharmaceutical therapy for many of these respiratory ailments has long been viewed as a cost-effective alternative to hospitalization. For example, proper adherence to a well-designed asthma treatment protocol has been shown to decrease hospitalization admissions and costs.[4,5] The nature of the relationship between pharmaceutical expenditures and savings in other medical areas makes cost-effectiveness analysis (CEA) and cost-benefit analysis (CBA) important decision-making tools. Thirdly, many managed care organizations view asthma and COPD as excellent candidates for the development of disease state management programs which integrate pharmaceutical care into the overall patient management strategy. The economic evaluation of the impact of these programs on economic, humanistic, and clinical outcomes is important. Finally, research indicates that successful therapeutic response is highly correlated with strict adherence to the patient's drug regimen. Improper administration of therapeutic agents, missed doses, and poor timing of doses generally result in worse health-related and economic outcomes. The use of pharmacoeconomic techniques to evaluate different adherence strategies, patient education programs, and long-term effectiveness of interventions has become increasingly important to providers and administrators. Difficulties in measuring outcomes in respiratory disease make these analyses challenging.[4,5]

CLINICAL CHARACTERISTICS OF RESPIRATORY DISEASES

Diseases of the respiratory system are diverse epidemiologically and pathologically. A discussion of these differences is important to the conceptualization and development of pharmacoeconomic strategies. We limit our discussion of pharmacoeconomic applications in this area to the respiratory diseases that lend themselves well to this type of analysis. These disease states include, airway diseases (including emphysema, chronic bronchitis, and asthma) and infectious diseases of the respiratory system (primarily pneumonias and influenza).

Airway Diseases

COPD and asthma are the two major airway diseases most amenable to pharmacoeconomic evaluation. Researchers and practitioners often consider asthma a chronic obstructive pulmonary disease. We will consider asthma separately from other obstructive processes due to its unique etiology and treatment strategies.

COPD is characterized by a limitation in airflow caused by bronchitis, bronchospasm, or emphysema. These disorders are generally chronic in nature[6] and have been estimated to afflict over 15 million Americans. Economic costs of COPD, including both direct and indirect medical expenses, has been estimated at about $12 billion/ year.[6] In the United States, 2.6% of annual deaths are attributed to the disease.[7] Smoking, in both its active and passive form, is the major risk factor for these respiratory illnesses. Approximately 80–90% of the risk of developing COPD is related to tobacco smoke.[8,9] There is a higher prevalence of COPD in men, even after controlling for smoking. White race and lower socioeconomic status are both risk factors for higher mortality. Air pollution, $alpha_1$-antitrypsin deficiency, and various occupational factors also contribute to the development of COPD.[3]

COPD is treated both pharmacologically and through other means. Mainstays of therapy include ipratropium as a first-line agent and inhaled beta-agonists as add-on therapeutic agents. Theophylline and /or corticosteroids may be added to treat severe COPD. Supplemental oxygen is reserved for the most severely ill.[7,10–12] Intervention by primary care providers, health management organizations, and health educators can be extremely important in controlling the human, clinical, and economic costs.[7,11] Proper management of the treatment algorithm, compliance improvement, and appropriate resource utilization can be instrumental in preventing complications of the illness and ameliorating the severe symptoms of COPD.[13] Figure 10-1 summarizes a common algorithm for the treatment of COPD.

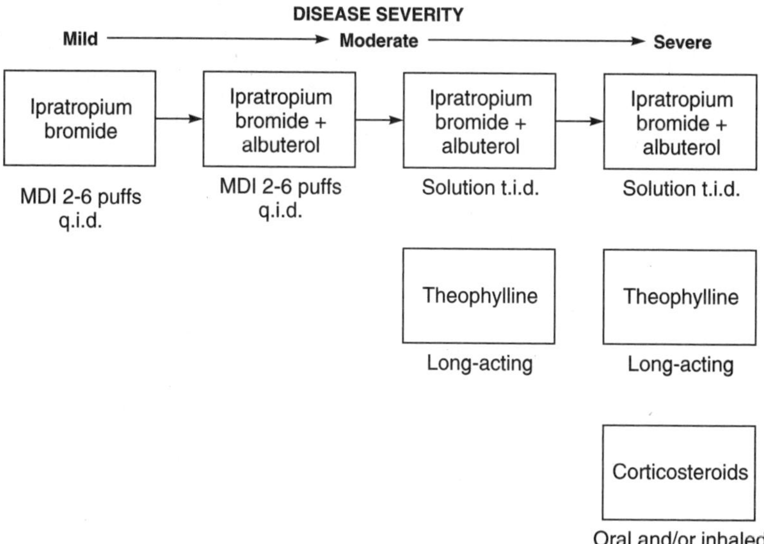

Figure 10-1. Treatment algorithm for COPD based upon disease severity. (Adapted from Friedman.[12])

While COPD is a relatively new public health problem, tracing its roots back to the introduction of tobacco in Europe in the late 1400s and the Industrial Revolution of the 1800s, asthma was recognized by Hippocrates over 2000 years ago.[6] A common characteristic of asthma is the narrowing of the airways in response to a negative stimulus.[10] The prevalence of asthma in children was over 6% in the United States in 1994, an increase from 3% in 1980.[2] Among children, boys are at 2× greater risk of having asthma than girls. Adult males and females are at similar risk of asthma.[14] Elevated levels of total serum immunoglobulin E (IgE), hyperresponsiveness, exposure to passive tobacco smoke, genetics, and diet are frequently cited as risk factors for the development of asthma.[1,2,6]

Therapeutic treatment for asthma can be dichotomized into agents that relieve symptoms of the disease and those that assist in preventing asthma attacks from occurring. Beta-agonists, ipratropium, and oral steroids are key agents for the treatment of an acute exacerbation of symptoms, while inhaled corticosteroids, leukotriene modifiers, salmeterol and other long-acting beta-agonists, theophylline, nedocromil, and cromolyn are useful in controlling asthma symptoms.[15] Undertreatment, poor compliance with a prescribed medication regimen, and/or inappropriate therapy are the major contributors to asthma morbidity and mortality.

The economic and human ramifications of therapeutic failure are very high. Asthma is the third leading cause of preventable hospital admissions in the country.[16] In the United States, the mean annual cost of asthma is estimated to be greater than $1000 per patient.[17] Smith et al. noted that 80% of asthma treatment resources were devoted to 20% of asthma patients, which they termed "high cost patients." These individuals cost approximately $2584 per year on average to treat, while the remaining asthma patients costs averaged $140 per patient per year. Total estimated costs in the United States in 1996 dollars were $5.8 billion, of which $5.1 billion were direct costs.[18] Many major medical providers recognize the opportunity to decrease the negative outcomes of asthma by offering comprehensive disease state management programs, case management, and patient education programs.[19,20] Figures 10-2 and 10-3 present a summary of treatment options for asthma patients.

Infectious Diseases

Respiratory infections acquired in the community or hospital have been major public health problems since recorded time began. A primary care physician treats most community acquired pneumonias (CAP) in an ambulatory setting. One major goal of treatment is to resolve the infection quickly to avoid hospitalization and prolonged patient disability. Incidence rates for CAP range from 4.7 to 11.6 per 1000 people per year. Of these individuals, 22–51% are hospitalized.[21,22] Age, institutionalization, poor nutrition, alcoholism, and

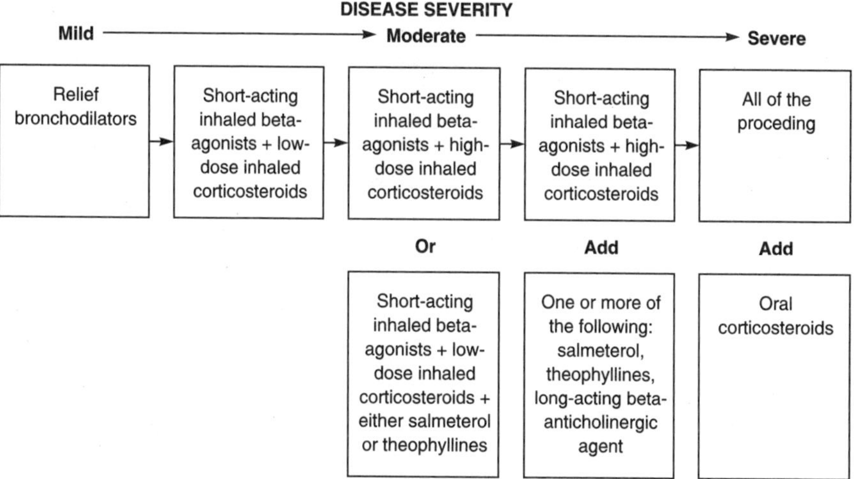

Figure 10-2. Step treatment algorithm for asthma based upon disease severity. (From British Thoracic Society.[15])

smoking are the key risk factors for pneumonia. These infections may be of bacterial, viral, or fungal origin with *Streptococcus pneumoniae* being the most commonly cultured pathogen. In at least half of the cases, the responsible organism cannot be accurately identified.[6] Unlike other respiratory disorders, these infections are usually considered to be acute rather than chronic disease processes.

Immediate treatment of bacterial CAP with an antibiotic is important for an early resolution of the illness and for limiting negative clinical and economic outcomes. This treatment should start before microbiologic results are available.[6] Treatment costs with antibiotics vary widely and have led many health providers and managers to make therapeutic decisions based upon the per unit or per therapy cost of the antibiotic agent. Often, the savings incurred by rapid resolution of the illness outweigh savings gained through the use of low cost per unit antibiotics. Appropriate CEA and CBA are of particular importance in developing treatment strategies and evaluating current treatment practices.

The rapid increase in the incidence of HIV infection has brought with it a commensurate increase in the incidence of viral and fungal respiratory infections in the immunocompromised host.[23] Influenza A and B are responsible for at least half of the viral pneumonias that infect these individuals. Pharmacologic therapy is relatively expensive, while effectiveness in patient populations is quite variable. The pharmaceutical industry is devoting ever-increasing resources to antiviral research and it is anticipated that more innovative, effective, and costly agents will be marketed in the near future.

Estimated Comparative Daily Dosages for Inhaled Steroids:

Adults

Inhaled Steroid	Low Dose	Medium Dose	High Dose
Beclomethasone dipropionate 42 mcg/puff 84 mcg/puff	168-504 mcg **4-12 puffs—42 mcg** **2-6 puffs—84 mcg**	504-840 mcg **12-20 puffs—42 mcg** **6-10 puffs—84 mcg**	>840 mcg **>20 puffs—42 mcg** **>10 puffs—84 mcg**
Budesonide DPI 200 mcg/dose	200-400 mcg **1-2 inhalations**	400-600 mcg **2-3 inhalations**	>600 mcg **>3 inhalations**
Flunisolide 250 mcg/puff	500-1,000 mcg **2-4 puffs**	1,000-2,000 mcg **4-8 puffs**	>2,000 mcg **>8 puffs**
Fluticasone **MDI:** 44, 110, 220 mcg/puff	88-264 mcg **2-6 puffs—44 mcg** or **2 puffs—110 mcg**	264-660 mcg **2-6 puffs—110 mcg**	>660 mcg **>6 puffs—110 mcg** or **>3 puffs—220 mcg**
DPI: 50, 100, 250 mcg/dose	**2-6 inhalations—50 mcg**	**3-6 inhalations—100 mcg**	**>6 inhalations—100 mcg** or **>2 inhalations—250 mcg**
Triamcinolone acetonide 100 mcg/puff	400-1,000 mcg **4-10 puffs**	1,000-2,000 mcg **10-20 puffs**	>2,000 mcg **>20 puffs**

Children ≤ 12 years

Inhaled Steroid	Low Dose	Medium Dose	High Dose
Beclomethasone dipropionate 42 mcg/puff 84 mcg/puff	84-336 mcg **2-8 puffs—42 mcg** **1-4 puffs—84 mcg**	336-672 mcg **8-16 puffs—42 mcg** **4-8 puffs—84 mcg**	>672 mcg **>16 puffs—42 mcg** **>8 puffs—84 mcg**
Budesonide DPI 200 mcg/dose	100-200 mcg	200-400 mcg **1-2 inhalations—200 mcg**	>400 mcg **>2 inhalations—200 mcg**
Flunisolide 250 mcg/puff	500-750 mcg **2-3 puffs**	1,000-1,250 mcg **4-5 puffs**	>1,250 mcg **>5 puffs**
Fluticasone **MDI:** 44, 110, 220 mcg/puff	88-176 mcg **2-4 puffs—44 mcg**	176-440 mcg **4-10 puffs—44 mcg** or **2-4 puffs—110 mcg**	>440 mcg **>4 puffs—110 mcg** or **>2 puffs—220 mcg**
DPI: 50, 100, 250 mcg/dose	**2-4 inhalations—50 mcg**	**2-4 inhalations—100 mcg**	**>4 inhalations—100 mcg** or **>2 inhalations—250 mcg**
Triamcinolone acetonide 100 mcg/puff	400-800 mcg **4-8 puffs**	800-1,200 mcg **8-12 puffs**	>1,200 mcg **>12 puffs**

- *Clinician judgment of patient response is essential to appropriate dosing.* Once asthma is controlled, medication doses should be carefully titrated to the minimum dose required to maintain control, thus reducing the potential for adverse effect.
- Data from *in vitro* and clinical trials suggest that different inhaled corticosteroid preparations are not equivalent on a per puff or microgram basis. However, few data directly compare the preparations. *The Expert Panel developed recommended dose ranges for different preparations based on available data.*
- Inhaled corticosteroid safety data suggest dose ranges for children equivalent to beclomethasone dipropionate 200-400 mcg/day (low dose), 400-800 mcg/day (medium dose), and >800 mcg/day (high dose).

For more information on managing asthma, see the *Practical Guide for the Diagnosis and Management of Asthma*, National Institutes of Health, pub no 97-4053, Bethesda, MD, 1997.

Figure 10-3. NEAPP stepwise approach to managing asthma long term for adults and children more than 5 years of age.[38]

Stepwise Approach to Managing Asthma Long Term for

Adults and Children More Than 5 Years of Age

Goals of therapy

- Minimal or no chronic symptoms day or night
- Minimal or no episodes
- No limitations on activities; no school/work missed
- PEF ≥ 80% of personal best
- Minimal use of inhaled short-acting beta$_2$- agonist (<1 per day)
- No or minimal adverse effects from medications

Clinical Features Before Treatment to Classify Severity

	Days With Symptoms	Nights With Symptoms	PEF or FEV$_1$ / PEF variability	Long Term Control—Daily Medications
Step 4 Severe Persistent	Continual	Frequent	≤60% / >30%	**Inhaled steroid—high dose*** plus **Long-acting inhaled beta$_2$-agonist**—adult 2 puffs (child 1-2 puffs) q 12 hours, sustained-release theophylline, or oral long-acting beta$_2$-agonists plus **Steroid tablets or syrup long term**; make repeated attempts to reduce oral steroids.
Step 3 Moderate Persistent	Daily	≥5/month	>60%-<80% / >30%	**Inhaled steroid—medium dose*** or **Inhaled steroid—low-to-medium dose*** plus **long-acting inhaled beta$_2$-agonist**—adult 2 puffs (child 1-2 puffs) q 12 hours, sustained-release theophylline or oral long-acting beta$_2$-agonists **If needed**, increase medications up to: Inhaled steroid—high dose plus long-acting inhaled beta$_2$-agonist, sustained-release theophylline, or oral long-acting beta$_2$-agonists
Step 2 Mild Persistent	3-6/week	3-4/month	≥80% / 20-30%	**Inhaled steroid—low dose*** or **Cromolyn**—adult 2-4 puffs (child 1-2 puffs) tid-qid, or 1 ampule by nebulizer tid-qid, or **Nedocromil**—adult 2-4 puffs (child 1-2 puffs) bid-qid Sustained-release theophylline to serum concentration 5-15 mcg/mL is an alternative, but not preferred, therapy. Zafirlukast or zileuton may also be considered for patients ≥12 years of age, although their position in therapy is not fully established.
Step 1 Mild Intermittent	≤2/week	≤2/month	≥80% / <20%	**No daily medications**

All Patients **2-4 puffs of short-acting inhaled beta$_2$-agonist for exacerbations.** Up to three treatments at 20-minute intervals or single nebulizer treatment, as needed. Course of oral steroids may be needed.

Starting Point
Gain control as quickly as possible. Either start with aggressive therapy (e.g., *add* a course of oral steroids or a higher dose of inhaled steroids to the therapy that corresponds to the patient's initial step of severity); or start at the step that corresponds to the patient's initial severity and step up treatment, if necessary.

Step Down
Review treatment every 1 to 6 months. If control is sustained for at least 3 months, a gradual stepwise reduction in treatment may be possible.

Step Up
If control is not maintained, consider step up. Inadequate control is indicated by increased use of short-acting beta$_2$-agonists and in: step 1 when patient uses a short-acting beta$_2$-agonist more than two times a week; steps 2 and 3 when patient uses short-acting beta$_2$-agonist on a daily basis OR more than three to four times in 1 day. But before stepping up: Review patient inhaler technique, compliance, and environmental control (avoidance of allergens or other precipitant factors). A course of oral steroids may be needed at any time and at any step.

Exercise-Induced Bronchospasm
Patients with exercise-induced bronchospasm should take two to four puffs of an inhaled beta$_2$-agonist 5 to 60 minutes before exercise.

Referral
Referral to an asthma specialist for consultation or co-management is *recommended* if there is difficulty maintaining control or if the patient requires step 4 care. Referral may be *considered* for step 3 care.

Notes on classifying severity:

- Patients should be assigned to the most severe step in which *any* feature occurs.
- Patients at any level of severity can have mild, moderate, or severe exacerbations.
- Two or more asthma exacerbations per week (i.e., progressively worsening symptoms that may last hours or days) indicates moderate-to-severe persistent asthma.

Patient Education/Environmental Control—Help patients identify and control precipitants of asthma episodes. Provide education on self-management.

* Use spacer/holding chamber and mouth rinsing after inhalation.

The stepwise approach presents general guidelines to assist clinical decision making. Asthma is highly variable; clinicians should tailor specific medication plans to the needs of individual patients.

U.S. DEPARTMENT OF HEALTH AND HUMAN SERVICES
Public Health Service • National Institutes of Health • National Heart, Lung, and Blood Institute NIH Publication No. 99-4055A June 1999

Figure 10-3 (*continued*)

Opportunistic lung infections associated with the HIV syndrome are of particular interest in the United States and the rest of the world. In addition to bacterial and viral (notably cytomegalovirus and herpes virus) infections, these individuals are susceptible to *Pneumocystis carinii* infection. This fungal pathogen infects over 4% of HIV-infected patients annually. The economic and humanistic costs of the infection are significant when applied to the 31 million HIV infected individuals worldwide.[24] In these patients, respiratory infections are treated as chronic conditions.[25] Multidrug regimens including trimethoprim/sulfamethoxazole, pentamidine, and corticosteroids are common, with frequent relapse characteristics of the course of the disease.[6,26] Drug interactions between these agents and the multidrug antiviral regimens consumed by an HIV-infected individual are common and may have an effect on the cost-effectiveness of the patient's therapy. These individuals are also subject to an increased likelihood of adverse reactions to these agents.[27]

Rhinitis and sinusitis are common ailments among both children and adults. These syndromes may be of either infectious or allergic origin, although it may be difficult to make the distinction between the two. Infectious sinusitis is often present as a component of the common cold. Bed rest, hydration, antihistamines, analgesics, and broad-spectrum antibiotics are often prescribed for this self-limiting condition. The chronic presence of infectious sinusitis may be treated surgically or through sustained antibiotic therapy.[6]

Allergic rhinitis afflicts 10–16% of the population. Dust mites, pollen, mold spores, animal dander, and other allergens are often responsible for triggering this condition in susceptible individuals.[28] Medical treatment involves allergen avoidance, immunotherapy to desensitize the patient, and pharmacologic therapy to suppress the allergic response. Topical corticosteroids, such as beclomethasone nasal spray, are often prescribed. Antihistamines, particularly nonsedating H_1-specific histamine receptor antagonists, are useful in alleviating the rhinorrhea, sneezing, and itching common to this type of allergic reaction.[28,29]

Preventive measures, notably vaccination, contribute significantly to lowering the incidence of many of the respiratory infections or to diminishing the severity of the course of the infection. Economic and clinical evaluation of treatment regimens is essential due to the rapid pace of the introduction of new anti-infective agents, particularly antivirals. Pharmacoeconomic evaluation is again an important tool for providing cost-effective treatment for these relatively common diseases.

Neoplastic Disease

Malignant tumors involving the respiratory system are the most common cause of cancer mortality in the United States and other developed countries. Lung cancer has long been the major cancer killer of men, and just recently assumed that distinction in women. The mortality rate in 1992 was approximately 70/100,000 and 30/100,000 for American men and women, respectively. This disease is of particular concern for researchers and practitioners due to its lethal nature. The 5-year survival rate is only 13%.[30] Tobacco smoke is the most significant risk factor for lung cancer. Approximately 85% of lung cancers occur in smokers or former smokers, while those exposed to second-hand smoke are at 1.2 to 2.0 times greater risk of the disease than those not exposed to this factor.[31] Air pollution, ionizing radiation (i.e., radon), genetic predisposition, and asbestos have also been shown to be risk factors for lung cancer. Interestingly, COPD has also been linked to a higher risk of developing this type of cancer.[32]

Lung cancer is primarily catagorized into two subgroups; small-cell carcinoma and nonsmall-cell carcinoma. These two types account for over 95% of observed cancers. The lethal nature of lung cancer is due primarily to its ability to metastasize to other organs, primarily the liver, adrenal glands, bone, and nervous system. Treatment for pulmonary tumors caught in earlier stages consists of surgery and/or radiation and chemotherapy. The clinical success of these options is still limited, while the economic and humanistic costs for treatment and hospitalization are quite high.[6]

Pharmaceutical treatment typically involves cycles of highly active oncology agents that pose a significant risk of adverse drug reactions and drug interactions. Older agents include cyclophosphamide, doxorubicin, and vincristine (CAV chemotherapy). Newer alternatives include cisplatin, etoposide, and paclitaxel. Later stages of both small-cell and nonsmall-cell cancers are difficult to treat successfully. For example, aggressive use of chemotherapeutic agents in stage 4 nonsmall-cell carcinoma of the lung add, on average, only 3–9 months of survival.[6] This area of respiratory disease is particularly well-suited for pharmacoeconomic analysis of treatment options and measurement of clinical and economic outcomes.

THE INPUT COSTS OF RESPIRATORY DISEASES

Pharmacoeconomic analyses can be used to track the costs and consequences of disease management programs. Essentially, costs of a disease management program refer to the resources consumed in the production of the program. This section describes the different categories of costs associated with an asthma disease management program. Costing schemes for specific resources are suggested. An asthma disease management program has been chosen as an example since these types of programs are the most common among respiratory disease management programs. The concepts addressed in the asthma disease management example below could be applied to any other respiratory disease.

Identification of the Target Population

It is well known that the most severe asthma patients consume the greatest resources.[33] In one asthma population, 5% of the patients accounted for about 46% of the total resources consumed.[34] Therefore, it would make sense in an asthma disease management program to concentrate on the most severe patients. The first task would be to identify the patients that need to be included in the disease management program.

Since most health systems have databases that include ICD-9-CM diagnoses codes, all asthma patients in the health system could be identified (ICD-9-CM 493.00).[35] The next step is to identify the most severe patients. From a health system perspective, patients consuming the greatest resources should be targeted. The major cost drivers among asthmatics are hospitalizations and emergency department visits.[33,34] Though drug therapy costs and scheduled physician office visits do contribute to the resources consumed by asthma patients, these components are not as costly as hospitalizations and emergency department visits. In fact, there is evidence that patients who have higher drug therapy and physician visit costs, have lower hospitalization and emergency department visit costs.[34] Therefore, patients with the highest number of hospitalizations and emergency department visits should be identified as the target population for an asthma disease management program.

Identification of Treatment Pathways

An important step in the disease management process is the establishment of treatment pathways. These pathways are clinical algorithms that are used by health care providers as step-wise guides in the treatment of patients. A treatment pathway can be developed from an existing pathway being used at another institution. For example, the University Health System Consortium (UHC) maintains information on clinical pathways that are voluntarily reported to the UHC by its members.[36] Additionally, some organizations have also developed their own asthma disease management programs.[34,37] Regardless of the source of the clinical pathway, it must always be modified for the institution in which it will be used.

Another option is to develop one's own disease management program from available literature and organization data. The UHC has provided guidelines in the development of disease management programs that can be useful in this process.[36] It is important to note that all asthma disease management programs are based on the National Asthma Education and Prevention Program Expert Panel Report II: Guidelines for the diagnosis and management of asthma (NAEPP).[38]

Identification of Disease State Management Program Costs

There are four basic types of costs involved with a disease: direct medical costs, direct non-medical costs, indirect costs, and intangible costs.[39] Direct medical costs are the costs incurred in the production and delivery of medical care, such as physician services, hospitalizations, and pharmaceutical therapy. Direct non-medical costs are costs necessary to enable patients to receive medical care, such as transportation to and from the site of medical care. Indirect costs are a measure of the patient's lost productivity. They are also a measure of the lost productivity of unpaid caregivers. Loss of productivity here refers to the inability to work. Intangible costs are the difficult to quantify costs of pain and suffering.

Review of the costs associated with an asthma disease management program

Prior to costing the different components for a disease management program it is important to consider the perspective from which the costing is being done.[39] For example, if the costs of an asthma disease management program are being calculated from the perspective of a particular institution, only direct medical costs will be included. Direct non-medical costs and indirect costs are not costs that the institution will incur, and consequently are not important from the institution's perspective. On the other hand, if a self-insured organization is costing an asthma disease management program, direct non-medical and indirect costs would be relevant costs to consider if an expenditure is incurred for these components.

After the perspective from which the costing will be done is determined, the ingredients of each type of cost need to be considered. Examples of the ingredients of each type of cost that might be considered in an asthma disease management program are discussed below.

Examples of direct medical costs for an asthma disease management program

Types of direct medical costs that are important to asthma disease management programs are presented in Table 10-1.[34,40] These direct medical costs are discussed briefly below.

Any physician services, hospitalizations, or emergency department visits that may arise after the asthma disease management program is implemented will consume resources and therefore be a cost of the program. With regard to physician education, it is extremely important that the clinical leadership at an institution supports the disease management program it is backing. Also, physicians need to be educated about the asthma treatment pathways that need to be followed. Communication with physicians is the key in this process. Costs

TABLE 10-1.

Examples of Direct Medical Costs in Asthma Disease Management Programs
Physician services
Hospital services
Emergency department visits
Physician education
Patient education and empowerment
Alternative health providers
Drug costs
Pharmaceutical care
Data acquisition and analysis

associated with physician buy-in and education should be considered direct medical costs since they are integral to the production of an asthma disease management program.[34,40]

Along with physician education, patient education is also a vital component in the disease management process.[40] Making educational materials available to patients has been shown to improve asthma self-management and compliance with therapeutic recommendations.[34] Any costs of patient education are treated as direct medical costs.

Often, asthma disease management programs will involve alternative health care providers such as nurse educators or case managers.[40] The costs of educating these practitioners, as well as the cost of their services are direct medical costs. Pharmacy-related costs, such as costs of drugs and costs of pharmaceutical care, would also be considered direct medical costs. Pharmaceutical care costs are important since they can potentially lead to better compliance with a therapeutic regimen, eventually leading to more appropriate use of drugs.

Finally, data about how practitioners are adhering to treatment pathways and therapeutic outcomes being achieved in the asthma disease management program need to be monitored. These data can be then used in further improvement of treatment pathways.[40] Maintaining a database and analyzing the results is an expensive proposition. However, since this an integral part of a disease management program, and helps in the production and continual upgrading of treatment pathways, it is considered a direct medical cost.

Direct non-medical, indirect, and intangible costs

Direct non-medical costs would include the costs such as those incurred by patients in traveling to the clinic to receive care for either scheduled visits or unscheduled visits for asthma exacerbations. Indirect costs would include costs of lost productivity. In other words, if an individual is required to miss work due to their asthma, this would be an indirect cost. The methods used to place a value on indirect costs are beyond the scope of this chapter. Readers are referred to the work of Luce and Elixhauser for a discussion on this topic.[41] Intangible costs are the costs of pain and suffering. Essentially, decrease in health-related quality of life (HRQOL) due to asthma will account for these costs.

As mentioned earlier, direct non-medical costs and indirect costs may not be important from the perspective of an institution or a managed care organization. However, these are important costs to self-insured organizations or from the perspective of society. Intangible costs are very difficult to quantify in monetary terms and are therefore generally omitted from pharmacoeconomic analyses.

Adjusting for the time value of money and uncertainty of costs

Once all the costs of the asthma disease management have been listed, it has to be determined whether the costs will be incurred over a single year, or over several years. If costs will be realized over several years, the costs of future years have to be discounted to reflect their current value. This is done since the current value of a dollar is more than what it will be worth in the future. This concept is called the "time value of money." Generally, discount rates of 5, 7, or 10% are used to adjust the value of future costs to present value. A detailed description of how multi-year cost streams are discounted to present value is presented by Larson.[42]

All cost estimates have some degree of uncertainty associated with them. Sensitivity analysis is conducted by varying cost estimates to cover a logical range of values. This process helps guard against some of the uncertainty in cost estimates. It is always advisable to perform sensitivity analysis for costing in any disease management program.[42]

Summary of Monitoring the Input Costs of Respiratory Disease Management Programs

1. Identify the population to be targeted with a disease management program.
2. Identify treatment pathways to be implemented in the disease management program.
3. List the resources that will be consumed by the disease management programs.
4. Classify the resources listed as direct medical costs, direct non-medical costs, indirect costs, and intangible costs.
5. Assign a dollar value to costs, taking into consideration the present value of a future stream of costs.
6. Identify a logical range for all cost estimates to guard against the uncertainty of the estimates.

CLINICAL OUTCOMES ASSOCIATED WITH TREATING RESPIRATORY DISEASES

The clinical outcomes of respiratory disease are commonly measured through a series of respiratory efficiency tests. The primary goal of these tests is to provide some quantification of the oxygen extraction ability of the respiratory system. These endpoints can be either intermediate or final endpoints. General measures used to assess a wide variety of respiratory diseases include forced expiratory volume in 1 second (FEV_1), airflow volume curves, single breath nitrogen washout (SBN2), and symptom limited oxygen consumption (SLVO2).[43–48]

Since the respiratory system and the cardiovascular system are highly integrated, many measures of cardiovascular functioning can also be used to assess the health of the respiratory system. For example, endurance tests, heart rate changes, and blood pressure changes can be applied to the clinical assessment of respiratory disease (Table 10-2).

Clinical outcomes that provide a more direct measure of the effect of a disease process on the patient include a quantification of symptom days, number of attacks over a defined time period, and episode-free days. These measures are especially useful to the health care provider treating the patient with emphysema, asthma, or rhinitis. These types of clinical measures can be used to approximate some of the more time-intensive HRQOL measures discussed later in this chapter. The accuracy of this approach is greatly dependent on the memory and/or record-keeping skills of the patient. The integration of these more subjective measures with pulmonary function tests is a useful strategy for assessing the extent and impact of these chronic respiratory ailments.

Lung cancer clinical assessment involves an additional set of measures that attempt to quantify the extent of disease progression. This often involves tumor biopsy and CT scans for tumor measurement, pathological tumor grading, disease staging, and response assessment. The lethal nature of lung cancer makes measurement of mortality rates particularly important. Clinical comparison of different treatment protocols typically incorporates both measures of morbidity (staging and grading) and mortality (mortality rate).

Pneumocystis carinii pneumonia (PCP), commonly found in immunocompromised patients, has been evaluated on the basis of the duration of anti-PCP therapy and the occurrence of drug toxicity or therapy failure.[49]

Finally, the measurement of adverse drug events among those being treated for both chronic and acute respiratory disease is important. The nature of therapy for these illnesses is such that misuse, under or over utilization, and/or misprescribing can have a significant impact on the outcomes of treatment. Most medications utilized in respiratory disease treatment can have important systemic effects that can greatly alter the cardiovascular and endocrine systems. Drugs such as the oral and inhaled corticosteroids, theophylline derivatives,

TABLE 10-2.

Commonly Utilized Clinical Outcome Measures for Patients with Respiratory Diseases

Clinical outcome measures	*Most pertinent disease(s)*
Forced expiratory volume in 1 second (FEV_1)	A,C
Histamine-induced airway responsiveness test	A,C
Frequency of symptoms (e.g., attacks/month)	A,C,R
Days of symptoms (e.g., days of symptoms/year)	A,C,R
Spirometry test	A,C
Airflow volume curves	A,C
Body plethysmography	A,C
Single breath nitrogen washout (SBN2)	A,C
Symptom limited oxygen consumption (SLVO2)	A,C
12-minute distance walk (12MW)	A,C
Occurrence of dyspnea	A,C
Minute ventilation (MV)	A,C
Endurance	A,C
Heart rate change	A,C
Blood pressure change	A,C
Inspiratory muscle work tolerance (IMWT)	A,C
Episode-free days (e.g., EFD/month)	A,C,R
Restricted activity days (e.g., RAD/month)	A,C,R
Mortality rate	Ca
Initial arterial O_2 tension (PAO_2)	A,C
Duration of anti-PCP therapy	I
Diagnosis confirmation	A,C,Ca,I,R
Extent of disease	A,C,Ca,I,R
Change in smoking habits	A,C,Ca

A, asthma; C, COPD; I, pneumonia/infection; Ca, cancer; R, rhinitis.

and chemotherapeutic agents are of particular concern for the clinician and researcher. Complicating this situation is the high occurrences of multidrug treatment protocols for the majority of respiratory illnesses.

ECONOMIC OUTCOMES ASSOCIATED WITH TREATING RESPIRATORY DISEASES

The measurement of the economic effects of respiratory disease is a particularly complex task. A complete model for economic outcomes would include the direct costs of a particular therapy, costs of related medical treatment, and economic costs to the patient and employee. Since the proper use of pharmaceuticals can have a significant influence on the economic outcomes associated with respiratory disease, the incorporation of a diverse set of measures can be important.

The perspective of the study mandates the type of economic outcome measures to use. A capitated pharmacy benefit manager or managed care organization would be most concerned with the cost of pharmaceuticals, while a provider responsible for a patient's total cost of care would want to quantify the downstream medical costs. Of particular importance for the chronic respiratory diseases is the cost of emergency room treatment (i.e., asthma), home respiratory treatment (i.e., COPD), and total outpatient costs. A well-designed economic assessment will measure medical cost savings that accrue to a particular outpatient treatment strategy through the avoidance of these medical expenditures (Table 10-3).[4,45,50]

TABLE 10-3.

Commonly Utilized Economic Outcome Measures for Patients with Respiratory Diseases

Economic outcome measures	*Most pertinent disease(s)*
School absenteeism	A,I,R
Work absenteeism	A,C,Ca,I,R
Change in work productivity	A,C,Ca,I,R
Outpatient treatment costs	A,C,R
Inpatient treatment costs	A,C,Ca,I,R
Emergency room visits	A,C
Hospital admissions	A,C,Ca,I,R
Home respiratory therapy expenditures	C
Hospice expenditures	Ca
Physician visits	A,C,Ca,I,R
Total cost of care	A,C,Ca,I,R
Travel expenses	A,C,Ca,I,R
Intensive care unit admissions	A,C,Ca

A, asthma; C, COPD; I, pneumonia/infection; Ca, cancer; R, rhinitis.

Economic expenditures related to treating lung cancer, PCP, and community-acquired pneumonias (CAP) are typically inpatient in nature. The economic impact of efforts to provide care for these patients in the home setting must also be considered.[49] Hospice costs are of particular concern when assessing lung cancer treatments.

The high prevalence of asthma, coupled with the acute debilitating exacerbations characteristics of this disease process, makes it a particularly expensive disease to treat from a patient's perspective. Changes in work productivity (i.e., work and school absenteeism rates) should be measured and quantified in a well-designed economic assessment. Related travel and out-of-pocket prescription costs are also important considerations.

HRQOL OUTCOMES ASSOCIATED WITH TREATING RESPIRATORY DISEASE

In addition to monitoring economic outcomes of health care products and services, documentation of HRQOL information is rapidly gaining importance.[51,52] HRQOL has been classified as a humanistic outcome since instruments used to measure this concept examine patients' perspectives about how a health care product or service has affected their lives. Measurement of HRQOL is especially important in patients with chronic diseases. Since chronic diseases cannot be cured, it is important that patients' experience improvements in quality of life as a result of the health care that they receive. Many respiratory diseases are chronic in nature, thus justifying the need to monitor HRQOL as an outcome in these patients.

While selecting a specific instrument to measure HRQOL outcomes, four concepts need to be understood and considered: (1) differences between generic and disease-specific HRQOL instruments; (2) the purpose for which an HRQOL instrument was constructed; (3) evidence for the validity, reliability, responsiveness, and acceptability for use of an HRQOL instrument; and (4) cultural or language adaptation of HRQOL instruments.

Generic Versus Disease-Specific HRQOL Instruments

The first concept that needs to be understood and considered is the issue of whether one requires a generic or disease-specific HRQOL instrument. Generic HRQOL instruments are used to measure overall health and well-being in patients without regard to a specific disease. Questions specific to a particular disease are not included in generic HRQOL instruments. On the other hand, disease-specific instruments comprise questions that are specific to a particular

TABLE 10-4.

Commonly Utilized Health-Related Quality of Life Measures for Patients with Respiratory Diseases

Disease/instrument	*Domains*	*Number of items*
Asthma		
Asthma Quality of Life Questionnaire—Juniper (AQLQ-J)	Activity limitations; symptoms; exposure to environmental stimuli; emotional function	32
Asthma Quality of Life Questionnaire—Marks (AQLQ-M)	Breathlessness; social factors; mood; concerns	20
Living with Asthma Questionnaire (LWAQ)	Social factors and leisure; sports; holidays; sleep; work and other activities; colds; mobility; effects on others; medication use; sex; dysphoric states and attitudes	68
COPD		
St. George's Respiratory Questionnaire	Symptoms; activity; impacts on daily life	76
Chronic Respiratory Disease Questionnaire	Dyspnea; fatigue; emotional function; mastery (feeling of being in control)	20

(*continued*)

Allergic rhinitis		
Rhinoconjuctivitis Quality of Life Questionnaire	Sleep; non-hay-fever symptoms; practical problems; nasal symptoms; eye symptoms; activities; emotions	
Rhinitis Quality of Life Questionnaire (RQLQ)	Sleep; emotional dysfunction; activities; nonrhinitis symptoms; practical problems; nasal symptoms	24
Rhinosinusitis Disability Index (RDI)	Emotional; functional; physical	30
Lung Cancer		
European Organization for Research and Treatment of Cancer Quality of Life Questionnaire Lung Cancer—13 (EORTC QLQ LC-13)	Coughing; hemoptysis; dyspnea; sour mouth or tongue; trouble swallowing; tingling hands and feet; hair loss; experience of pain; pain medication	13
Lung Cancer Symptom Scale (LCSS)	Loss of appetite; fatigue; cough; dyspnea; hemoptysis; pain	15

disease or condition. They measure the impact of a specific disease on the patient's normal daily functioning.[53]

The advantage of generic HRQOL instruments are that they can be used to compare the health status of individuals or groups across diseases. However, since generic HRQOL instruments do not contain questions specific to a particular disease, they may not be sensitive to changes in quality of life. This problem is overcome by using disease-specific instruments. The disadvantage with disease-specific instruments is that they can only be used to compare patients or groups that have the same disease.

Examples of disease-specific HRQOL instruments for asthma, COPD, allergic rhinitis, and lung cancer are presented in Table 10-4.[53–63] The Nottingham Health Profile and the SF-36 are examples of generic HRQOL instruments that have been used as outcome measures of respiratory disease interventions.[64,65]

Purpose for which the HRQOL Instrument was Constructed

Here are three purposes for which HRQOL instruments are constructed: discriminative, evaluative, and predictive. Selection of a specific HRQOL instrument should be based on the purpose for which an instrument was originally developed (Table 10-5).[66,67]

Discriminative instruments are used to measure HRQOL at one point in time. Therefore, these instruments can be used to describe the health status of an individual or a group at a point in time. For example, the health care professional can assess the impact of COPD on a patient during a consultation with the patient. It follows that discriminative instruments can also be used to compare the HRQOL of individuals or groups at one point in time. Therefore, for example, an asthma-specific HRQOL instrument could be used to compare the quality of life of two groups of patients at a point in time.

Evaluative instruments are developed to measure change in HRQOL in an individual or group over time. These instruments can be useful to clinicians in monitoring the progress of individual patients. They can also be used in clinical trials or community interventions to monitor changes in HRQOL. Since the main focus of health care professionals is to evaluate patient progress, most HRQOL instruments are constructed to be evaluative in nature. For example, the Rhinitis Quality of Life Questionnaire, the ITG-Asthma Short Form, the Asthma Quality of Life Questionnaire—Juniper, and the St. George's Respiratory Questionnaire have been used to measure HRQOL change in patients with allergic rhinitis, asthma, and COPD, respectively.[56,68,69]

The purpose of predictive instruments is to classify individuals into groups at risk of developing a particular disease or severity of disease. For example, an asthma-specific HRQOL instrument may be used to classify patients into severity categories based on the NEAPP guidelines.[70] The question one might ask, is

TABLE 10-5.

Purposes for Which Health-Related Quality of Life Instruments are Constructed

Purpose	*Explanation*
Discriminative	Used to distinguish among individuals or groups at one point in time. Can be used to distinguish among communities based on their health status
Evaluative	Used to measure changes in quality of life of an individual or a group over time. The benefit of treatment during a clinical trial or a community intervention are determined using evaluative instruments
Predictive	Used to classify individuals into predefined categories when a "gold standard" is available. Generally used as screening or diagnostic tests to identify which individuals have or will develop a specific condition or outcome

why should an HRQOL instrument be used if a "gold standard" like the NEAPP guidelines exist to classify asthma patients by severity. The answer might lie in the fact that measuring HRQOL may be a less elaborate and a reliable way to classify patients. Very little, if any, research has been performed to develop HRQOL instruments for predictive purposes in the respiratory disease area. As a result, the use of HRQOL instruments for predictive purposes remains an untapped area.

Evidence for the Validity, Reliability, Responsiveness, and Acceptability of an HRQOL Instrument

The third set of considerations in the choice of a specific HRQOL instrument are psychometric in nature. Validity is the extent to which an instrument measures what it purports to measure.[70] The validity requirements differ according to the purpose of the instrument. Evidence for the validity of a discriminative instrument constitutes correlating scores on the HRQOL instrument with scores on theoretically related concepts at a single point in time.[66,67] This property of a discriminative instrument is termed cross-sectional construct validity. When changes in scores on an evaluative instrument correlate with changes in scores on another instrument in a theoretically consistent manner, evidence of longitudinal construct validity for an evaluative HRQOL instrument is obtained. Evidence for the validity of a predictive instrument is obtained by relating scores on the instrument with a "gold standard."

Reliability refers to the degree to which an HRQOL instrument measures the true variation in scores while minimizing the measurement of variation in scores due to random error.[71] When an instrument measures true variation, it can be expected that scores on the instrument are very close to each other at two points in time. Reliability is measured by different types of reliability coefficients which range from 0 to 1 (1 being ideal). A reliability coefficient of at least 0.7 is considered an adequate indication of reliability.[70]

For discriminative instruments the most commonly calculated reliability coefficients are Cronbach's alpha, the intra-class correlation coefficient, or the test–retest correlation coefficient.[66] In evaluative instruments, scores for patients who are clinically stable should not change between two points in time. However, patients whose HRQOL improves or deteriorates should have changed HRQOL scores. To be reliable, predictive instruments should have the ability to classify individuals into the same disease categories at multiple points in time. In other words, agreement in scores among replicate measurements is required. The intra-class correlation coefficient and test–retest reliability coefficient are used to determine the reliability of predictive HRQOL instruments.

Responsiveness is the property of an HRQOL instrument to detect change in scores over time. In other words, the instrument should be sensitive enough to detect changes in HRQOL across two points in time.[66] Typically, responsiveness is measured by comparing changes in scores of patients who have either clinically improved or deteriorated with those of patients who have remained clinically stable. Evaluative instruments should have good responsiveness.

Finally, the HRQOL instrument being chosen should be acceptable to both patients and researchers. Acceptability from the patient's perspective means that the instrument is understandable and not too long. When an instrument satisfies these properties, it is said to have an acceptable "respondent burden." From the researcher's perspective, an HRQOL instrument should be easy to use, score, and interpret.[53]

An Example of Instrument Evaluation and Selection

Sen et al. used the intended purpose and psychometric criteria mentioned above to evaluate three of the most widely used asthma-specific HRQOL instruments: the Asthma Quality of Life Questionnaire—Juniper (AQLQ-J), the Asthma Quality of Life Questionnaire—Marks (AQLQ-M), and the Living with Asthma Questionnaire (LWAQ).[66] The AQLQ-J was found to satisfy the criteria for its stated purpose of being an evaluative instrument. The AQLQ-M was developed as both a discriminative and evaluative instrument. Though the AQLQ-M satisfied the criteria for a discriminative instrument, it did not perform well on the criteria for evaluative instruments. The LWAQ was also developed as both a discriminative and evaluative instrument. It did satisfy criteria for discriminative instruments, but had not yet been tested for its evaluative properties.

The results presented by Sen et al. indicate that the AQLQ-J can be used as an evaluative measure to monitor changes in asthma-specific HRQOL patients. On the other hand, the AQLQ-M and the LWAQ may be used as discriminative instruments to measure the impact of asthma on patients at a point in time. The difference between the AQLQ-M and the LWAQ was that while the AQLQ-M consists of 20 items, the LWAQ contains 68 items. From the patient's perspective, the former instrument presents a less "respondent burden."[66]

Cultural Adaptation of HRQOL Instruments

Recently, the issue of validity of an HRQOL instrument in specific cultures or groups of patients has received attention.[72] Several HRQOL instruments for respiratory diseases have undergone language and cultural adaptations. For example, the AQLQ-J has been adapted for use in France and the AQLQ-M has been modified for use in Spain.[73,74] Instruments have also been adapted for specific cultures. Gupchup et al. have modified the AQLQ-M for use in Native American adults.[75]

With regard to generic HRQOL instruments, the SF-36 has been adapted for several cultures through the International Quality of Life Assessment project (IQOLA Project).[76] The lesson to be learned from the language and cultural adaptations that have been performed on HRQOL instruments is that an instrument can be used with more confidence when it has been adapted for a specific population. Since the adaptation process is very intricate, it is suggested that practitioners use validated cultural adaptations of HRQOL instruments when they are available. Also, these adapted instruments should have been developed for the intended purpose (i.e., discriminative, evaluative, or predictive).

Summary of Steps in the Selection of HRQOL Instruments in Respiratory Diseases

1. Determine whether a generic and/or disease-specific HRQOL questionnaire is needed for your purpose of monitoring HRQOL.
2. Select an instrument that has been developed for a purpose consistent with your purpose of monitoring HRQOL (i.e., discriminative, evaluative, or predictive).
3. Determine whether the selected HRQOL instrument meets the validity, reliability, responsiveness, and acceptability criteria for the purpose that you will use the instrument.
4. In case you expect to monitor HRQOL in a population that has unique cultural or language requirements, look for an instrument that is validated in that population.

Case Study: Asthma

The following case studies allow readers the opportunity to apply the information presented in this chapter in a pharmacoeconomic pharmacy practice situation.

A recent audit completed by your health maintenance organization (HMO) showed that asthma was one of the most expensive disease states in terms of hospitalizations and outpatient clinic visits. The adult asthma population that is seen in your HMO can be broken down into the following categories established by the National Asthma Education and Prevention Program (NAEPP) Guidelines for the Diagnosis and Management of Asthma: 15% have mild intermittent asthma, 35% have mild persistent asthma; 35% have moderate persistent asthma; and 15% have severe persistent asthma. The patients in the moderate and severe persistent groups experience 85% of the hospitalizations for asthma. A disease management team has been organized to help determine what is causing the high costs and how to reduce the costs of asthma management.

What factors may be contributing to the high hospitalization rate in these patients?

- incorrect medications (e.g., not using a long-term controller medication when indicated)
- incorrect dosing of medications (e.g., receiving a sub-optimal dose of an appropriate medication)
- lack of patient education (e.g., patient has not been taught the basic pathophysiology of the disease or goals of therapy)

- incorrect use of medications (e.g., using a long-term controller medication for the immediate relief of symptoms)
- incorrect techniques used in medication administration (e.g., not understanding the different techniques necessary to deliver medication from a dry powder inhaler and a metered dose inhaler).

What factors contribute to the costs of a hospitalization?

- pharmacy (e.g., the cost of the medication)
- hospital charge (e.g., room charge)
- physician (e.g., physician cost)
- nursing (e.g., cost for administration of medications)
- respiratory therapist (e.g., cost for carrying out pulmonary function tests)
- procedures (e.g., cost of administering nebulized medications).

The disease management committee decides that the best way to decrease the number of hospitalizations is to address the way that asthma is managed in the outpatient setting.

What issues need to be addressed in the outpatient clinic to assure that patients are getting complete asthma care?

- correct diagnosis
- correct severity classification of the disease
- correct medication choice for disease severity
- education regarding disease pathophysiology
- education regarding medications used in the treatment
- education regarding correct administration of the medication
- education regarding the use and interpretation of the peak flow meter
- formation of a partnership with the patient for understanding the goals of therapy.

The disease management team concludes that the fastest and easiest way to decrease costs is to develop a formulary guiding health care providers to use the most cost-efficient medications available. The committee agrees that agents that help prevent asthma symptoms from occurring must be made available and, in addition, agents that quickly relieve symptoms must also be made available. While developing the formulary, several issues regarding availability of different agents on the formulary have emerged.

What considerations must be taken into account when deciding which long-term controller medications should be made available?

- cost
- HRQOL
- dosing frequency

- efficacy
- adverse event profile
- severity of disease of the patients being treated
- route of administration
- age of patients being treated.

After lengthy discussions, the disease management committee decides that an inhaled corticosteroid should be made available; however, several agents are currently available.

What issues need to be addressed when deciding which agent to make available?

- cost
- efficacy
- comparison of systemic to topical activity
- device used for administration
- dosing frequency
- HRQOL.

After developing a formulary, the disease management team decides that other measures must be instituted in order to help decrease costs. What additional steps may be taken to help reduce asthma costs?

- establish case managers for patients with two or more emergency department visits or hospitalizations in the last 6 months (return of investment should be assumed)
- identify high-risk patients and institute educational programs
- establish a critical pathway treatment protocol for both emergency department and inpatient care of acute severe asthma
- develop a system-wide patient educational program for the moderate to severe persistent asthmatics.

Which of the above mentioned strategies can be completed without the addition of new resources or reallocation of existing resources?

- establishing critical pathways requires only education of existing personnel.

Case Study: Allergic Rhinitis

Your HMO, after concluding that allergic rhinitis only amounts to 0.5% of their total expenditures, minimal hospitalizations, and low mortality, wants to reevaluate the use of prescription medications for the disease.

What factors are considered when looking at the direct costs for allergic rhinitis?

- physician visits (e.g., cost of seeing the physician)
- prescription drug costs (e.g., antihistamines, intranasal steroids)
- non-prescription drug costs (e.g., over-the-counter antihistamines)
- immunotherapy (e.g., cost of extracts).

What factors are considered when looking at the indirect costs associated for allergic rhinitis?

- missed work days
- missed work days to care for a child
- decreased productivity at work.

Your HMO is considering having only over-the-counter antihistamines available on the formulary.

What considerations must be accounted for when choosing an appropriate antihistamine?

- cost
- effectiveness
- adverse effects
- dosing frequency
- symptoms relieved
- HRQOL.

REFERENCES

1. Centers for Disease Control and Prevention: *Morbidity and Mortality Weekly Report* 1994;43:917.
2. Centers for Disease Control and Prevention: *Morbidity and Mortality Weekly Report* 1995;43:952–955.
3. American Thoracic Society: Cigarette smoking and health. *Am J Respir Crit Care Med* 1996;153:861–865.
4. Bryan S, Buxton MJ: Economic evaluation of treatments for respiratory disease. *Pharmacoeconomics* 1992;2:207–218.
5. Maille AR, Kaptein AA, de Haes JC, et al.: Assessing quality of life in chronic non-specific lung disease—a review of empirical studies published between 1980 and 1994. *Qual Life Res* 1996;5:287–301.
6. Albert RK, Spiro SG, Jett JR: *Comprehensive Respiratory Medicine*. St Louis: Mosby; 1999.
7. Hafner JP, J Ferro T: Recent developments in the management of COPD. *Hosp Med* 1998;34:29–30,32–38.
8. Sherrill DL, Lebowitz MD, Burrow B: Edpidemiology of chronic obstructive pulmonary disease. *Clin Chest Med* 1990;11:375–388.
9. US Surgeon General: The health consequences of smoking: chronic Obstructive Lung Disease. DHSS publication # 84-502051984.
10. American Thoracic Society: Standards for the diagnosis and care of patients with chronic obstructive pulmonary disease. *Am J Respir Crit Care Med* 1995;152:S77–121.
11. Ferguson GT, Cherniack RM: Management of chronic obstructive pulmonary disease [see comments]. *N Engl J Med* 1993;328:1017–1022.
12. Friedman M: Changing practices in COPD. A new pharmacologic treatment algorithm. *Chest* 1995;107:194S–197S.
13. Sondergaard B, Rasmussen H, Rasmussen M: COPD education reduces consumption of healthcare services. *Pharmacoeconomics* 1993;3:175–177.
14. Pedersen PA, Weeke ER: Allergic rhinitis in Danish general practice. Prevalence and consultation rates. *Allergy* 1981;36:375–379.
15. British Thoracic Society: The British asthma guidelines on asthma management. *Thorax* 1997;52(Suppl. 1):S1–21.
16. Pappas G, Hadden WC, Kozak LJ, et al.: Potentially avoidable hospitalizations: inequalities in rates between US socioeconomic groups. *Am J Public Health* 1997;87:811–816.
17. Lenney W: The burden of pediatric asthma. *Pediatr Pulmonol Suppl* 1997;15:13–16.
18. Smith DH, Malone DC, Lawson KA, et al.: A national estimate of the economic costs of asthma. *Am J Respir Crit Care Med* 1997;156:787–793.

19. Jin RL, Choi BC: The 1996 and 1997 national survey of physician asthma management practices: background and study methodology. *Can Respir J* 1999;6:269–272.
20. Kolbe J: Asthma education, action plans, psychosocial issues and adherence. *Can Respir J* 1999;6:273–280.
21. Woodhead MA, Macfarlane JT, McCracken JS, et al.: Prospective study of the aetiology and outcome of pneumonia in the community. *Lancet* 1987;1:671–674.
22. Jokinen C, Heiskanen L, Juvonen H, et al.: Incidence of community-acquired pneumonia in the population of four municipalities in eastern Finland. *Am J Epidemiol* 1993;137:977–988.
23. Glezen WP: Serious morbidity and mortality associated with influenza epidemics. *Epidemiol Rev* 1982;4:25–44.
24. Agostini C, Zambello R, Trentin L, et al.: HIV and pulmonary immune responses. *Immunol Today* 1996;17:359–364.
25. Levine AM: AIDS-related malignancies: the emerging epidemic. *J Natl Cancer Inst* 1993;85:1382–1397.
26. Tirelli U, Vaccher E, Spina M: Other cancers in HIV-infected patients. *Curr Opin Oncol* 1994;6:508–511.
27. Biggar RJ, Rabkin CS: The epidemiology of acquired immunodeficiency syndrome-related lymphomas. *Curr Opin Oncol* 1992;4:883–893.
28. Mackay I, Durham S: Perennial rhinitis. *Br Med J* 1998;316:917–920.
29. International Rhinitis Management Working Group: International consensus report on the diagnosis and treatment of rhinitis. *Eur J Allergy Clin Immunol* 1994;49(suppl.)
30. American Cancer Society: Cancer facts and figures. ACS website, 1999.
31. Janerich DT, Thompson WD, Varela LR, et al.: Lung cancer and exposure to tobacco smoke in the household [see comments]. *N Engl J Med* 1990;323:632–636.
32. Tockman MS, Anthonisen NR, Wright EC, et al.: Airways obstruction and the risk for lung cancer. *Ann Intern Med* 1987;106:512–518.
33. Serra-Batlles J, Plaza V, Morejon E, et al.: Costs of asthma according to the degree of severity. *Eur Respir J* 1998;12:1322–1326.
34. DaSilva RV: A disease management case study on asthma. *Clin Ther* 1996;18:1374–1382.
35. Practice Management Information Corporation, United States. Health Care Financing Administration: ICD-9-CM: *International Classification of Diseases*, 9th revision, clinical modification, 5th edition, color coded, volumes 1, 2, and 3, 1998. Los Angeles, Calif.: PMIC (Practice Management Information Corp.) 1997;viii:1700 (3 vols in 1).
36. University Health System Consortium O, IL: Clinical Process Improvement Manual, 1997.
37. Summers KH: Measuring and monitoring outcomes of disease management programs. *Clin Ther* 1996;18:1341–1348.

38. National Heart Lung and Blood Institute. *NAEPP: Expert Panel Report II: Guidelines for the Diagnosis and Management of Asthma.* NIH publication. Bethesda, Md.: National Institutes of Health National Heart Lung and Blood Institute; 1997.
39. Johnson NE: Cost measurement. In: Johnson NE, Nash DB, eds, *The Role of Pharmacoeconomics in Outcomes Management.* Chicago: American Hospital Pub.; 1996;97.
40. Soucy B, Sidorov J: Asthma disease management: history and development within an integrated health care system. *Dis Manage* 1998;1:228–259.
41. Luce BR, Elixhauser A, Culyer AJ: *Standards for the Socioeconomic Evaluation of Health Care Services. Health Systems Research.* Berlin: Springer-Verlag, 1990;xi:184.
42. Larson L: Cost determination and analysis. In: Bootman JL, Townsend RJ, McGhan WF, eds, *Principles of Pharmacoeconomics.* Cincinnati, OH: H. Whitney Books Co., 1991;v:162.
43. Loss RW, Hall WJ, Speers DM: Evaluation of early airway disease in smokers: cost effectiveness of pulmonary function testing. *Am J Med Sci* 1979;278:27–37.
44. Reina-Rosenbaum R, Bach JR, Penek J: The cost/benefits of outpatient-based pulmonary rehabilitation. *Arch Phys Med Rehabil* 1997;78:240–244.
45. Rutten-van Molken MP, Van Doorslaer EK, Jansen MC, et al.: Cost effectiveness of inhaled corticosteroid plus bronchodilator therapy versus bronchodilator monotherapy in children with asthma. *Pharmacoeconomics* 1993;4:257–270.
46. Rutten-van Molken MP, Van Doorslaer EK, Jansen MC, et al.: Costs and effects of inhaled corticosteroids and bronchodilators in asthma and chronic obstructive pulmonary disease. *Am J Respir Crit Care Med* 1995;151:975–982.
47. Rutten-van Molken MP, van Doorslaer EK, Till MD: Cost-effectiveness analysis of formoterol versus salmeterol in patients with asthma. *Pharmacoeconomics* 1998;14:671–684.
48. Friedman M, Serby CW, Menjoge SS, et al.: Pharmacoeconomic evaluation of a combination of ipratropium plus albuterol compared with ipratropium alone and albuterol alone in COPD. *Chest* 1999;115:635–641.
49. Nicolau DP, Ross JW, Quintiliani R, et al.: Pharmacoeconomics of *Pneumocystis carinii* pneumonia in HIV-infected and HIV-noninfected patients. *Pharmacoeconomics* 1996;10:72–78.
50. Goldstein RS, Gort EH, Guyatt GH, et al.: Economic analysis of respiratory rehabilitation. *Chest* 1997;112:370–379.
51. Testa MA, Simonson DC: Review articles: assessment of quality-of-life outcomes. *N Engl J Med* 1996;334:835–840.

52. Patrick DL, Erickson P: Health status and health policy: quality of life in health care evaluation and resource allocation. New York: Oxford University Press, 1993;xxv:478.
53. Bootman JL, Townsend RJ, McGhan WF: *Principles of Pharmacoeconomics*. Cincinnati, OH: H. Whitney Books Co., 1991;v:162.
54. Juniper EF, Guyatt GH: Development and testing of a new measure of health status for clinical trials in rhinoconjunctivitis. *Clin Exp Allergy* 1991;21:77–83.
55. Juniper EF, Guyatt GH, Epstein RS, et al.: Evaluation of impairment of health related quality of life in asthma: development of a questionnaire for use in clinical trials. *Thorax* 1992;47:76–83.
56. Juniper EF, Guyatt GH, Andersson B, et al.: Comparison of powder and aerosolized budesonide in perennial rhinitis: validation of rhinitis quality of life questionnaire. *Ann Allergy* 1993;70:225–230.
57. Hyland ME, Finnis S, Irvine SH: A scale for assessing quality of life in adult asthma sufferers. *J Psychosom Res* 1991;35:99–110.
58. Marks GB, Dunn SM, Woolcock AJ: A scale for the measurement of quality of life in adults with asthma. *J Clin Epidemiol* 1992;45:461–472.
59. Jones PW, Quirk FH, Baveystock CM, et al.: A self-complete measure of health status for chronic airflow limitation. The St. George's Respiratory Questionnaire. *Am Rev Respir Dis* 1992;145:1321–1327.
60. Guyatt GH, Berman LB, Townsend M, et al.: A measure of quality of life for clinical trials in chronic lung disease. *Thorax* 1987;42:773–778.
61. Hollen PJ, Gralla RJ, Kris MG, et al.: Quality of life assessment in individuals with lung cancer: testing the Lung Cancer Symptom Scale (LCSS). *Eur J Cancer* 1993;29A:S51–8.
62. Benninger MS, Senior BA: The development of the Rhinosinusitis Disability Index. *Arch Otolaryngol Head Neck Surg* 1997;123:1175–1179.
63. Bergman B, Aaronson NK, Ahmedzai S, et al.: The EORTC QLQ-LC13: a modular supplement to the EORTC Core Quality of Life Questionnaire (QLQ-C30) for use in lung cancer clinical trials. EORTC Study Group on Quality of Life. *Eur J Cancer* 1994;5:635–642.
64. Guyatt GH, King DR, Feeny DH, et al.: Generic and specific measurement of health-related quality of life in a clinical trial of respiratory rehabilitation. *J Clin Epidemiol* 1999;52:187–192.
65. Prieto L, Alonso J, Ferrer M, et al.: Are results of the SF-36 health survey and the Nottingham Health Profile similar? A comparison in COPD patients. Quality of Life in COPD Study Group. *J Clin Epidemiol* 1997;50:463–473.
66. Sen SS, Gupchup GV, Thomas J, 3rd: Selecting among health-related quality-of-life instruments. *Am J Health Syst Pharm* 1999;56:1965–70; quiz p. 1971.

67. Kirshner B, Guyatt G: A methodological framework for assessing health indices. *J Chronic Dis* 1985;38:27–36.
68. Wenzel SE, Lumry W, Manning M, et al.: Efficacy, safety, and effects on quality of life of salmeterol versus albuterol in patients with mild to moderate persistent asthma. *Ann Allergy Asthma Immunol* 1998;80:463–470.
69. Gallefoss F, Bakke PS, Rsgaard PK: Quality of life assessment after patient education in a randomized controlled study on asthma and chronic obstructive pulmonary disease. *Am J Respir Crit Care Med* 1999;159:812–871.
70. Nunnally JC: *Psychometric Theory*. McGraw-Hill Series in psychology. New York: McGraw-Hill; 1967;xiii:640.
71. Kerlinger FN: *Foundations of Behavioral Research*. New York: Holt Rinehart and Winston; 1986;xviii:667.
72. Guillemin F, Bombardier C, Beaton D: Cross-cultural adaptation of health-related quality of life measures: literature review and proposed guidelines [see comments]. *J Clin Epidemiol* 1993;46:1417–1432.
73. Leroyer C, Lebrun T, Proust A, et al.: Knowledge, self-management, compliance and quality of life in asthma: a cross-sectional study of the French version of the Asthma Quality of Life Questionnaire. *Qual Life Res* 1998;7:267–272.
74. Perpina M, Belloch A, Marks GB, et al.: Assessment of the reliability, validity, and responsiveness of a Spanish Asthma Quality of Life questionnaire. *J Asthma* 1998;35:513–521.
75. Gupchup G, Teel M, Singhal P: Development of an Asthma Quality of Life Questionnaire for Native American Adults (AQLQ-NAA). *Value Health* 1999;2:178.
76. Spilker B: Quality of life and pharmacoeconomics in clinical trials. Philadelphia: Lippincott-Raven; 1996;xlv:1259.

CHAPTER

11

Guidelines and Information Requirements

C. Daniel Mullins
and
Sanjay Merchant

THE STANDARDS DEBATE

The debate on standards for pharmacoeconomic guidelines has been around almost as long as the field of pharmacoeconomics. There have been several conferences on the topic of guidelines, including those sponsored by the University of North Carolina, Duke University, and the International Society for Pharmacoeconomics and Outcomes Research (ISPOR). There are many articles, monographs, and even a book dedicated to this topic.[1] As the field of pharmacoeconomics continues to evolve, it is useful to review new proposals for improving methodologies and standardizing the way in which studies are conducted. At the same time, there is a danger in providing "cook book" rules that simplify the process of performing studies but do not provide the scientific rigor and flexibility to address concerns of medical decision makers.

An underlying issue driving the need for the development of methodological and ethical guidelines is the potential for bias in cost-effectiveness research.[2] Bias may be introduced throughout the entire process of conducting an economic evaluation; it may be intentional or unintentional. Creating a set of standardized methods to be used when performing an economic evaluation may help to limit the introduction of bias into the evaluation as well as assure the reader that the evaluation is methodologically and ethically sound. Furthermore, standardization increases the comparability among analyses, therefore rendering them more useful to the user.

Are Standards Necessary?

Before addressing the issue of how standards for pharmacoeconomic should be developed, it is worth asking whether they are necessary. Rittenhouse[3] questions the need for standardized methods for economic evaluation of medicines in his introductory comments to the 1995 Conference on "Standards for Economic Evaluation of Drugs." His argument is that the relevant economic concern is not whether or not there is a benefit to standards, but rather whether the benefits of implementing standards outweigh the costs. In addition, he delineates the differences among the concepts of "principles," "guidelines," and "standards." "Principles" may suggest a list of issues to be addressed, while "guidelines" are more prescriptive in how analysis should be done. Finally, "standards" imply that failure to adhere to recommendations is inherently "wrong." Thus, in deciding whether or not standards are necessary, it is important to consider the extent to which standards will dictate how analysis should be performed. In general, there seems to be consensus that certain key elements should be addressed in any pharmacoeconomic study, but it may still be premature to assume that a universal set of standards should be used to measure the validity of studies.

If there appears to be a need for standards, the next concern is whether appropriate methods have evolved to allow for implementation at this point in time or whether it is better to defer to a future date. In the mid 1990s Luce argued that, "although the outcomes research field is in need of general guidelines for some elements . . . it is not ready for standards for evaluating outcomes."[4] Since that time, there has been convergence of opinions in certain areas, but considerable debate continues on other key topics.[5] Resolution on some of the basic tenets of pharmacoeconomic analysis must occur in order for standards to receive wide acceptance. Part of the challenge is getting researchers from various backgrounds and disciplines to come to a common understanding.

Where Have we Been?

One of the earlier discussions of the foundations of cost-effectiveness analysis in health was published in the *New England Journal of Medicine* by Weinstein and Mason in 1977.[6] At the time, there was very little published literature addressing pharmacoeconomic guidelines and cost-effectiveness in medicine, and few empirical drug studies included a health economics component. Over the last two decades there has been an explosion in the number of empirical and theoretical articles focussed on cost-effectiveness and pharmacoeconomics. In 1978, the year after Weinstein and Mason's publication, only seven articles on cost-effectiveness of drugs/pharmacoeconomics were published in journals indexed by MEDLINE. Twenty years later, in 1998, there were several thousand articles. This exponential increase is attributable to the scope of journals that are publishing articles on these topics and the number of articles being published in those journals.

We performed MEDLINE searches using the subject terms "pharmacoecon*" or "cost-effective*" and "drug*" to determine the increase in the number of periodicals that published articles on these topics. The results are displayed in Figure 11-1. In 1978, only six journals met the search criteria. In 1983 and 1988 the number of journals increased to 22 and 38, respectively. By 1993, the number of journals publishing articles on these topics tripled the number 5 years earlier, rising to 113. Finally, between 1993 and 1998, the number almost doubled again to 220 journals. A summary of the literature from 1979 to 1990 was presented by Elixhauser and colleagues[7] in the early 1990s and updated for the years 1991–1996 in the late 1990s.[8] More recently, Diener et al. have reviewed health care contingent valuation studies.[9] These authors find similar increases in the number of published articles.

The source of much of the debate and frustration has been the search for a common metric.[10] In one camp, there are economists who are trying to resolve which methods provide the best analytical framework. In another, there are clinicians who are trying to determine when it is appropriate to compare two different medical technologies or interventions which may have different indications and outcomes. On a positive note, researchers from a wide variety of disciplines have begun to work together to address these concerns. This combined effort brings a more rational approach to health technology assessment.[11]

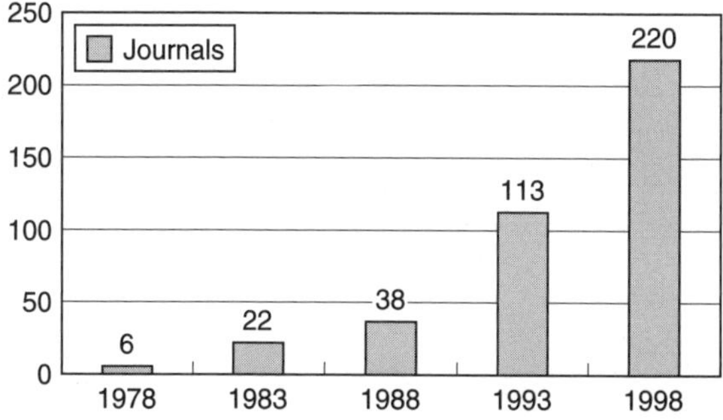

Figure 11-1. Number of journals publishing pharmacoeconomics articles by year.

Where are we Headed?

While some researchers would argue for waiting until the ideal methodology is developed, others are beginning to advocate for compromise and balance between the rigidity of clinical trials and the flexibility and practicality of modeling. Drummond explains that clinical trials have high internal validity but low external validity (generalizability), while models provide a means of exploring real world environments.[12] The future of guidelines may differ by audience. Researchers may have one set of objectives that differ from those of decision makers. If the future is anything like the past, a new series of textbook-type guidelines will not significantly impact health care decisions and are unlikely to receive approval from a broad audience.[13]

As journal reviewers and health technology decision makers become more knowledgeable, the methodological weaknesses that appeared in previously published articles will no longer be tolerated. In their discussion of pharmacoeconomics in the new millennium, Thwaites and Townsend argue that there will be greater challenges with improved methods, but the rewards will be greater access to markets and improved value for money in health care.[14] Corporations who provide financial support for studies will require increased credibility in terms of modeling techniques, selection of type of evaluation, and assumptions. In order to meet the demands of customers, the pharmaceutical industry will work with their clients to produce locally initiated prospective studies with real world populations.[14]

What are the Controversies?

Considerable attention has been focussed on the potential for bias in pharmacoeconomic studies, particularly those funded by the pharmaceutical industry.[15] Although outcomes research studies are funded by the same companies that fund clinical trials of products, financial support from the industry is viewed as significantly more controversial for pharmacoeconomic analyses than it is for randomized, controlled clinical trials. This skepticism is likely to continue until a generally accepted set of guidelines is produced.

Another controversy stems from divergent expectations among those who produce and those who interpret pharmacoeconomic studies. Researchers aim to describe the relative cost-effectiveness of products, while decision makers often seek to determine if new therapies will reduce total costs.[16] Assessment of economic outcomes without consideration for health outcomes (i.e., what happens to patients) may lead to inefficient decisions that save money in the short run but have negative long-term health consequences. This difference in focus between those who perform research and those who are fiscally responsible for health care spending may reflect confusion or mistrust on behalf of users of pharmacoeconomic information who must interpret volumes of published studies with differing perspectives, methodologies, and sources of data. The widespread and highly visible disagreement among leading researchers in the field may contribute to the external skepticism of outcomes research studies with economic components. End users may be reluctant to rely upon studies that they do not understand, particularly when they are aware of disagreement among those who conduct such studies.[12] The challenge for developers of guidelines is to resolve the controversial issues regarding study design and interpretation, while keeping in mind the fact that the goal of outcomes research is to inform decision makers.[16]

Who Benefits from Standardization?

Governments, the pharmaceutical industry, researchers, health care decision makers, and patients have a vested interest in the development of standardized guidelines which can be implemented and used for decision making. Governments that provide national health insurance may have an interest in standardization of drug economic evaluation when such "methodological standards" provide a mechanism for controlling expenditures on pharmaceuticals. In addition, economic studies can play a role in pricing decisions in countries that have universal health care coverage.[17] In the United States, pharmacoeconomics is valuable for Medicaid and other government-supported health programs' formulary considerations.

A University of Arizona conference on "Facilitating Collaboration among Academic Institutions, Managed-Care Organizations (MCOs), and the Pharmaceutical Industry" described the potential benefits for such collaborative efforts among three key players.[18] The challenge for MCOs is to develop and support clinical and economic databases with support and advice from academic colleagues; at the same time, the pharmaceutical industry must be sensitive and responsive to MCO concerns. The solutions proposed at the conference focused on overcoming barriers by (1) developing trust; (2) recognizing common ground; (3) sharing risk; (4) promoting communication and understanding; and (5) designing research sensitive to corporate objectives.

Pharmaceutical companies believe that the evidence of "value for money" spent on pharmacoeconomic studies may be increased by guidelines, especially when a premium price needs to be justified in terms of economic benefits such as savings in health care resources or improved quality of life.[19] On the other hand, mandatory guidelines may constitute an additional hurdle for the pharmaceutical industry, over and above the demand to demonstrate efficacy, safety, and quality. This may lead to consumption of time and costly resources for the pharmaceutical industry and may delay the drug development and approval process.

Researchers may benefit from guidelines by formalizing, and perhaps simplifying, the way in which analyses should be conducted. Guidelines will provide an accepted procedure for carrying out pharmacoeconomic analyses, thereby increasing the acceptance of study methodology. The downside is that standardization might unnecessarily stifle methodological developments.[20]

Health care decision makers such as physicians, pharmacists, or formulary committees often base their decisions on the basis of clinical and pharmacoeconomic studies. Guidelines for the conduct and reporting of pharmacoeconomics and research provide a common platform for health care decision makers to evaluate pharmacoeconomic studies. It gives the decision makers an assurance about the quality of the studies on the basis of which they make their decisions.[17] Private insurers and MCOs will also have an assurance since they often make formulary decisions on the basis of pharmacoeconomic studies. Such standardized procedures ultimately may provide benefits to patients who purchase and consume the medications.

REVIEW OF GUIDELINES WORLDWIDE

The first, and most widely discussed pharmacoeconomic guidelines, are from Australia.[21–25] In addition, guidelines have been developed for Canada,[26–28] Denmark,[29] Italy,[30] Spain,[31] the United Kingdom,[32,33] the United States,[34,35] and the European Community.[36] There have also been articles published on the influence of pharmacoeconomics in Belgium,[37] France,[38] Germany,[39] Japan,[40] the Middle East,[41] the Netherlands,[42] Norway[43] and Sweden.[44]

In most countries, national guidelines are general in nature and do not make prescriptive criteria for pharmacoeconomic information as a requirement for formulary listing.[45] In Australia, however, the Commonwealth Department of Health, Housing, and Community Services introduced, in August 1992, Guidelines for the Pharmaceutical Industry on Preparation of Submissions to the Pharmaceutical Benefits Advisory Committee (PBAC).[46] The purpose of the guidelines was to "provide a means for identifying and formatting the necessary basic information, and provide guidance on the most appropriate form of economic analysis in a particular instance."[46] The Australian guidelines, which were revised in November 1995, not only were the first guidelines to be published, but also set mandatory evidentiary standards for all pharmaceutical companies wishing to make submissions to the PBAC for national formulary listing under the Pharmaceutical Benefits Scheme. Given Australia's national health system, economic guidelines have become mandatory for a pharmaceutical product to be reimbursed.

In 1994, Canada became the second country to release national guidelines for the economic evaluation of pharmaceuticals.[47] The Canadian Coordinating Office for Health Technology Assessment (CCOHTA)—a non-profit organization, funded by the federal, provincial, and territorial governments in

Canada—published the first edition of guidelines for economic evaluation of pharmaceuticals in 1994. The second edition of the guidelines was published in 1997.[48] Each of the provinces in Canada is free to adopt the guidelines with or without modifications. The intent of the guidelines was "to provide guidance to doers and users of studies, by laying out general state-of-the-art regarding methods and by providing specific methodological advice on many matters."[48] The aim was to improve the scientific quality and integrity of studies, and to enhance consistency and comparability across studies.

Other countries such as Spain, Italy, and the United Kingdom have developed guidelines. In Italy, researchers have proposed guidelines to homogenize studies to alleviate pressures on decision makers to evaluate health care programs. In the United Kingdom, guidelines have been developed because both the Department of Health and the industry want to ensure value for money. The guidelines were intended to add to the existing mechanisms in place in the United Kingdom to monitor purchasing and prescribing decisions.

Unlike Australia, the United States does not have a national set of guidelines for pharmacoeconomic studies. Furthermore, there are no pharmacoeconomic requirements for pharmaceutical reimbursement. However, most pharmaceutical companies carry out pharmacoeconomic studies to enhance the "value" of their product. There have been several proposed pharmacoeconomic guidelines for use in the United States, but their purpose is mainly to provide a set of voluntary principles to guide researchers to carry out the pharmacoeconomic analysis. The Food and Drug Administration (FDA)—the administrative body that overlooks drug approvals in the United States—has published a draft guidance, enumerating the principles for reviewing pharmacoeconomic claims.[49] The purview of the FDA, however, is merely to ensure that the pharmacoeconomic information being disseminated by the pharmaceutical companies is not false or misleading. The FDA does not routinely use this information for approval or labeling and the FDA has no jurisdiction over drug pricing. A discussion of the FDA draft guidelines is provided in a later section.

The major difference between Australia and the United States is that Australia has a national health system. This means that pharmaceutical companies seeking recommendation for national formulary listing and subsidization need to provide a detailed economic analysis to support their case. The United States, on the other hand, does not have a national health system. Rather, the health system is dominated by Medicare, Medicaid, and various MCOs. Pharmacoeconomic studies have been used by various pharmaceutical companies to convince the managers of health plan purchasers to include their products in the plan's formulary. Pharmacoeconomic guidelines have been used in the United States mainly as a means of providing a format for carrying out the analyses and for purposes of standardizing pharmacoeconomic studies.

Readers who are interested in a description of the differences across various countries are referred to a publication by Genduso and Kotsanos, where an excellent summary is provided.[50] In this chapter, we provide a general overview of several key aspects of guidelines instead of reiterating the main points for each country. We now briefly describe various aspects of the guidelines along with highlights that summarize where there is agreement or controversy.

Type of PE Evaluation

Cost-effectiveness analysis (CEA) is the most popular form of empirical analysis. Mark Pauly has argued that cost-benefit analysis (CBA) may be superior to CEA from a theoretical perspective for a variety of reasons.[51] CBA arguably incorporates *all* aspects of a program, whereas CEA may incorporate only a unidimensional metric for outcomes assessment. This concern for incorporating many different outcome variables in health economics research may explain the increasing popularity of cost-consequence analysis (CCA) models.[52] CCAs incorporate a matrix of outcomes, which may provide more complete clinical information; unfortunately, this information cannot easily be used to calculate a cost-consequence ratio. CCA is required in Canada whenever comparative therapies do not result in equivalent consequences (i.e., whenever cost-minimization analysis (CMA) is inappropriate).

When preferences are assessed and cost-utility analysis (CUA) is used, many pharmacoeconomic researchers prefer the use of quality-adjusted life years (QALYs) over simple life years gained. In particular, the Panel on Cost-Effectiveness recommends the use of QALYs in the denominator and prefers the use of community preferences.[50]

Perspective

Most government payers prefer the use of the public payer perspective, which is very close to the societal perspective but with less emphasis on indirect costs and benefits. The public payer also places less emphasis on the value (utility) to family members and individuals other than the patient. In the United States, there is an empiric preference for a managed care perspective, principally because this is the intended audience for most industry-sponsored studies.

The patient perspective is almost never mentioned as a preferred option; however, patient preferences are incorporated when quality or utility measures are presented as part of a CUA study.

Comparators and data sources

Most payers prefer comparisons with standard of care rather than placebo, yet the empirical literature still contains a great deal of pharmacoeconomic studies based on randomized, controlled clinical trial (RCT) data which compare active treatment to placebo. This is true for government payers and MCOs. Recently, Grabowski and Mullins reported similar findings for pharmacy benefit managers (PBMs) in the United States.[53] For a discussion of differences between cost-efficacy from RCTs versus cost-effectiveness from retrospective analysis see O'Brien.[54] The *British Medical Journal* recognizes that data sources and comparators may need to be jointly determined.

Data Analysis

One topic which has not received a great deal of attention in the literature until recently is the issue of estimating the variability of the cost-effectiveness ratio using statistical methods. The most common means of assessing the variability of the ratio is sensitivity analysis. However, there are two significant limitations associated with sensitivity analysis. One is that the individual researcher chooses which variables are subjected to sensitivity analyses as well as the range of estimates used. The other limitation is that there are no criteria which can be used to objectively determine if a cost-effectiveness ratio is considered robust. During the last couple of years, a growing number of articles have been published concerning the application of statistical methods to pharmacoeconomics. Specifically, most of the literature relates to assessing the variability of cost-effectiveness ratios, calculating confidence intervals, and formal hypothesis testing with cost-effectiveness ratios. This body of literature is likely to continue to evolve and may develop into an area of much debate among a broader constituency of pharmacoeconomic researchers.

Costs

The preferred approach for reporting costs includes documentation of unit costs rather than just aggregate cost figures, and marginal costs as well as total costs. Empirically, there are still a number of studies that report average rather than marginal costs, although this appears to be changing as the discipline becomes more sophisticated. Recently, a great deal of emphasis has been placed on reporting frictional costs (also known as transaction or transitional costs) to assure that all societal costs are reported and to avoid double counting. When reporting cost-effectiveness ratios, appropriately assigning costs to the numerator or denominator is equally important as accurately measuring those costs which are reported. The Panel on Cost-Effectiveness has recommendations on the topic of "Components Belonging to the Numerator and the Denominator" on page 306 of their book.[50]

The net present value of future costs is dependent on both the discount rate and the time horizon of the study. The discount rate and time horizon are addressed below. One of the most controversial issues in cost-effectiveness research is whether to include unrelated future costs of health care. This issue centers on the argument of whether it is appropriate to incorporate costs that occur in years of life added (or subtracted) due to the intervention under study. The opinions of leaders in the field reflect this polemic issue.

Weinstein and Stason[6] and Drummond et al.[55] have argued for their inclusion, while Russell[56] has argued for their exclusion. In light of these arguments, the Panel on Cost Effectiveness in Health and Medicine could not come to agreement on the issue. They recommend that individual researchers use their own judgment when deciding whether to include or exclude these costs. They go on to recommend that if these costs are small relative to the magnitude of the cost-effectiveness ratio, they can be excluded. If these costs are relatively large, they recommend using a sensitivity analysis to assess the influence of these costs.

Outcomes

The presentation of consequences or outcomes in most empirical studies uses a single metric with "add on" information about other positive and negative effects. Two examples are:

- Mark et al. published a cost-effectiveness article comparing thrombolytic therapy with tissue plasminogen activator (t-PA) or streptokinase for the treatment of acute myocardial infarction.[57] The primary outcome measure used was the cost per year of life saved. A significant side effect of treatment with t-PA is an increased risk of hemorrhagic strokes. Because this side effect was not incorporated into the denominator of the cost-effectiveness ratio, additional information was needed to inform readers about the additional risks and benefits associated with the treatment.
- Hlatky et al. recently published a cost-effectiveness analysis based on a large randomized trial of patients with multivessel coronary disease treated with either angioplasty or coronary bypass surgery at 5 years of follow up.[58] The primary outcome measure used was the cost per year of life added. In this case, only changes in survival are captured in the cost-effectiveness ratio. Thus, differences in rates of subsequent revascularization procedures and measures of quality of life and relief of angina were presented separately.

Many studies use surrogate or intermediate endpoints and the time horizon is sometimes dictated by the availability of data rather than what appears theoretically appropriate from a clinical viewpoint. There are no general guidelines for which particular outcomes should be included in an analysis—the implication being that outcomes should be selected based on the disease state; however, there is a preference for developing lists of outcome measures that are disease-specific rather than drug-specific in order to provide greater comparability across studies.

The Panel on Cost-Effectiveness states that outcomes should be utility-weighted in the form of QALYs.[50] The guidelines from the *British Medical Journal* state that indirect benefits should be reported in a separate section which describes the relevance of the indirect benefits to the study objective.[59]

Modeling

A great deal of emphasis is placed on designing models that bridge the gap between efficacy and effectiveness. There are few standards at this point but a unanimous recommendation that all assumptions should be based on published, peer-reviewed literature and supplemented by current medical expert knowledge. All assumptions and the model itself should be justified in any publication.

Markov modeling has become increasingly popular and is supported by a variety of computer software packages. These models allow greater complexity of assumptions which have the potential to more accurately reflect disease progression, but are only as good as the corresponding assumptions. Many published cost-effectiveness studies use stochastic models that address the issue of state-dependent transition probabilities but do not account for changes in the probability matrix over time; that is, the models have no "memory" of previous information that would appear relevant from a clinical perspective. In some cases, the models are complex but offer little benefit over existing information from RCTs when the objective is to predict real world effectiveness. Furthermore, the data used in these models are generally not available for critical review. Often the greatest contribution that results from current published pharmacoeconomic models is their ability to document a range of plausible outcomes and ratios using sensitivity analysis.

Time horizon

The general rule is that the time horizon should be long enough to capture the full effects of the intervention. The appropriate length is not always well defined a priori, however, especially when the effectiveness study itself provides information regarding the length of follow-up required to capture long-term effects. An unresolved issue related to the time horizon is how to incorporate the effect of interventions on illnesses other than the principal focus of the study (e.g., how cardiovascular therapy may effect diabetes as well). It is well known that interventions that extend life will result in costs and benefits that are unrelated to the specific disease being examined and have only to do with the aging process itself. There is general consensus that it is not necessary to model these costs and benefits associated with extended life into a cost-effectiveness study (see also the discussion in Costs section above).

Discounting

The discount rate is one of the areas with greatest consensus. The general rule is to discount at either 3% or 5% and carry out sensitivity analysis between 0% and 10%. The upper limit becomes more important when the study costs or outcomes occur in the distant future or when patterns of resource consumption vary between alternatives being compared.

The majority opinion is that the costs and benefits should be discounted at the same rate;[60] however, there are some pharmacoeconomic experts who feel that outcomes should be discounted at a different rate or should not be discounted at all. Some of the arguments on both sides can be supported by widely accepted economic principles.

Uncertainty

Sources of uncertainty include projections of parameter estimates based on similar studies or expert opinion, the study's time horizon, and sampling errors. Several approaches have been recommended to deal with the issue of uncertainty in outcomes studies. Studies should address and minimize sampling error as a source of uncertainty. Because study results and related sampling errors depend on the quality of data, researchers should describe all data sources and their associated weaknesses and limitations; the type of data (e.g., randomized control trial, cohort study, expert opinion); and, where appropriate, the power of the study.

Modeling is often used to address the uncertainty of outcomes or cases for which the data are insufficient to evaluate. Modeling allows a range of outcomes to be mapped out using a variety of parameters under differing circumstances. The nature and objectives of the study will determine whether researchers use stochastic models, for which probabilities do not vary across time, or deterministic models, where previous events influence future probabilities.

Decision trees are one of the simplest means of modeling uncertainty. Often they describe or predict short-run outcomes by addressing choices and uncertainties associated with diagnosis and treatment decisions. Decision-tree modeling involving the use of Markov processes has become increasingly popular, especially for chronic illnesses. Markov chains and processes are used to predict longer-term, more complex outcomes of a particular treatment. Markov chains model sequences of events or states and incorporate probability matrices which describe the likelihood of transferring from one state to another.

The value of pharmacoeconomic models lies partly in their ability to predict "real world" cost-effectiveness under a variety of assumptions. This value can be strengthened with appropriate sensitivity analysis. Sensitivity analysis should be used to determine the robustness of study results and outcomes when assumptions and parameter estimates are varied.

Disclosure

There is consensus that disclosure of any relationships between investigators and sources of funding should be clearly described to ensure independence and integrity. Most journals require the disclosure of funding sources and financial relationships. Some publications also request disclosure related to payments and cost of the study, conflict(s) of interest, and any other affiliations that may be interpreted as potential bias(es) of a study.

Generalizability

Studies should use appropriate and comparable analyses so that the results can be generalized to meet the needs of a particular user or audience. Study results should be modifiable to account for variations in populations, treatment, and practice environments. Results should be presented such that they are both transparent and replicable. Studies results should not, however, be so general that they become inapplicable to any specific user or audience.

REVIEW OF CHECKLISTS FOR PUBLICATIONS

As the number of pharmacoeconomic studies being published in various health journals rises, so do concerns about the quality of pharmacoeconomic studies that have been published in these journals.[61,62] In a study by Schulman and colleagues, editors of 15 major medical journals were surveyed to assess the publication process that may influence the quality of the health economics and ethics literature.[63] Of the 12 editors who responded, only two reported having health economists among their editors. The editors reported knowing little about the formal training of their reviewers in the disciplines of statistics, economics, and ethics. Disclosure of the financial contract between the author and the sponsor was requested by nine journals; however, only four requested information regarding publication rights of the researcher. Various journals now have published checklists or have listed restrictions that will be applied to pharmacoeconomic studies before they can be accepted for publications in those journals. Notable among those are the *New England Journal of Medicine* (NEJ) and the *British Medical Journal* (BMJ).

The *New England Journal of Medicine* Guidelines

NEJ published a controversial policy relating to pharmacoeconomic studies in 1994. NEJ's main concern appears to be the influence of pharmaceutical companies on these studies, and the fact that these pharmaceutical companies may influence the analyses to favorably portray their products.[64] The journal's policy is in response to the lack of standard approaches to pharmacoeconomic evaluation; the fact that methodologies used to carry out cost-effectiveness analyses vary from author to author; the fact that data used for the analyses may be derived from either a single randomized controlled clinical trial or from various sources; and the fact that sources for cost data used to carry out the analyses vary from one study to another. These inconsistencies may lead to the introduction of bias into some studies. The marketing objectives of the pharmaceutical companies that fund these studies may further create an incentive of bias. As a result, the journal has created a policy that it will utilize for review of any cost-effectiveness study for the purpose of publication into the journal.

As a background, the journal has a long-standing policy on authors' financial conflicts of interest in other types of articles submitted to the NEJ.[64] Any author who submits scientific articles to the journal is required to disclose any financial connection with a company that makes the product under study (or its competitors). In contrast, the journal does not even consider review articles or editorials by authors with any financial connections to the companies whose products are featured prominently in the article (or their competitors). The journal feels that cost-effectiveness analyses have some of the features of both "original scientific articles" and those of "review articles." CEAs are similar to original articles in that the methods and data are explicit and the conclusions are based on the data presented. On the other hand, like review articles, the assumptions made in constructing a model of the outcomes of alternative treatment and the data used in CEA are usually chosen from the literature, and the choices could be biased. In keeping with its policy on the authors' financial conflicts of interest with respect to original scientific articles, the journal will not exclude such cost-effectiveness studies from consideration if they are supported by a grant from industry to a nonprofit organization. Furthermore, as with NEJ's policy towards review articles, the journal will not to even consider review articles or editorials by authors with any financial connections to the companies whose products are featured in the article.

NEJ adds that authors submitting cost-effectiveness studies for publication should provide information that will allow the journal to judge whether bias exists. First, the grant must be made to a not-for-profit entity such as a hospital or a university and not to an individual or groups of individuals. Secondly, the journal must receive a written assurance that the author(s) have complete freedom in the study design, interpretation of data, report writing, and decision making regarding publication, regardless of the results of the analysis. Finally, the manuscript must include a description of all data used in the analysis, all assumptions made, and the model (if any) that was used in the analysis. This will ensure that the study can be assessed or replicated by readers.

The NEJ policy has been looked upon with criticism from some health researchers and pharmaceutical companies. Many people feel that the pharmaceutical industry is a good source of funding for pharmacoeconomic studies. If the NEJ policy were to be used by most major journals, there would be a vast reduction in the number of pharmacoeconomic studies that would be published. Rather than using the NEJ policy of not accepting pharmacoeconomic articles for publication if they are funded by pharmaceutical companies, many health journals have adopted a policy that requires full disclosure of any financial interests or contractual arrangements with pharmaceutical companies. This means that the authors need to make a disclosure of any kind of funding from pharmaceutical companies when submitting an article for publication.

British Medical Journal Guidelines

The BMJ set up a working party on economic evaluation to improve the quality of submitted and published economic articles.[59] The working party's task was to produce guidelines for economic evaluation, together with a comprehensive supporting statement which could be easily understood by both specialist and non-specialist readers, produce a checklist for use by referees and authors, and produce a checklist for use by editors.

The BMJ guidelines contain 10 sections that are further grouped under three headings. The guidelines are designed for use in conjunction with other more general guidance to the authors from the BMJ and the BMJ guidelines on statistical methods. The three main headings are study design, data collection, and analysis and interpretation of the results. The list of the 10 sections with a brief description of each section follows.

Study design

(1) Study question This includes the hypothesis being tested or the research question, the importance of the research question, and the perspective or the viewpoint of the economic evaluation; that is, whether the study is being done from the perspective of the physician, the hospital, the patient, or the insurer.

(2) Selection of alternatives This section should include the rationale for the choice of alternative programs/interventions and a brief description of the alternative interventions.

(3) Form of evaluation The type of analysis used (CMA, CBA, CEA, or CUA) should be stated along with a justification for the use of that particular type of analysis.

Data collection

(4) Effectiveness data If the effectiveness data is based on a single effectiveness study, such as a clinical trial, details of the design and results of the study should be given; that is, it should include the selection of study population, method of randomization of the subjects, whether analyzed by intention to treat or evaluable cohort, and effect size with confidence intervals. If the economic evaluation is based on a number of effectiveness studies, details should be given of the method of synthesis or meta-analysis of evidence (e.g., search strategy, criteria for inclusion of studies).

(5) Benefit measurement and valuation The primary outcome measure(s) for the economic evaluation should be clearly stated (e.g., number of cases detected, life years, QALYs, willingness to pay). If a dollar amount has been attached to a health benefit, details of the methods used should be furnished (e.g., time trade-off, standard gamble, contingent valuation). If indirect benefits are included in the study, they should be reported separately and their relevance to the study question must be discussed.

(6) Cost information Quantities of resources should be reported separately from the prices (unit costs) of those resources. This will help the reader judge their relevance to his/her setting. The methods used for estimation of the quantities and prices (unit costs) should be given. The dates of both the estimates of resource quantities and prices should be recorded, along with details of any adjustments to a more recent price level.

(7) Modeling Details about any modeling technique used in the analysis, such as a decision-tree model, regression model, or epidemiologic model should be provided. A justification for the use of the model should also be included.

Analysis and interpretation of results

(8) Adjustments for timing of costs and benefits The time horizon over which costs and benefits are measured should be given. The discount rate used in the study, for adjustment of differences in the timing of costs, should be specified along with a justification for the specific rate used in the study. If costs and benefits are not discounted, a justification should be provided for not adjusting for differences in the timing of costs and benefits (e.g., all relevant costs and benefits occur within 1 to 2 years).

(9) Allowance for uncertainty Three broad types of uncertainty are possible: uncertainty related to observed data inputs; uncertainty relating to extrapolation; and uncertainty relating to analytical methods. The last two types of uncertainty are usually handled by sensitivity analysis. When a sensitivity analysis is performed, details should be given for the approach used (e.g., univariate, multivariate, threshold analysis, analysis of extremes, probabilistic sensitivity analysis). The researchers should provide justification for selection of variables used for carrying out the sensitivity analysis and the ranges over which the assumptions were varied.

(10) Presentation of results Results should be reported as incremental analyses (e.g., incremental cost per life saved). Major outcomes, such as impact on quality of life, should be presented as disaggregated as well as aggregated data. The answer to the original study question should be provided and any conclusions made should follow clearly from the data reported and should be accompanied by appropriate qualifications and/or limitations.

Besides providing guidelines for economic evaluation, the BMJ working party also created two checklists: one for use by the referees and the authors, and the other for use by editors. The checklist for the referees and the authors is a 35-item list, based on the three broad headings and the 10 sections that are described in the preceding list. Each of the 35 items are stated in the form of a question and the answers are to be marked as "Yes," "No," "Not Clear," or "Not Appropriate." The *study design* section contains questions pertaining to the research question and its appropriateness, the perspective used, the alternatives/comparisons used, and the form of economic evaluation (CBA, CEA, CUA). The *data collection* section contains questions pertaining to the sources of effectiveness estimates, whether the primary outcomes(s) are clearly stated, methods used to value health states, whether quantities of resources are reported separately from their unit costs, adjustment for inflation, and details of models used in the economic analysis. The *analysis and interpretation of results* section contains questions pertaining to discounting and discount rates used, details of statistical tests and confidence intervals, use of sensitivity analysis, whether incremental analysis was reported, whether the study question was answered, and whether conclusions follow from the data reported.

The checklist for the editors contains a short checklist and a partial evaluation checklist. *The short checklist* consists of four questions that are to be answered as "Yes," "No," or "Not Clear." The four questions in this checklist include whether the research question is stated, whether the sources of effectiveness claims (single study or multiple study) are clearly stated, whether the primary outcome(s) are clearly stated, and whether the methods used for estimation of quantities and unit costs are described.

The partial evaluation checklist contains six questions that pertain to whether the research question is important, whether the topic is of interest to BMJ, whether there is enough economic detail to allow peer review, whether the economic content is sound enough, and whether it is publishable (based on the design and the results of the analysis). The BMJ working party has stated that the working party "did not intend to be unduly prescriptive, rather their objectives were to improve the quality of submitted and published economic evaluations by agreeing acceptable methods and their systematic application, before, during, and after peer review."

Sacristán et al. published a checklist for evaluation of pharmacoeconomic studies in the *Annals of Pharmacotherapy*.[65] The checklist was created from the perspective of the hospital, the local government, and the pharmaceutical industry. The checklist contains 12 main sections, each of which is further divided into sub-sections. Each of the checklist item may be marked as "correct," "acceptable," "doubtful," "incorrect," or "not applicable." The following points are covered in the checklist: Does a well-defined question exist? Are the perspectives and the alternatives well-defined? Is the sample selection appropriate? Are the alternatives analyzed correctly? Are the costs up to date and is there an adjustment made for the costs? Is the type of analysis (e.g., CBA, CEA) correct? Is marginal analysis performed? Are the assumptions and limitations of the study discussed? Finally, are the conclusions justified and are they generalizable?

There have been criticisms regarding the use of a checklist for pharmacoeconomic studies. Joel Hay has questioned the applicability of checklists to economic studies.[66] Hay states that checklists are convenient in determining whether a routine procedure has been performed according to a standard protocol, as in a clinical trial or an experiment. However, pharmacoeconomic studies do not have standard protocols, and hence checklists will never be applicable to such studies. With reference to the checklist published by Sacristán et al. in the *Annals of Pharmacotherapy* (discussed in the previous paragraph), Hay claims that nothing in the checklist helps the reader determine whether the calculations presented in the study are correct, even if all of the items in the checklist are done. Hay gives the example of the Australian guidelines to support his position. According to Hay, the Australian guidelines for pharmacoeconomic studies are designed primarily with the political objective of constraining the rapid growth in government expenditure on new drugs rather than in guaranteeing that drugs and other health care resources are used equitably and efficiently by the population. He argues that if Australia had been truly interested in medical efficiency considerations, the same economic guidelines would have applied to existing drug therapies, including older generic drugs that are often being used in questionable circumstances. Hay suggests that the Australian government would be better off taxing drug manufacturers, rather than having drug manufacturers spend huge amounts of money to meet the Australian pharmacoeconomic approval process. Hay goes to the extent of calling checklists "a waste of time."

The debate on the value and applicability of standards and checklists is likely to continue.[67] It appears that at the current time most checklists required by various journals are basically derived from the 10 basic steps of pharmacoeconomics that were proposed by Bootman et al.[68] The 10 steps essentially are: establish a perspective; specify the treatment alternatives; specify outcomes for each treatment; specify the health care resources consumed; assign dollar values; specify and monitor non-health care resources consumed; specify the unit of outcome measurement; specify the non-economic attributes of the alternatives; analyze the data; and perform a sensitivity analysis. The checklists proposed by various journals are modifications of these 10 basic steps of pharmacoeconomics. Adherence to these basic steps will make any economic study a more acceptable one.

PRESENTING PE INFORMATION FOR FORMULARY DECISION MAKING

In the past few years, the health care industry in the United States has seen a dramatic rise in the managed care industry. Managed care companies, by their sheer size, can strategically negotiate drug prices. This has led pharmaceutical companies to shift emphasis away from the traditional marketing campaigns aimed at health care providers toward campaigns aimed at health plan purchasing managers.[69] The pharmacoeconomic study is one such tool that has been increasingly used by pharmaceutical companies to demonstrate that their product provides the best value for money. This is evidenced by the fact that by 1994 an average of 24 pharmacoeconomic studies were being conducted by pharmaceutical companies compared with fewer than two studies 6 years prior to 1994.[69]

Pharmacoeconomic studies generally compare a pharmaceutical therapy's costs and outcomes to those of an alternative intervention. Health care decision makers use this information to make decisions about pharmaceutical therapies. However, as more economic evaluations have been published, particularly in medical journals, a number of concerns have been raised. Hillman et al. suggested that there were a number of potential biases in industry-sponsored economic evaluations and suggested a tentative code of conduct.[2] Drummond suggested that the pharmaceutical industry needed to decide whether it regarded economic evaluations a science or merely a new marketing ploy.[19] The draft guidelines for submissions to the Drug Quality and Therapeutic Committee in Ontario, Canada, suggested that not only should the methods of economic evaluations be scrutinized but the ways in which the studies are commissioned and conducted should also be scrutinized.[17]

The Role of the FDA

Pharmacoeconomic studies may be considered as scientific information if their purpose is merely to provide information to health care providers or decision makers. However, when the same studies are used for promotional purposes, such as presenting the results of the study to managed care plans for formulary approval, they may fall into the class of promotional activities. This is where the FDA steps in, given its responsibility that decisions regarding pharmaceuticals and other medical products be based on "truthful and nonmisleading information" and to ensure that only "truthful and nonmisleading information" is passed on to the health care decision makers. In spring 1995, the FDA's division of Drug Marketing, Advertising, and Communications (DDMAC) issued draft guidelines, enumerating the principles it will use in reviewing pharmacoeconomic claims.[49] A pharmacoeconomic claim is defined in the draft as "pharmacoeconomic statements emanating from manufacturers or their agents in any of a wide variety of vehicles regulated by FDA as promotion, e.g. advertisements, formulary kits, publications distributed by the sales force." The guidelines state that pharmacoeconomic studies fall under the FDA's existing statutory authority, as per the FDA's jurisdiction to regulate and prohibit the misuse of drug labeling and advertising.[49] The guidelines stipulate that pharmacoeconomic claims should be compatible with existing rules prohibiting false and misleading promotion and must be consistent with, and not contrary to, approved product labeling. All comparative claims would be required to provide substantial evidence, typically demonstrated by two adequate and well-controlled studies. These include placebo, active, and historical controlled studies. The results of these studies should be presented in terms of physical units that represent resources utilized. The perspective of the study should be clearly specified.

Pharmacoeconomic studies would also be required to produce an adequate level of precision, scientific rigor, and validity (internal and external) to support the resulting claims and take into account both the positive and negative effects of the drug. Since the issuance of the proposed FDA guidelines, DDMAC has softened its position and has yet to publish the revised guidelines.

Regence BlueShield Requirements for Submission of Economic Data

While the FDA has resisted pressures to publish final guidelines, formulary decision makers are now requiring drug manufacturers to demonstrate economic evaluations for drug approvals into their formulary. Regence BlueShield, University of Washington, provides health care coverage to over one million members.[70] In December 1997, Regence BlueShield Pharmacy Services published guidelines for submission of economic data supporting formulary consideration. The purpose of the guidelines was to outline a format for manufacturers to identify, organize, and present data and supporting literature for evaluation. The guidelines, meant to be effective January 1998, require pharmaceutical manufacturers to submit safety, efficacy, and effectiveness information (including summaries of data, reprints of key published articles) in a standardized format and include outcomes modeling in the submission document. The modeling should include both medical outcomes (e.g., how many patients actually got well), as well as cost outcomes (impact of the drug on total drug costs, and on total medical claims costs). Regence pharmacy services staff, working with leading pharmacoeconomists, will conduct independent assessments of the modeling.

Regence BlueShield added that the purpose of the guidelines was not the simple reduction in drug costs, but rather the optimization of drug utilization given the environment of limited resources. The guidelines were produced in recognition of the fact that data from pharmacoeconomic studies were meant to aid in decision making, and not to replace the decision-making process. Regence BlueShield also states that the submission of economic evaluations does not guarantee approval of a product on the Regence BlueShield drug formulary.

GUIDANCE ON MEASURING QOL/PATIENT CONCERNS

The term quality of life (QOL) is described as the evaluation, by the patient, of the combination of factors that promotes a full life. It is the combination of the social, economic, physiological, functional, and psychological domains. It also encompasses the underlying factors that affect quality of life such as pain reduction/tolerance, activities of daily living, and sexual function.[71] QOL instruments follow standard procedural protocols or guidelines that assist the researcher to assess patient responses to questions about their current health status or function. The instruments are usually self-administered, given under the supervision of a health care provider, or in the case of the terminally or chronically ill, a surrogate may be responsible for the completion of these forms. Investigators may hire telephone interviewers to assist in capturing complete and accurate data.[72] Health care administrators are interested in quality of life assessments in order to negotiate the high-cost expenditures of some of their patients. These high-cost patients are usually the chronically ill. Therefore, it is noted that payers are interested in a method to measure the quality of care and clinical effectiveness in relation to their reimbursement decisions.[72]

Outcomes researchers utilize both generic instruments (i.e., general health profiles and utility assessments) and specific instruments (i.e., disease-specific assessments) to measure QOL. Health profile type instruments are either discriminative (they examine patient differences at a particular point in time) or evaluative (they examine the patient's change in a longitudinal manner).[72] The single numeric scores reported are used in economic-based cost analyses, usually referred to as CUA, the results of which may be presented in terms of cost-utility ratios, where the numerator incorporates the total incremental cost of care and the denominator equals the increased gain in QOL.

The CUA assists the decision-making process for program development and adoption of new health interventions by comparing program costs to the gain in the number of QALYs.[73] Although there are other methods to determine states of health—for example, the healthy-years equivalent (HYE)[74] and the willingness to pay approach,[75] QALY is the most popular method for economic evaluation.[76]

CUA instruments follow two usual formats. In one type, when a response is obtained, patients are classified into categories and assigned a score, one that has been calculated from a previous group or study.[77] A second instrument, known as the standard gamble,[78] is based directly on the fundamental axioms of the von Neumann–Morgenstern (vNM) utility theory.[79] This approach asks the patient to choose between remaining in his/her own current health state or taking a gamble which involves a chance of attaining full health for the remainder of his/her life along with a risk of immediate death.[76] A simpler instrument is the time trade-off method, which asks the patient to determine the number of years of life in a compromised state of health that is equivalent to a set number of years of complete health.[78] In general, utility scores obtain the measurement of the patient's defined health status and health values.[72]

General assessment instruments, such as the Sickness Impact Profile (SIP), have been used in many specific studies such as total hip joint arthroplasty[80] and treatment of back pain.[81] The SIP has a physical dimension, a psychosocial dimension, and five independent categories that include eating, work, home, management, sleep, and rest, and recreations and pastimes.[77] The McMaster Health Index Questionnaire[82] identifies three dimensions: physical, emotional, and social. A well-respected instrument is the Medical Outcomes Study (MOS) 36-item Short-Form Health Survey (SF-36).[83] It is a comprehensive, yet non-taxing questionnaire that is designed to measure eight scales: physical functioning, role limitation (physical), social function, body pain, general mental health, role limitations (emotional), vitality, and general health perceptions. This instrument is easy to administer and is balanced in its construction with equally weighted scales. The questionnaire has been extensively validated and measures have been found to be applicable for a wide range of populations. Broad health concepts and precision of data collection is its trademark. Within the MOS SF-36, there are five (MHI-5) scales that have been used extensively to discriminate between patients with depression, severe affective disorders, and anxiety. The physical scales have been found to be discriminative for medical conditions with a high degree of confidence and have been generalizable both within and across various combinations of medical and psychiatric conditions.[84] However, this instrument does have its limitations, particularly within certain subgroups (e.g., the aged, the minorities, the less educated and lower income individuals). Instruments with larger type size and the use of easily understood words may assist data collection in these populations. In addition, the use of a telephone survey may be a more practical solution for certain population groups.[85]

Instruments that capture disease-specific data assist the investigator because they target therapeutic interventions that compare different interventions for specific medical conditions. Investigators that use a target population find that the response rate has a potential for increased responsiveness. In addition the results may be more easily analyzed by the clinician.[72] However, specific instruments have the disadvantage of not being comprehensive and cannot be used to compare across conditions or programs.[86]

A special area of concern facing the United States as we enter the new millennium is the quality of life for the very old and sick members of society. Generic assessments can be used as a preliminary measure to assist health professionals as they evaluate costs and quality of treatments for the chronically ill;[72] however, generic measures may not reflect the multiple changes occurring in elderly patients' lives. Examples of these changes are loss of status, loss of income, change in relationships (i.e., becoming dependent on those who may not appreciate the levels of personal adjustment that the elderly person is facing on a daily basis). In order to make a proper determination for the assignment of resources (financial, medical, social), the research community must address the needs of the elderly, noting any necessary accommodations required to capture accurate and complete data. This process is three-fold and requires careful planned use of the instruments during construction, administration, and interpretation phases.

QOL instrument construction for the elderly, and especially for those with advanced cancer and signs of depression, needs to follow specific guidelines. As noted in the LEIPAD,[87] an internationally applicable instrument to assess quality of life in the elderly, a multidimensional evaluation instrument is most useful with this special population. This study suggests the following for the construction of this type of instrument: (1) be short in length, but include a variety of QOL domains; (2) use a subjective approach; (3) contain a cross-cultural validity; (4) use separate modular subscales for the domains; (5) be aware of individual personality characteristics; and (6) be sensitive to changes brought about by medical or social treatment. The LEIPAD team suggests that a study for the elderly must be developed for use in multiple setting: private homes, hospitals, rest homes, and transcultural settings. Specific domains suggested for inclusion in a questionnaire include mental status, social and occupational status, pain, and the more subjective domains of self-esteem, optimism, anxiety, depression, and mood disorders.

The following is a list of a few other instruments that have been found to be appropriate for the elderly. The UNISCALE,[88] which uses single-item visual-analog scales, requests that the patient places an X on a horizontal rectangle that rates his/her QOL for the past week.[89] The FLIC[90] is a 22-item Likert visual-analogy self-reporting scale. The items are scored from 1 to 7, with different anchors for each item such as "always = 1" to "never = 7" or "not at all = 1" to "a great deal = 7."[86] The Quality of Life Index (QLI) was the first instrument to rate individuals on their view of personal well-being.[85] This five-item instrument offers the respondent the choice of choosing "0" (positive), "1" (neutral), or "2" (negative) for each item. The Zung Self-Rating Depression Scale (ZSDS)[91] is a 20-item questionnaire that rank responses from 1–4 on how the person felt during the previous week. The questionnaire has cut-off scores that break into four categories. This instrument does depict items of clinical significance, even though the scores do not necessarily correspond to the DSM-IV (ed 4).[92] The FACT is multidimensional and has specific subscales that assess patient status and augment patient interviews. In addition, the FACT-G can provide a global measure of HRQOL, while the specific subscales provide information into functional, physical, social, and emotional dimensions that may affect perceived outcome and rehabilitation.[93]

The administrative processing of these instruments should facilitate the completion of the forms by the elderly. For best results, data collection should be requested just before a health assessment.[89] If multiple questionnaires are presented, as in the case of a randomized clinical trial, the questionnaire with the most relevance to the other arms of the study should be presented first. This will aid in data collection, especially if the respondent tires easily and would not be able to complete the other assessment tools. The questionnaire should be presented in an attractive, easy-to-read language, possibly with large print, and should not appear to overburden the respondent. There is anecdotal information noted that if patients have 15 minutes to wait to be seen by the doctor, the administration of an instrument may be a good anxiety reducer.

A recurring theme concerning the accurate interpretation of QOL measures has been noted in studies involving the patient–physician relationship.[89] Physicians are focused on the physical aspects of QOL while the patient focuses on the psychosocial aspects of coping with their disease. In a study involving 25 ambulatory oncology clinics affiliated with Community Cancer Care, Inc., Indiana, physicians were able to recognize mild depression in their patients; however, physicians accurately classified only 20 of 159 moderately to severely depressed patients, and rated 78 of these patients as having essentially no depressive symptoms.[92] This lack of recognition has an impact on the assignment of resources for mental health. If physicians are not aware of the needs of their patients, the medical records are inaccurate. As hospital administrators make recommendations for the allocation of funds, using these same medical records, there is a chance that the funding will prove to be inaccurately assessed. This error in data collection is an example of the purpose of the QOL instruments—to accurately assess the needs of the patients in order to allocate funds, and to determine which therapeutic methods are giving the greatest relief to the population in question.

When selecting an inventory for a research study, items such as patient cognitive function, literacy, the patient's time involvement, and the method of test administration need to be addressed. How are instruments selected for administration to a particular group? There are three methods available to the researcher.[75] Usually a judgment is made using expert opinion or by the use of a convenience sample. Researchers then proceed with a sensitivity analysis to determine the robustness of the conclusions. A second method is to use existing utility values available in the literature. Here the researcher must match the sample in question with subjects from a previous sample. Frequently, researchers can examine disease-specific instruments to assist with this process. The third method is for the researcher to obtain current utility measures. An example of this process is to make a classification system, to select a sample population, to develop a rating-scale, and to perform sensitivity analyses on the utility. Assessments undertaken using a combination of disease-specific and general health profile QOL instruments offer greater insight as to the treatment impact on QOL than when only a disease-specific or a general QOL tool is used.[94]

For further information on QOL assessment instruments, begin your search on the internet at http://www.glamm.com/ql/url.htm. This internet source is an excellent example of how information technology can assist physicians, administrators, and consumers increase their knowledge in the area of QOL. This site also increases the awareness of the need to understand the value of rigorous scientific methods in research and development. At this site visitors will find assessment instruments, a listing of major organizations and research groups, information on disease, symptoms and special populations, methodology, listings of journals, and a variety of directories.

GENERAL VERSUS DISEASE-SPECIFIC GUIDELINES

It may be unreasonable to assume that any set of guidelines will address all drugs, diseases, and populations. Acute and chronic conditions might require different methodologies since the relevant time frame and ability to influence future events may vary. Similarly, low-prevalent, high-cost illnesses might require different forms of evaluation than high-prevalent, low-cost diseases. Finally, illnesses that have significant impact on patient subjective measures but low impact on managed care bottom lines may be analyzed differently than those that have significant impact on provider expenditures and profits. In all of these cases, there is reason to question whether disease-specific guidelines would be preferable to universal "one stop shopping" guidelines, especially since general guidelines tend to be vague.

Each disease may require its own set of guidelines for pharmacoeconomic evaluation. Alternatively, a set of principles could be developed that would provide general guidance. Then, more prescriptive guidance could be developed that would suggest variation or extension from those general principles for applications to specific diseases. In the extreme, guidelines could be developed at the therapeutic class level; however, at some point, the development and approval of guidelines at the micro level begins to approach the standard review process for published literature. Economic efficiency argues that guidelines should not approach the boundary of replacing peer review.

Psychopharmacology is one example of a class of agents where disease-specific methods have been applied to CEA. Evaluation of pharmacologic therapies for major depression should be tailored to address the impact of treatment on patient functioning and well-being, and the comparators and complimentary treatment modalities that may affect patient outcomes. This latter concern would include outpatient primary care and psychiatrist services, medications, emergency room and inpatient services, electroconvulsive therapy, psychological counseling, and laboratory services.[95] The focus on antipsychotic medications stems from their controversial premium prices, litigation, and extensive press coverage regarding the bundling of clozapine with weekly white cell monitoring, and increased prior authorization requirements for drugs like clozapine and risperidone.[96]

Other illnesses where disease-specific guidance has been proposed include acute myocardial infarction,[97] cancer,[98,99] coronary heart disease,[100] duodenal ulcers,[101] gastroesophageal reflux disease,[102,103] NSAID-induced gastropathy,[104] and other illnesses. Class specific cost-effectiveness has been examined for ACE inhibitors in patients with chronic heart failure[105] and for calcium channel blockers for patients with reduced left ventricular function.[106]

CONCLUSION

Many guidelines for outcomes research and pharmacoeconomic studies have been developed. There are common themes that are covered in most published sets of recommendations; however, a number of controversies continue to be discussed. The lack of agreement has led to skepticism on the part of certain decision makers, but has provided a format for debate which may likely result in improved methodologies. As the disciplines of outcomes research and pharmacoeconomics continue to evolve, enhanced guidelines will need to address both the scientific rigor of studies and the usefulness of analysis and results to decision makers. In the past, guidelines have addressed broad topics with few specific recommendations. Future guidelines may emerge for disease-specific methodologies.

REFERENCES

1. Gold MR, Siegel JE, Russell LB, et al., eds: *Cost-Effectiveness in Health and Medicine*. New York: Oxford University Press; 1996.
2. Hillman AL, Eisenberg JM, Pauly MV, et al.: Avoiding bias in the conduct and reporting of cost-effectiveness research sponsored by pharmaceutical companies. *New Engl J Med* 1991;324(19):1362–1365.
3. Rittenhouse BE: Is there a need for standardization of methods in economic evaluations of medicine? *Med Care* 1996;34(12):DS13–DS22.
4. Luce BR: Working toward a common currency: is standardization of cost-effectiveness analysis possible? *J Acq Immune Def Syndr Hum Retrovirol* 1995;10(Suppl 4):S19–S22.

5. Mullins CD, Ogilvie S: Emerging standardization in pharmacoeconomics. *Clin Therap* 1998;20(6):1194–1202.
6. Weinstein MC, Stason WB: Foundations of cost-effectiveness analysis for health and medical practices. *New Engl J Med* 1977;296(13):716–721.
7. Elixhauser A, Luce BR, Taylor WR, et al.: Health care CBA/CEA: an update on the growth and composition of the literature. *Med Care* 1993;31(Suppl 7):JS1–JS11, JS18–JS149.
8. Elixhauser A, Halpern M, Schmier J, et al.: Health care CBA and CEA from 1991 to 1996: an updated bibliography. *Med Care* 1998;36(Suppl 5):MS1–MS9, MS18–MS147.
9. Diener A, O'Brien B, Gafni A: Health care contingent valuation studies: a review and classification of the literature. *Health Econ* 1998;7(4):313–326.
10. Luce BR: Cost-effectiveness analysis: obstacles to standardisation and its use in regulating pharmaceuticals. *Pharmacoeconomics* 1993;3(1):1–9.
11. Guyatt G, Drummond M, Feeny D, et al.: Guidelines for the clinical and economic evaluation of health care technologies. *Soc Sci Med* 1986;22(4):393–408.
12. Drummond MF: The future of pharmacoeconomics: bridging science and practice. *Clin Therap* 1996;18(5):969–978; discussion 968.
13. Pausjenssen AM, Detsky AS: Guidelines for measuring the costs and consequences of adopting new pharmaceutical products: are they on track? *Med Decision Making* 1998;18(2):S19–S22.
14. Thwaites R, Townsend RJ: Pharmacoeconomics in the new millennium. A pharmaceutical industry perspective. *Pharmacoeconomics* 1998;13(2):175–180.
15. Neumann PJ: Paying the piper for pharmacoeconomic studies. *Med Decision Making* 1998;18(2):S23–S26.
16. Cahill NE: Caveats in interpreting and applying pharmacoeconomic data. *Am J Health-Syst Pharm* 1995;52(Suppl 4):S24–S26.
17. Drummond MF: Guidelines for pharmacoeconomic studies: The ways forward. *Pharmacoeconomics* 1994;6(6):493–497.
18. Draugalis JR, Coons SJ: Pharmacoeconomic research—facilitating collaboration among academic institutions, managed-care organizations, and the pharmaceutical industry: a conference report. *Clin Therap* 1995;17(1):89–108, discussion 88.
19. Drummond MF: Issues in the conduct of economic evaluations of pharmaceutical products. *Pharmacoeconomics* 1994;6(5):405–411.
20. Drummond M, Brandt A, Luce B, et al.: Standardizing methodologies for economic evaluation in health care. *Int J Technol Assess Health Care* 1993;9(1):26–36.

21. Freund DA: Initial development of the Australian guidelines. *Med Care* 1996;34(12 Suppl):DS211–DS215.
22. Langley PC: The role of pharmacoeconomic guidelines for formulary approval: The Australian experience. *Clin Therap* 1993;15(6):1154–1176; discussion 1120.
23. Anonymous: Speaking from experience: Australia. *Med Care* 1996;34(12 Suppl):DS233–DS235.
24. Mitchell A: Update and evaluation of Australian guidelines: Government perspective. *Med Care* 1996;34(12 Suppl):DS216–DS225.
25. Hailey D: Australian economic evaluation and government decisions on pharmaceuticals, compared to assessment of other health technologies. *Soc Sci & Med* 1997;45(4):563–581.
26. Canadian Coordinating Office for Health Technology Assessment: *Guidelines for Economic Evaluation of Pharmaceuticals: Canada*, 1st edn. Ottawa, Ontario: CCOHTA; November 1994.
27. CCOHTA. Report from the Canadian Coordinating Office for Health Technology Assessment (CCOHTA): Guidelines for economic evaluation of pharmaceuticals: Canada. *Int J Technol Assess Health Care* 1995;11(4):796–797.
28. Menon D, Schubert F, Torrance GW: Canada's new guidelines for the economic evaluation of pharmaceuticals. *Med Care* 1996;34(12 Suppl):DS77–DS86.
29. Alban A, Gyldmark M, Pedersen AV, et al.: The Danish approach to standards for economic evaluation methodologies. *Pharmacoeconomics* 1997;12(6):627–636.
30. Garattini L, Grilli R, Scopelliti D, et al.: A proposal for Italian guidelines in pharmacoeconomics. *Pharmacoeconomics* 1995;7(1):1–6.
31. Badia X, Rovira J, Segu JI, et al.: Economic assessment of drugs in Spain. *Pharmacoeconomics* 1994;5:123–129.
32. Lovatt B: The United Kingdom guidelines for the economic evaluation of medicines. *Med Care* 1996;34(12 Suppl):DS179–DS181.
33. Drummond M, Cooke J, Walley T: Economic evaluation under managed competition: evidence from the U.K. *Soc Sci & Med* 1997;45(4):583–595.
34. Hillman AL: Summary of economic analysis of health care technology: a report on principles. *Med Care* 1996;34(12 Suppl):DS193–DS196.
35. PhRMA: Methodological and conduct principles for pharmacoeconomic research. Washington, DC: Pharmaceutical Research and Manufacturers of America (PhRMA); 1995.
36. Rovira J: Standardization of the economic evaluation of health technologies: European developments. *Med Care* 1996;34(12 Suppl):DS182–DS188.

37. Annemans L, Crott R, De Clercq H, et al.: Pricing and reimbursement of pharmaceuticals in Belgium. *Pharmacoeconomics* 1997;11(3):203–209.
38. Le Pen C: Pharmaceutical economy and the economic assessment of drugs in France. *Soc Sci & Med* 1997;45(4):635–643.
39. Schulenburg J: Economic evaluation of medical technologies: from theory to practice—The German perspective. *Soc Sci & Med* 1997;45(4):621–633.
40. Ikeda S, Ikegami N, Oliver AJ, Ikeda M: A case for the adoption of pharmacoeconomic guidelines in Japan. *Pharmacoeconomics* 1996;10(6):546–551.
41. Harron DW: Pharmacoeconomics: quality use of quality medicines and its impact on the Middle East. *Int Pharm J* 1995;9:161–163.
42. Elsinga E, Rutten F: Economic evaluation in support of national health policy: the case of the Netherlands. *Soc Sci & Med* 1997;45(4):605–620.
43. Grund J, Husbyn H: Role of pharmacoeconomics in health policy and management in Norway. *Pharmacoeconomics* 1995;7:475–483.
44. Jönsson B: Economic evaluation of medical technologies in Sweden. *Soc Sci & Med* 1997;45(4):597–604.
45. Johnson JA, Friesen E: Reassessing the relevance of pharmacoeconomics analyses in formulary decisions. *Pharmacoeconomics* May (Part 1) 1998;13:479–485.
46. Langley PC: The FDA and pharmacoeconomic guidelines. *Drug Benefit Trends* 1997;9(1):17–20,25.
47. Torrance GW, Blaker D, Detsky A: Canadian guidelines for economic evaluation of pharmaceuticals. Canadian Collaborative Workshop for Pharmacoeconomics. *Pharmacoeconomics* Jun 1996;9(6):535–539.
48. Canadian Coordinating Office for Health Technology Assessment: *Guidelines for Economic Evaluation of Pharmaceuticals: Canada*, 2nd edn. Ottawa: CCOHTA; 1997.
49. DDMAC: *Principles for the Review of Pharmacoeconomic Promotion.* Division of Drug Marketing, Advertising and Communications (DDMAC) Draft Report. Rockville, MD: Food and Drug Administration (FDA); March 20 1995.
50. Genduso LA, Kotsanos JG: Review of health economic guidelines in the form of regulations, principles, policies, and positions. *Drug Inform J* 1996;30:1003–1016.
51. Pauly MV: Valuing health care benefits in money terms. In: Sloan FA, ed., *Valuing Health Care.* New York: Cambridge University Press; 1995; 99–124.
52. Stergachis A: Overview of cost-consequence modeling in outcomes research. *Pharmacotherapy* 1995;15(5 pt 2):40S–42S.

53. Grabowski HG, Mullins CD: Pharmacy benefit management, cost-effectiveness analysis and drug formulary decisions. *Soc Sci & Med* 1997;45(4):535–544.
54. O'Brien B: Economic evaluation of pharmaceuticals: Frankenstein's monster or vampire of trials? *Med Care* 1996;34(12):DS99–DS108.
55. Drummond MF, Stoddart GL, Torrance GW: *Methods for the Economic Evaluation of Health Care Programmes*. Oxford: Oxford University Press; 1987.
56. Russell LB: *Is Prevention Better than Cure?* Washington, DC: Brookings Institution; 1986.
57. Mark DB, Hlatky MA, Califf RM, et al.: Cost effectiveness of thrombolytic therapy with tissue plasminogen activator as compared with streptokinase for acute myocardial infarction. *New Engl J Med* 1995;332:1418–1424.
58. Hltaky MA, Rogers WJ, Johnstone I, et al.: Medical care costs and quality of life after randomization to coronary angioplasty or coronary bypass surgery. *New Engl J Med* 1997;336(2):92–99.
59. Drummond MF, Jefferson TO: Guidelines for authors and peer reviewers of economic submissions to the BMJ. *Br Med J* 1996;313:275–283.
60. Viscusi WK: Discounting health effects for medical decisions. In: Sloan FA, ed., *Valuing Health Care*. New York: Cambridge University Press; 1995;125–147.
61. Udvarhelyi S, Colditz GA, Rai A, et al.: Cost-effectiveness and cost-benefit analysis in the medical literature: are the methods being used correctly? *Ann Intern Med* 1992;116:238–244.
62. Bradley CA, Iskedjian M, Lanctôt KL, et al.: Quality assessment of economic evaluations in selected pharmacy, medical, and health economics journals. *Ann Pharmacother* 1995;29:681–689.
63. Schulman K, Sulmasy DP, Roney D: Ethics, economics, and the publication of policies of major medical journals. *J Am Med Assoc (JAMA)* 1994;272(2):154–156.
64. Kassirer JP, Angell M: The journal's policy on cost-effectiveness analyses. *New Engl J Med* 1994;331(16):669–670.
65. Sacristán JA, Soto J, Galende I: Evaluation of pharmacoeconomic studies: utilization of a checklist. *Ann Pharmacother* 1993;27:1126–1233.
66. Hay JW: Comment: evaluation of pharmacoeconomic studies: utilization of a checklist. *Ann Pharmacother* 1994;28(4):539.
67. Jefferson T, Smith R, Yee Y, et al.: Evaluating the BMJ guidelines for economic submissions: prospective audit of economic submissions to BMJ and the *Lancet*. *J Am Med Assoc (JAMA)* 1998;280(3):275–277.

68. Bootman JL, Townsend RJ, McGhan WF: *Principles of Pharmacoeconomics*. Cincinnati, OH: Harvey Whitney Books Company; 1991.
69. Neumann PJ, Zinner DE, Paltiel AD: The FDA and regulation of cost-effectiveness claims. *Health Affairs* 1996;15(3):54–71.
70. Sullivan S, Mather D, Augenstein D, et al.: Regence BlueShield Pharmacy Services: *Guidelines for the Submission of Clinical and Economic Data Supporting Formulary Consideration*. Regence BlueShield, University of Washington, Version 1.3, December 1997.
71. Spilker B, ed.: *Quality of Life and Pharmacoeconomics in Clinical Trials*, 2nd edn. Philadelphia, PA: Lippincott-Raven Publications; 1996.
72. Guyatt GH, Feeny DH, Patrick DL: Measuring health-related quality of life. *Ann Inter Med* 1993;118(8):622–629.
73. Freund DA, Dittus RS: Principles of pharmacoeconomic analysis of drug therapy. *Pharmacoeconomics* 1992;1(1):20–29.
74. Mehrez A, Gafni A: Quality-adjusted life-years, utility theory, and healthy-years equivalents. *Med Decision Making* 1989;9(2):142–149.
75. Thompson MS: Willingness to pay and accept risk to cure chronic disease. *Am J Publ Health* 1986;76(4):392–396.
76. Drummond M: The role and importance of quality of life measurements in economic evaluations. *Br J Med Econ* 1992;4:9–16.
77. Jaeschke R, Guyatt GH, Cook D: Quality of life instruments in the evaluation of new drugs. *Pharmacoeconomics* 1992;1(2):84–93.
78. Torrance GW: Measurement of health state utilities for economic appraisal: a review. *J Health Econ* 1986;5:1–30.
79. Mehrez A, Gafni A: Evaluating health related quality of life: an indifference curve interpretation for the time trade-off technique. *Soc Sci & Med* 1990;31(11):1281–1283.
80. Liang MH, Larson MG, Cullen KE, et al.: Comparative measurement efficiency and sensitivity of five health status instruments for arthritis research. *Arthritis and Rheumatism* 1985;28:542–547.
81. Deyo RA, Diehl AK, Rosenthal M: How many days of bed rest for acute low back pain? A randomized clinical trial. *New Engl J Med* 1986;315:1064–1070.
82. Sacket DL, Chambers LW, MacPherson AS, et al.: The development and application of indices of health: general methods and a summary of results. *Am J Publ Health* 1977;67(5):423–428.
83. Ware JE, Sherbourne CD: The MOS 36-Item Short-Form Health Survey (SF-36). I. Conceptual framework and item selection. *Med Care* 1992;30(6):473–483.
84. McHorney CA, Ware JE, Raczek AE: The MOS 36-Item Short-Form Health Survey (SF-36): II. Psychometric and clinical tests of validity in

measuring physical and mental health constructs. *Med Care* 1993;31(3):247–263.

85. McHorney CA, Ware JE, Lu JFR, et al.: The MOS 36-item Short-Form Health Survey (SF-36): III. Tests of data quality, scaling assumptions, and reliability across diverse patient groups. *Med Care* 1994;32(1):40–66.
86. Bombardier C, Ware J, Russel IJ.: Auranofin therapy and quality of life in patients with rheumatoid arthritis: results of a multicenter trial. *Am J Med* 1986;81:565–578.
87. De Leo D, Diekstra RFW, Lonnqvist J, et al.: LEIPAD, internationally applicable instrument to assess quality of life in the elderly. *Behav Med* 1998;24:17–27.
88. Spitzer WO, Dobson AJ, Hall J, et al.: Measuring the quality of life of cancer patients. A concise QL-index for use by physicians. *J Chron Dis* 1981;34:585–597.
89. Sloan JA, Laprinzi CL, Kuross SA, et al.: Randomized comparison of four tools measuring overall quality of life in patients with advanced cancer. *J Clin Oncol* 1998;16(11):3662–3673.
90. Pocock SJ, Simon R: Sequential treatment assignment with balancing for prognostic factors in the controlled clinical trial. *Biometrics* 1975;31:103–115.
91. Zung WWK: A self-rating depression scale. *Arch Gen Psych* 1965;12:63–70.
92. Passik SD, Dugan W, et al.: Oncologists' recognition of depression in their patients with cancer. *J Clin Oncol* 1998;16(4):1594–1600.
93. D'Antonio LL, Long SA, Zimmerman GJ, et al.: Relationship between quality of life and depression in patients with head and neck cancer. *The Laryngoscope* 1998;108:806–811.
94. Boyer JG, Townsend RJ: Quality of life: methodologies in pharmacoepidemiologic studies. In: Hartezema AG, Porta MS, Tilson HH, eds., *Pharmacoepidemiology: An Introduction*, 2nd edn. Cincinnati, OH: Harvey Whitney Press; 1991.
95. Revicki DA, Luce BR: Pharmacoeconomics research applied to psychopharmacology development and evaluation. *Psychopharmacol Bull* 1995;31(4):45–53.
96. Hargreaves WA, Shumway M: Pharmacoeconomics of antipsychotic drug therapy. *J Clin Psych* 1996;57(Suppl 9):66–76.
97. Castillo PA, Palmer CS, Halpern MT, et al.: Cost-effectiveness of thrombolytic therapy for acute myocardial infarction. *Ann Pharmacother* 1997;31(5):596–603.
98. Arikian SR, Suver J, Einarson T, et al.: Economic and quality of life outcomes: the four-step pharmacoeconomic research model. *Oncology* 1995;9(11 Suppl):33–36.

99. Bishop JF, Macarounas-Kirchman K: The pharmacoeconomics of cancer therapies. *Sem Oncol* 1997;24(6 Suppl 19):S19-106–S-19-111.
100. Szucs TD: Pharmacoeconomic aspects of lipid-lowering therapy: is it worth the price? *Eur Heart J* 1998;19(Suppl M):M22–M28.
101. O'Brien B, Goeree R, Hunt R, et al.: Cost effectiveness of alternative *Helicobacter pylori* eradication strategies in the management of duodenal ulcers. *Can J Gastroenterol* 1997;11(4):323–331.
102. Bate CM, Richardson PD: Clinical and economic factors in the selection of drugs for gastroesophageal reflux disease. *Pharmacoeconomics* 1993;3(2):94–99.
103. Sadowski D, Champion M, Goeree R, et al.: Health economics of gastroesophageal reflux disease. *Can J Gastroenterol* 1997;11(Suppl B):108B–112B.
104. Goldstein JL, Larson LR, Yamashita BD, et al.: Management of NSAID-induced gastropathy: an economic decision analysis. *Clin Therap* 1997;19(6):1496–1509.
105. McMurray J, Davie A: The pharmacoeconomics of ACE inhibitors in chronic heart failure. *Pharmacoeconomics* 1996;9(3):188–197.
106. Goldberg Arnold RJ, Kaniecki DJ, Frishman WH: Cost-effectiveness of antihypertensive agents in patients with reduced left ventricular function. *Pharmacotherapy* 1994;14(2):178–184.

C H A P T E R

12

Pharmacoeconomic Applications

Peter Mok
and
F. Randy Vogenberg

PHARMACOECONOMIC APPLICATIONS IN PRACTICE

Now that pharmacoeconomic methods and various applications have been discussed, we would like to bring together these concepts and apply them in practice.

Most of us are practitioners, not researchers or economists focused only on economic analysis. This fact, however, does not prevent us from using economic tools to make decisions in our practice settings.

Practitioners in health care understand the term "outcome," best described by Donabedian[1] as the end product resulting from the processing by providers of structured inputs and resources. Readers of the US Public Health Service publication, *Morbidity and Mortality Weekly Report* (*MMWR*) can also find many guidelines and examples of outcome assessment from a public health perspective. In this chapter we create some examples to help our reader understand how outcomes evolve as a result of pharmacoeconomic assessment of the impact of medications in different health care environments.

In the following application examples, we illustrate assessment concepts and quantitative relationships to review concepts without the in-depth discussion of statistical techniques covered elsewhere in this book:

1. Cost-minimization analysis.
2. Cost of illness (or disease) analysis.
3. Cost-effectiveness analysis.
4. Cost-benefit analysis.
5. Meta-analysis.
6. Cost-utility analysis.

BASIC STEPS OF ASSESSMENTS

We use the following steps in each example:

1. *Identify the outcome measurement we want as our metric.* How are we going to show improvement or establish an appropriate baseline from which we can measure periodic changes in a patient care outcome? The measure chosen must be easily obtained from our practice setting, reproducible over time, and appropriately relate to the clinical practice being studied.
2. *Establish the assumptions we are making and the conditions of practice in which the measurements are made.* Certain variables will be assigned with an arbitrary estimate. These values can be based on information we have measured in our own practice, on referenced publications, or on reasonable estimates, e.g., by key members of the Pharmacy and Therapeutics Committee. These values can be argued, because our practice settings are all different. Our objective is to show how the outcome evolves based on our own situations and assumptions. Also, depending on the perspective one takes, these values and estimates will also differ. For example, CDC usually looks at societal costs, which have much broader and deeper implications than the cost to one individual institution. One could also take the consumer's perspective in cost estimates and arrive at very different results from both of the above perspectives. For all our examples, we limit our cost estimates to the viewpoint of the provider or providing organization, e.g., a managed care group.
3. *Calculate the variables.* Identification of the issues (variables) to be addressed that may alter or change our results needs to be carried out. Quantification of those variables and how it/they may impact our outcome assessment must be done.
4. *Arrive at the outcome measurements we desire.* This is the result of our study and corresponding calculations which takes us to the final step.

5. *Find out what the outcome is*: the interpretation of the outcome measurement results.

EXAMPLES OF ASSESSMENT

Example 1. Cost-Minimization Analysis

This assessment model is comparable to how most of us do comparisons shopping for daily use items. We try to compare different products for a purpose (outcome) primarily based on package and handling costs.

In this example, we pick a simple health care or therapeutic problem to make it easier to understand. Let us do a cost-minimization analysis by comparing the costs of eardrops in treating patients with impacted earwax.

Outcome measurements desired Cost minimization for common eardrops used for the removal of impacted earwax for 500 outpatients.

Assumptions and conditions

1. Treatment is for patients with impacted earwax, with no history of perforated eardrums.
2. Adverse outcome is averted; i.e., impacted earwax was removed successfully without problems.
3. Number of outpatients treated is 500.
4. Duration for treatment is less than 5 days.
5. No compliance and failure problems are found.

Medication alternatives compared:

Rx a	polypeptide oleate mixture (6 ml)
Rx b	carbamide peroxide (15 ml)
Rx c	mineral oil and hydrogen peroxide USP (15 ml of each prepackaged separately)

	Rx a	Rx b	Rx c*
Acquisition cost	$21.26	$1.25	$0.06
Dispensing costs (parts & labor)	$6.00	$6.00	$7.00

(Rx c requires filling the liquids in two containers; thus we assign an extra cost.)

Calculations

	Rx a	Rx b	Rx c
Total cost per Rx	$37.26	$7.25	$7.06

Outcome measurements

Total cost 500 Rx's	$18,630.00	$3,625.00	$3,530.00

Outcome findings

Rx C leads to cost minimization.
Rx A is 527% of the cost of Rx C.

Example 2. Cost of Illness/Disease Analysis

For this exercise, let us estimate the cost of an illness to our institution. We will use impacted earwax as our example.

Let us estimate the total cost of resolving the problem of impacted earwax for 500 patients if the problem is untreated by medications. The problem will eventually require physical removal of the cerumen (earwax). This will include direct and indirect costs.

Outcome measurements desired To estimate the total cost of the problem of impacted earwax without medications: i.e., physical removal of earwax for 500 patients.

Assumptions

1. The earwax will need to be removed by syringe and/or curettage in a special appointment. The cost of the appointment, including time, labor, and materials will be $90 for each patient. This is the direct cost.
2. For every 500 patients going through this procedure, one will result in an accidental perforation of the eardrum. This will require extra time, evaluation and care, resulting in time and follow-up costs of $2000. This is the indirect cost.

Calculations

Direct costs = 500 patients × $90/patient = $45,000

Indirect costs = $2,000

Outcome measurement

Total costs of resolving illness for 500 patients = $47,000

Example 3. Cost-Effectiveness Analysis

Let us apply the earwax treatments to a cost-effectiveness analysis:

Cost-effectiveness = net cost/net effectiveness (or adverse outcomes averted)[2]

Let us define our net effectiveness as averting impacted earwax for 500 patients with medication therapy. We define our net cost in achieving this as the sum of the costs of drugs and costs due to side effects and noncompliance treatments.

Outcome measurements desired Estimating cost-effectiveness for three common eardrops used for the resolution of impacted earwax in 500 outpatients in our organization.

Assumptions and conditions

1. Medications and packaged costs are the same as in Example 1.
2. Assumptions 1–3 are the same as in Example 1.
3. Costs of treatment depends on the effectiveness of each choice—direct side-effect costs and noncompliance costs are to be included as follows:

Side effects Side effects require extra visits. Costs are $70 per visit:

Visits caused by local irritation

	Rx a*	Rx b	Rx c
Per 500 patients	30	5	5

*Rx a has been reported to cause more irritations

Compliance failures Compliance failures require extra prescriptions to re-treat. Repeat prescriptions for re-treating non-adherence are:

Per 500 patients	25	50	100

(Note: Mineral Oil and Peroxide Rx c are used p.m. and a.m. respectively; i.e., more difficult to comply. Polypeptide oleate (Rx a) requires the least applications.

Calculations

	Rx a	Rx b	Rx c
Side effect costs:			
Extra visits/500 patients	30	5	5
Cost of visits @ $70	$2,100	$350	$350
Compliance failure costs:			
Repeat Rx's/500 patients	25	50	100
Cost per Rx (from Example 1)	$37.26	$7.25	$7.06
Cost of repeat Rx's	$931.50	$362.50	$706.00

Net costs

Drug costs for 500 patients	$18,630.00	$3,625.00	$3,530.00
+ side effect costs	$2,100.00	$350.00	$350.00
+ compliance failure costs	$931.50	$362.50	$706.00
	$21,661.50	$4,337.50	$4,586.00

Outcomes measured

Cost-effectiveness or net costs for resolving impacted earwax for 500 patients in our organization are $21,661.50 $4,337.50 $4,586.00

Interestingly, from Example 2, cost of illness (untreated) was $47,000.00, so the medication intervention gave us cost savings of (subtracting from above) $25,338.50 $42,662.50 $42,414.00

Outcome findings Cost-effectiveness of the three eardrops by ratio

Rx a	Rx b	Rx c
$21,661.50	$4,337.50	$4,586.00
4.99	1.00	1.06

Rx b is the most cost-effective; Rx a is the least cost-effective. However, it is still saving $25,338.50 compared with cost of illness. Note that Rx C, the cost-minimization champion in Example 1, is not the most cost-effective. We should now appreciate how outcomes differ with the use of different models for drug impact analysis.

Example 4. Cost-Benefit Analysis

In this example, we would like to go through an exercise of comparing the cost-benefits of two medication regimens for resolving an infection.

Outcome measurement desired To compare the costs/benefits of two regimens of antibacterials in resolving an infectious disease in a 30-bed unit of our hospital. One regimen uses parenteral antibacterials only; the other regimen uses a combined regimen of parenteral and oral antibacterial.

Assumptions

1. This was in a hospital with 30 beds in a unit fully used for each regimen.
2. Total hospital costs per bed-day were:
   (a) $700 for combination therapy
   (b) $720 for parenteral therapy
3. The combination therapy resulted in an average hospital stay of 8 days, and parenteral therapy resulted in an average hospital stay of 12 days.
4. The combination regimen was found to produce a cure rate of 88%, a failure rate of 5%, and partial resolutions of 7%. The parenteral regimen had a cure rate of 90%, a failure rate of 7%, and partial resolutions of 3%.

Calculations The benefits (cure rate or problem resolution) of the two regimens were so close that, for the purpose of our discussion, we consider them equal without going into statistical discussions. Thus, the denominators in the equations that follow are equal:

Cost-benefit ratio for combination therapy

$= 8$ days $\times$ 30 beds $\times$ \$700/bed-day = \$168,000/benefit

Cost-benefit ratio for parenteral therapy

$= 12$ days $\times$ 30 beds $\times$ \$720/bed-day = \$259,2000/benefit

Comparing the cost-benefit ratios of the two regimens

Combination : parenteral = 168,000 : 259,200

Outcome measurements Our cost-benefit analysis shows that combination therapy compares favorably to parenteral therapy in the ratio of 168,000/259,200, or 0.648 to 1.00, in our service unit for treating 30 patients.

Note that if the benefits (outcome of treatment for the two regimens) were not equal, we would need to calculate the benefits in each denominator for each regimen to allow us to express them as ratios. Obviously, this would be more complex and is beyond the scope of this introductory exercise.

Example 5. Meta-Analysis

In this example we would like to use multiple studies or published references to find out how three competing angiotensin converting enzyme (ACE) inhibitors compare in overall costs to a managed care plan. We will consider the cost of each medication, and the three most common side effects that lead to extra costs in managing the illness.

Outcome measurement desired To compare three common ACE inhibitors—Drug A, Drug B, and Drug C—focusing on the costs of the medications, and the extra costs caused by the three most common side effects associated with each medication. This is for cost estimates for 1000 patients for 6 months in our managed care plan.

Assumptions and conditions Our meta-analysis includes public data from standard references[3,4] and each manufacturer's FDA-approved side effect profile. In meta-analysis, multiple studies/references can be used, as well as each manufacturer's package insert. We will use the data from these studies for the percent incidence per user data for the three most common side effects: cough, dizziness, and headache.

1. Let us estimate costs for a 6-month period for 1000 outpatients.
2. Patients were successfully maintained in a normotensive range for mild to moderate hypertension.
3. Patients have normal or mild renal dysfunction, creatinine clearance > 30 ml/min or serum creatinine < 3 mg/dl with no proteinuria.
4. Drug A requires 20 mg/day: the monthly cost is \$29.72.
   Drug B requires 40 mg/day: the monthly cost is \$31.00.

Drug C requires 20 mg/day: the monthly cost is $29.49.

5. Our managed care organization dispenses its own medications, so dispensing costs and overheads are not different between the three medicines.
6. Side-effect costs are estimated as follows:
   - Cough—may result in cough medicine use, request for extra visits for dose adjustments, or discontinuation. The per incidence cost of this is estimated to be $200.
   - Dizziness—may result in use of medication for dizziness, extra provider time to rule out other causes, or change in therapy. The per incidence cost of this is estimated to be $240.
   - Headache—may result in use of analgesics, extra provider time for ruling out other disorders, and change of therapy. The per incidence cost of this is estimated to be $280, since headaches require more caution.
7. Based on referenced studies the percent incidence per user for side effects are reported to be:

	Drug A	Drug B	Drug C
Cough	2.7%	2.2%	3.7%
Dizziness	3.3%	1.6%	6.3%
Headache	5.0%	3.2%	5.3%

Calculations

Side effect costs/user = cost/incidence × incidence/user

	Cough	Dizziness	Headache
Drug A	$200 × 2.7/100	$240 × 3.3/100	$280 × 5.0/100
Drug B	$200 × 2.2/100	$240 × 1.6/100	$280 × 3.2/100
Drug C	$200 × 3.7/100	$240 × 6.3/100	$280 × 5.3/100

Costs for 1000 users

Drug A	$5,400.00	$7,920.00	$14,000.00
Drug B	$4,400.00	$3,840.00	$8,960.00
Drug C	$7,400.00	$15,120.00	$14,840.00

Drug costs for 1000 users in 6 months

1000 users × 6 months × drug cost/user-month

Cost: Drug A = 1000 × 6 × $29.72 = $178,320.000
Drug B = 1000 × 6 × $31.00 = $186,940.000
Drug C = 1000 × 6 × $29.49 = $176,940.000

Outcome measurements Total costs (side-effect costs + drug cost) for 1000 users for 6 months:

$$\begin{aligned}
\text{Drug A} &= \$(5400 + 7920 + 14{,}000) + (178{,}320) = \$205{,}640 \\
\text{Drug B} &= \$(4400 + 3840 + 8960) + (186{,}940) = \$204{,}140 \\
\text{Drug C} &= \$(7400 + 15{,}120 + 14{,}840) + (176{,}940) = \$214{,}300
\end{aligned}$$

Note: Comparing drug cost alone, Drug C costing $176,940.00 was the least expensive, and Drug B, costing $186,940.00, was the most expensive. However, when side effects are included in the meta-analysis, Drug B, costing $204,140 became the least expensive, and Drug C, costing $214,300, became the most expensive.

Example 6. Cost-Utility Analysis

In this example, we want to express the net benefit of a drug, named Wonder X, in a utility unit, rather than by dollars.

Let us use quality-adjusted life years (QALYs) as the utility unit. Let us take the example of an anticancer drug. Let us assume that, based on expert meta-analysis, our drug can extend patients' lives by 8 years. However, this drug is so toxic that it produces a great deal of serious side effects that are miserable to the patient. So the question of the quality of life in using the drug is of real concern to the patient, in terms of how worthwhile it is to live with the drug and its side effects. QALYs is a meaningful unit for us to use in this situation. This value is subjective (based on the patient's response):

$$\begin{aligned}
&\text{QALYs produced by the drug} \\
&= \text{the unadjusted life years saved by the drug} \\
&\quad + \text{the morbidity reduced by the drug} \\
&\quad - \text{the side effects caused by the drug}
\end{aligned}$$

Outcome measurement desired To find the mean QALYs saved by our Drug, Wonder X, in treating our patients.

Assumptions

1. We take life years as our utility unit.
2. We collect our patients' subjective responses, based on their experience with taking Wonder X. Let us assume we did this with 500 patients over a 5-year period.
3. Let us assume that the mean values found from the responses were as follows:
   - Patients are willing to forego 1 year of their lives for every 4 years if they do not have to suffer from the morbidity caused by the cancer.

- Patients are willing to forego 1 year of their lives for every 2 years if they do not have to suffer from the severe side effects of Wonder X.

Calculations

Unadjusted life years saved = 8

Morbidity in life years = 8 years/(4 years/life year) = 2

Side effect adjusted life years = 8 years/(2 years/life year) = 4

Outcome measurements

$$\text{QALYs saved} = 8 + 2 - 4 = 6$$

Outcome findings Adjusting for quality of life, the original 8 years of life extended by the drug is only worth a net of 6 QALYs.

SUMMARY

In this chapter, we have used simple examples to apply commonly used economic tools to assess the impact of drugs on outcomes. We also observed how outcomes evolved, based on the tools we used and the assumptions we made in a variety of settings that involved everyday problems. We saw how we can apply them to estimate or project cost outcomes in selecting or recommending therapeutic choices based on clearly defined assumptions that can vary but simulate realistic conditions in our practice. In addition, selection of common measures can facilitate ease of pharmacoeconomic evaluation in various practice settings. Familiarity with these concepts can empower us to apply them to make more reliable and more comprehensive assessments of drug impact on health care costs and outcomes.

REFERENCES

1. Donabedian A: The quality of care: how can it be assessed? *J Am Med Assoc* 1988;260:1743–1748.
2. *The Morbidity and Mortality Weekly Report (MMWR) Series*. Center for Disease Control and Prevention. Atlanta, GA: Public Health Service; 1992; Vol. 41/No. RR-3
3. Hebel SK: *Drug Facts and Comparisons*. St. Louis, MO: Facts and Comparisons Publishing; 1998; p. 165 e–f.
4. Greenberg SB, ed.: *Physicians' Desk Reference*. Montvale, NJ: Medical Economics Co., Inc.; 1998.

CHAPTER

13

Government Regulation of Health Care Economic Information

Stephen J. Kogut,
Eleanor M. Perfetto
and
E. Paul Larrat

INTRODUCTION

Pharmacoeconomic information is increasingly in demand by professionals in a variety of health care settings.[1–7] Decision makers in managed care organizations can no longer rely solely upon volume discounting, contract pricing, or cost minimization when selecting preferred medications from therapeutic classes for inclusion on a formulary. Drug acquisition cost is only one factor used to ascertain the total cost of drug therapy.[8] Other direct costs, including laboratory monitoring or administration costs, can be important determinants of total cost incurred. Evaluation of indirect costs, such as productivity lost due to illness, can also be an important component of the pharmacoeconomic analysis, particularly when taking a societal perspective.[9] Policymakers in public and private agencies desire valid and applicable pharmacoeconomic information that can improve the value realized from pharmacy expenditures.

Drug manufacturers are eager to provide this information. Health economic studies have become a fundamental component of marketing a new medication or a new indication for an existing product.[10] No longer is it sufficient to promote differences in clinical parameters. Persuasive studies will include other differentiating advantages, such as improved daily functioning or a reduction in days lost from work. Pharmacoeconomic studies are used to distinguish a new medication from competing therapies.

Currently, however, a lack of standardization and comparability limits the utility of health economic research. Users of pharmacoeconomic information must compare studies that measure different outcomes from diverse populations. The use of disparate methods and measurement tools also can be complicating. Further, market competition can induce manufacturers to promote pharmacoeconomic claims generated from dubious research techniques. Even those skilled in evaluating health economic information can have difficulty ascertaining a study's validity.[11]

Despite these drawbacks, escalating expenditures for prescription medications have created a need for information that describes the economic effects of drugs. Growth in prescription drug spending has ranged between 9 and 14% during the latter half of the 1990s,[12,13] with double-digit growth projected to continue.[14,15] Total retail spending for prescription drugs exceeded $78 billion in 1997.[13] The number of prescriptions dispensed per year has also continued to increase,[16] likely resulting from expanded third-party prescription drug coverage.[13] New drugs contribute to accelerating costs considerably; products brought to market after 1992 accounted for over 30% of total drug costs in 1997.[13] The development of effective strategies for managing pharmacy costs will ultimately depend upon the availability and utility of pharmacoeconomic research.

THE ROLE OF THE GOVERNMENT

What is the government's role in regulating health economic information? Are cost-effectiveness studies an extension of clinical trials, and thus subject to similar rigors and scrutiny? Or can pharmacoeconomic research be defined and guided by the needs of its users, without the necessity of regulatory barriers that impede the dissemination of useful information.

It is important to differentiate among the different layers of potential government involvement related to the use or production of pharmacoeconomic information: registration, marketing and advertising, reimbursement, and pricing. Most government bodies of industrialized countries have put into place requirements that must be met for a drug to receive regulatory approval for sale in that country. This is referred to as market approval or registration. Routinely, a demonstration of safety and efficacy is required to gain market approval. Health economic information is not commonly a part of the dossier that government regulatory bodies review when making a determination regarding regulatory approval.

Once a product is approved, there are usually additional governmental requirements restricting what can be said during the marketing and advertising of that product. These restrictions are intended to protect the uninitiated public from being given false or misleading information about pharmaceutical products by the manufacturer. In this regard, governments can control the health care economic claims made in advertising and promotion.

In countries where the government is the primary purchaser of pharmaceutical products, health care economic information may be required for a product to gain listing on a national formulary or reimbursement list.[17] A product can gain regulatory approval but not gain listing on the formulary (or reimbursement approval). In this case, though approved or registered, the product may never be sold in that country. The governments in Australia and Canada, for example, require manufacturers to submit health economic information when requesting reimbursement listing in those countries.[18,19]

Additionally, many government purchasers also negotiate price with manufacturers, particularly when they are the primary purchaser buying most of the drugs in the country.[20] This can mean that even after clearing the registration and reimbursement processes, gaining both market approval and reimbursement listing, a manufacturer can be required to submit health care economic information when negotiating the drug price. Some countries will award a product a preferential pricing status based upon its uniqueness or its cost-effectiveness.[20]

Depending upon the country and circumstance, any or all of these processes can come into play. In the US, the issues regarding promotion are most relevant. Health care economic information is not required for registration. Reimbursement listing and pricing are negotiated with individual purchasers such as insurers, employers, or state Medicaid programs.[21] Thus, this chapter discusses US governmental regulation of health economic information, focusing upon the jurisdiction of the Food and Drug Administration (FDA) as it pertains to the regulation of pharmacoeconomic advertising and claims.

THE US FOOD AND DRUG ADMINISTRATION: A CENTURY OF REACTIVE LEGISLATION

The US government has historically intervened in response to drug manufacturing and marketing issues that have the potential to impact public health and safety. Since the Drug Importation Act of 1848, numerous food and drug laws have been enacted, paralleling the advancement of medical therapies.[22] A brief review of the evolution of US drug law can assist in understanding how current regulatory structures have developed.

The US government has regulated the pharmaceutical industry for over a century. Major regulatory interventions occurred during the early 1900s, when rampant quackery and a lack of product labeling were public concerns.[23] The Pure Food and Drug Act of 1906 helped to establish standards for pharmaceuticals, and contained some provisions that have been incorporated into current law.[24] Importantly, the Act mandated that all traded drug products were to include labeling indicating the quantity of active agent contained in the preparation. *Misbranding* was a crime punishable by law, with penalties later established by the Shirley Amendment of 1912.[22]

In 1914, the Harrison Narcotic Act established upper limits on prepared quantities of cocaine, opium, and heroin, and banned the use of cannabis.[25] The US government controlled considerable regulatory oversight over how medicines were prepared and marketed. Most importantly, the government could penalize firms who did not adhere to Federal requirements.

The Food and Drug Administration soon evolved as a regulatory body and became responsible for implementing and enforcing pharmaceutical legislation. Manufacturers hired additional chemists to ensure that their products were made to legal standards, and many scientists were recruited from leading universities, bringing along research projects that resulted in the development of new compounds. Two breakthrough antibiotics, sulfanilamide and penicillin, were brought to market. These agents were used in the treatment of many diseases, including syphilis, pneumonia, and meningitis.[26–28]

In 1937 over 100 children were fatally poisoned from a sulfanilamide elixir that contained the solvent diethylene glycol. Toxicity testing was only required for active ingredients, and the manufacturer had tested the solvent only for taste.[29] It became evident that standards for inert ingredients were necessary, and both consumers and industry sought regulatory assistance. The 1938 Food, Drug, and Cosmetic Act was enacted, requiring all drug products and vehicles to be tested for safety. Compliance with this act required increased expenditures for research and development by pharmaceutical manufacturers. The Wheeler–Lea Act, enacted the same year, assigned the Federal Trade Commission oversight of advertising of medical devices.[22]

Many important medications were brought to market during the next two decades. New anesthetics, antibiotics, and vitamins enhanced therapies, mitigated diseases, and prevented countless deaths. However, the complexity and number of various pharmacologic treatments became a concern. The Durham–Humphrey Amendment of 1951[30] established the requirement of a physician's prescription for certain medications, thus decreasing the risk of harm resulting from the unsupervised use of potentially dangerous drugs. This new prescription system fostered the growth of many US pharmaceutical firms, as manufacturers often charged a premium for prescription class drugs. As prescription drug prices increased, the public and the medical community began to question the effectiveness of some pharmaceuticals. Drug advertisements often described benefits that were seldom apparent, causing some to claim that firms were taking advantage of the ignorance of the consumer.[31]

In the early 1960s, a marked increase in tragic birth malformations was attributed to the use of thalidomide, a medication frequently prescribed as a sedative during pregnancy. Thousands of western European children exposed to the drug *in utero* were born with phocomelia, a condition resulting in shortened or absent extremities.[32] The FDA, led by medical officer Dr Frances Kelsey, was lauded for preventing thalidomide from entering the US market. Backed by strong support for additional drug legislation, Congress advanced a new initiative that responded to concerns relating to prescribed medications. The regulatory authority of the FDA would be significantly broadened, with the Agency committed to protecting the public from harm from prescription drugs (Table 13-1).

REGULATING EFFICACY

The Kefauver–Harris Amendments of 1962[33] required that drug manufacturers demonstrate efficacy in addition to safety. Firms seeking FDA approval of a new drug were required to provide studies that supported claims of effectiveness. The authority of the FDA to regulate efficacy was challenged by some drug firms that argued that a history of safe use of a medication could be cause for demonstrating efficacy. However, in 1970, the US Court of Appeals ruled in Upjohn *v.* Finch that drug efficacy and safety cannot be inferred from previous commercial success.[22]

The FDA required drug manufacturers to provide "substantial evidence" that a medication is efficacious. This included "adequate and well-controlled investigations, including clinical investigations, ... that the drug will have the effect it purports or is represented to have under the conditions of use prescribed, recommended, or suggested."[34] The FDA has regularly interpreted substantial evidence as requiring a minimum of two efficacy trials, each convincing on its own, and of adequate size and design.[35]

The efficacy standards established by Kefauver–Harris continue to guide the drug approval process. Manufacturers must provide at least two clinical trials to satisfy the FDA requirement of substantial evidence of efficacy necessary to gain market approval. The large, complex clinical trials obligatory for FDA approval of a new drug product contribute to an estimated total development cost exceeding $500 million for each marketed entity.[36]

TABLE 13–1.

Major Legislation Affecting Drug Marketing

Year	*Government intervention*	*Significance*
1906	Pure Food and Drug Act	Established standards for traded drug products
1912	Sherley Amendment	Prohibited false or misleading therapeutic claims intended to defraud
1914	Harrison Narcotic Act	Established upper limits for prepared quantities of narcotics
1938	The Federal Food, Drug, and Cosmetic Act	Required all drug products and vehicles to be tested for safety
1944	Public Health Service Act	Addressed anti-infective and biological product concerns
1951	Durham–Humphrey Amendment	Restricted the sale of certain pharmaceuticals by requiring a prescription from a licensed practitioner
1962	Kefauver–Harris Drug Amendments	Required substantial evidence of drug efficacy
1966	Fair Packaging and Labeling Act	Required honest and informative labeling of all consumer products
1983	Orphan Drug Act	Allowed FDA to promote marketing and research of therapies for rare conditions
1992	Prescription Drug User Fee Act	Drug approval process expedited through fees collected from manufacturers
1997	Food and Drug Administration Modernization Act	Included various provisions enacted to update regulations established in the 1938 Act. Promotion of health economic information directly addressed
1999, 2000	Food and Drug Administration *v.* Washington Legal Foundation	Addressed the FDA prohibition of promotional claims related to off-label drug use[62,64]

Source: *Milestones in US Food and Drug Law History*. Rockville, MD: 1999. US Food and Drug Administration, FDA backgrounder #BG99-4.

REGULATING ADVERTISING

The primary duty of the US Federal Trade Commission (FTC) is to deter harmful deceptive promotion while not impeding the dissemination of accurate and truthful claims.[37] Initial activities of the FTC relating to the pharmaceutical industry focused upon compliance with existing drug labeling requirements, such as the disclosure of effects, contraindications, and effectiveness of advertised drug products. In 1971 a working agreement between the FTC and FDA was formally acknowledged, with the FDA assuming primary responsibility of prescription drug advertisements.[38] The FTC continues to regulate over-the-counter drug advertising. Recently the FDA has claimed jurisdiction over nearly all information disseminated by a drug's manufacturer.[39]

Manufacturers have traditionally advertised drug products directly to health professionals in pages of medical journals, in face-to-face visits by company representatives, and at continuing education seminars. The FDA has delineated the type of clinical information that must accompany such advertisements and other disseminated promotional printed materials.[40] However, the emergence of managed care formulary systems and associated prescribing guidelines have limited physician's prescribing authority.[41]

Drug companies have increasingly directed advertising towards the consumer, attempting to drive demand for medications through prospective users.[42] The FDA regulates direct-to-consumer television and radio advertising through regulatory standards that prohibit false or misleading advertising.[40] Consumer-directed advertisements must include a *major statement* disclosing the medication's foremost risks, as described in the product labeling. The FDA also requires that all marketing communications pertaining to the product's indication be in consumer-friendly language and that *adequate provision* exists for the distribution or availability of product labeling associated with the advertised drug.

Federal prescription drug advertising regulations also state that a "*fair balance*" of potential therapeutic benefits and adverse effects is required for direct-to-consumer broadcast advertisements.[43] This equal balance must be present even in instances where a medication's side effects are minimal or inconsequential. Some have criticized this "fair balance" requirement, claiming that overemphasis of minor side effects may cause alarm, or hinder some patients from seeking treatment.[44] Manufacturers are also responsible for ensuring that advertised claims are not false or misleading. This includes the need to state that the advertised medication is available only by prescription, and may be prescribed only when deemed appropriate by a health care professional.

REGULATION OF HEALTH ECONOMIC INFORMATION

The increasing demand for health economic information has resulted in the conduct of economic research that has been of variable quality and utility.[45] Standards for research methods have been discussed and proposed by scientific advisors and expert panels,[46,47] yet the evolving nature of the field requires flexibility in strategies and design.[48] Additionally, the ability of many users of health economic information to evaluate pharmacoeconomic studies critically has been questioned.[49]

By the mid-1990s, the FDA reacted to increasing pressures to provide guidance on the dissemination of pharmacoeconomic information. Though many medical journals published economic studies, drug companies were hesitant to promote them until the FDA defined the criteria for evaluating health economic studies. However, the FDA had little experience critiquing this kind of data. In March of 1995, the FDA sponsored a 2-day meeting for public discussion of the issues, to gather expert advice, and to present current FDA policy as a backdrop to future policy development. During this meeting, a document entitled, "Principles for the Review of Pharmacoeconomic Promotion,"[50] was distributed by the Division of Drug Marketing, Advertising, and Communications (DDMAC), a sub-division of the FDA. It was specifically stated that this was not the release of a formal guidance by the FDA, but a draft simply released for comment only.

The draft discussed the degree of substantiation necessary to support comparative pharmacoeconomic claims. The standard required was similar to requirements for demonstrating efficacy during the approval process. Specifically, comparative pharmacoeconomic claims were subject to the "substantial evidence" burden, generally interpreted by the FDA as substantiated by "adequate and well-controlled studies." Promotional claims that included effectiveness were to be held to the FDA's highest standard of accountability.

The DDMAC document also described research techniques to be used in health economic studies. The perspective of the analysis was to be clearly stated, resources utilized should be measured in terms of "physical units, and resources affected by a drug's material effects must be included." These conditions were generally inherent in most pharmacoeconomic studies. Additional stipulations, however, were more directive. Randomized studies were considered best for comparative effectiveness trials, and studies were to be applicable to "the broad range of other settings, measurements, time periods, and patient populations." Further, all studies should include comprehensive economic measures of all therapeutic and adverse effects. Modeling of outcomes was acceptable only in cases where conducting adequate and well-controlled studies was not practical or possible. In summary, the type of pharmacoeconomic study appropriate for promotion had been defined. The Administration appeared poised to extend its regulatory authority over pharmacoeconomic promotional information.

The FDA's perspective was foreseeable. Health economic research is greatly subject to biases and error resulting from the use of "real world" populations.[49,51] Claims inappropriately derived can be inaccurate or have the potential to mislead. Many health economic studies are sponsored or directly conducted by drug companies, further increasing the potential for suspected bias. Importantly, the intense demand for pharmacoeconomic research caused an inundation of studies of differing validity and quality. Rigorous FDA standards would ensure that comparative cost-effectiveness data were reasonably accurate.

However, critics argued that these standards may provide reasonably accurate answers to unimportant, irrelevant, or mistimed questions.[11] Critics also argued that these proscriptive guidelines would impede the flow of health economic information.[52] Of particular concern was the requirement of "substantial evidence" to support effectiveness-based claims. Researchers contended that the traditional randomized, placebo-controlled trial was not always appropriate for determining effectiveness in health economic studies.[53,54] Retrospective studies that examine drug effects in populations cannot be randomized, and placebo-controlled trials are unethical when effective therapies are available. The FDA's clinical efficacy standards were deemed by many to be excessively rigorous for the purpose of cost-effectiveness comparisons. Most health economic studies, substantiated by administrative or epidemiologic-based data, would be insufficient to support promotional claims. The FDA considered modeling acceptable "only if well-controlled trials are not available," a position that was deemed inconsistent with the need to make decisions in uncertain circumstances.[55]

The FDA solicited input during various public hearings, in an attempt to develop policy that maintained evidence standards without inhibiting the flow of useful information.[56] The Federal Trade Commission, responsible for enforcing against deceptive marketing practices, provided considerable insight. Addressing the issue of requirements for substantiation of effectiveness claims, the FTC suggested that the FDA consider a more flexible position. Specifically, the FTC recommended a standard of "competent and reliable" evidence, determined retrospectively and dependent on the type of claim promoted.[37] The FDA may still require controlled trials in instances where efficacy claims are included, but may consider other types of information appropriate for substantiation of particular claims. The FTC was encouraging the FDA to adopt a position that would be more adaptable to the diverse types of studies used to support health economic claims.

The FDA was also concerned about the audience for health care economic information. Beyond misleading claims or factual inaccuracies, health economic information has the potential for misuse by those unskilled in interpreting such research.[57] Poor decisions resulting from the misinterpretation of health economic claims could result in increased costs and unnecessary disruptions in therapy. Misuse of this information in managed care settings may also result in inappropriate treatment protocols that compromise patient health. The FTC urged the FDA to recognize the special considerations specific to the audience receiving promotional health economic information.[37]

Many critics from the pharmaceutical industry argued that a tiered approach should be taken. They voiced the belief that managed care formulary committees and other formal decision-making bodies were more sophisticated users than the average consumer or typical, individual practitioner. These critics envisioned a system where more information could be shared with these discerning users, but that the standard restrictions would still be needed for a general audience.[58]

THE FOOD AND DRUG MODERNIZATION ACT OF 1997

Responding to a number of issues in pharmaceutical industry regulation, Congress passed the Food and Drug Administration Modernization Act (FDAMA) of 1997.[59] The Act amended or repealed sections of the Federal Food, Drug, and Cosmetic Act, providing a wide range of regulatory updates. The Prescription Drug User Fee Act of 1992 was re-authorized, continuing the policy of exacting fees from industry to be applied toward expediting the drug approval process. Provisions encouraging the study of drugs in pediatric populations were included. Other sections of the FDAMA addressed the need for accelerated study and approval of fast-track drugs and expanded access to investigational therapies. The Act also encouraged the submission of supplemental indications for marketed products

The dissemination of health care economic information was specifically addressed by the FDAMA (Figure 13-1). Apparently heeding the advice of the FTC, industry, and other experts, Congress appeared to have relaxed the standards required to substantiate comparative effectiveness claims. However, the Act increased regulatory authority by defining who may receive health economic information and by limiting the types of claims that may be promoted. In sum, the Act attempted to minimize FDA obstruction, yet provide standards that ensure accountability and reduce the potential for misuse by unqualified recipients.

According to the FDAMA, "competent and reliable scientific evidence" could now be used to substantiate health economic claims. This new standard, employed by the FTC in the evaluation of over-the-counter drug promotions, was perceived by many as a rational compromise. Clinical claims were still to be held to the substantial evidence standard, requiring well-controlled randomized trials as previously discussed. But, the FDAMA recognized that such

(a) In General.—Section 502(a) (21 U.S.C. 352(a)) is amended by adding at the end the following: "Health care economic information provided to a formulary committee, or other similar entity, in the course of the committee or the entity carrying out its responsibilities for the selection of drugs for managed care or other similar organizations, shall not be considered to be false or misleading under this paragraph if the health care economic information directly relates to an indication approved under section 505 or under section 351(a) of the Public Health Service Act for such drug and is based on competent and reliable scientific evidence. The requirements set forth in section 505(a) or in section 351(a) of the Public Health Service Act shall not apply to health care economic information provided to such a committee or entity in accordance with this paragraph. Information that is relevant to the substantiation of the health care economic information presented pursuant to this paragraph shall be made available to the Secretary upon request. In this paragraph, the term 'health care economic information' means any analysis that identifies, measures, or compares the economic consequences, including the costs of the represented health outcomes, of the use of a drug to the use of another drug, to another health care intervention, or to no intervention."

Figure 13-1. Food and Drug Administration Modernization Act of 1997, Sec. 114: Health Care Economic Information.

methods were impractical and often inappropriate for promoting cost-effectiveness and other comparative claims. This new "competent and reliable scientific evidence" standard potentially allowed for modeling of the effectiveness component of pharmacoeconomic studies. The Act also permitted claims originating from non-randomized "real world" study populations, such as insured managed care enrollees and other observational data sets.

Section 114 of the FDAMA specifically defined the audience for health economic information, identifying formulary committees and like entities as the appropriate recipients of promotional claims. The policy sought to enhance the availability of useful and truthful information while minimizing potential for misuse or misinterpretation. The Act recognized the increasing reliance on health economic information by groups responsible for managing the pharmacy benefit of insured populations. However, the new substantiation standards did not apply to claims promoted to individual heath practitioners or consumers. The regulatory language was interpreted as allowing drug companies and managed care groups to share information, provided that such information was to be used in the selection of medications by an organization or group entity.

Consistent with its policy on restricting activities regarding the off-label use of medications, the FDAMA applied only to the promotion of claims directly related to an approved indication. Dissemination of information relating to the off-label use of a medication remained prohibited.

In sum, the Food and Drug Administration Modernization Act of 1997 contained important provisions that could potentially enhance the exchange of useful health economic information. The acceptance of "competent and reliable scientific evidence" to support economic claims was endorsed by major stakeholders. However, certain ambiguous components of the legislation required elucidation, and other sections were outright contested by its intended users.

ISSUES ARISING FROM THE FOOD AND DRUG ADMINISTRATION MODERNIZATION ACT OF 1997

The "competent and reliable" evidence standard adopted from the FTC was deemed sufficient for the substantiation of economic claims, though clinical claims remained subject to the substantial evidence standards required for demonstrating efficacy. However, the difference between clinical and economic claims, though apparent in some instances, may in other cases be difficult to determine. Cost-effectiveness, for example, is determined by dividing relevant costs by a measure of therapeutic effect, the intended outcome. The effect could be specific, as in the complete relief of pain, or perhaps more general, such as ability to be employed. Would such analyses be subject to economic or clinical substantiation standards? The criteria for distinguishing between a straightforward clinical claim and the effectiveness component (the outcome) of a cost-effectiveness evaluation was not well elucidated by the FDAMA.

Also at issue is the restricting of the audience of health economic information. The law's apparent intent was not to impede the dissemination of useful and truthful information to groups engaged in the drug selection process. However, the FDAMA attempted to prevent the misuse of health economic information by unskilled reviewers. It has been assumed that the defined audience has the expertise required to properly analyze and evaluate sophisticated health economic information. Though many responsible for drug selection have not been formally trained, continuing education and other published reviews can assist in providing basic proficiencies.[60] Additionally, some have questioned the FDA's jurisdiction, noting that the restriction of communication that is neither false nor misleading is prohibited by the First Amendment of the US Constitution.[61]

The FDAMA also requires that promoted health economic claims be directly related to an approved indication. It has long been the policy of the

FDA to prohibit drug companies from distributing unsolicited information regarding the off-label use of medications. This policy serves to encourage manufacturers to submit applications for additional indications. The FDA has expressed concern that the unregulated distribution of off-label information would obviate the company's need to apply for an additional indication. Physicians may prescribe a medication, even when its use for that condition is not FDA approved. Prescribers may also request information about off-label uses of medications from manufacturers. However, drug firms are prohibited from distributing information regarding the off-label use of medications, regardless of whether the claims are clinical or economic in nature. The FDAMA sought to sustain the policy of limiting promotional claims to approved uses.

Also subject to interpretation is the phrase "directly related to an (FDA) approved indication." Health economic claims often measure important practical outcomes that may indirectly relate to an approved FDA use. For example, an antihypertensive medication may purport the additional benefit of reducing morbidity, perhaps as measured by decreased incidence of stroke during treatment. Is such a study promotable, given the absence of FDA approval for stroke prevention? Under the current law, the answer would be "no" given the product is not approved for stroke prevention. The FDAMA failed to identify the types of outcomes considered to directly relate to an approved indication.

The Food and Drug Administration Modernization Act seemingly sought to improve the flow of health care economic information from manufacturers to decision makers responsible for drug selection in populations. Reducing the degree of substantiation required for health economic claims could result in an increase in potentially useful cost-effectiveness studies. However, further elucidation of the distinction between clinical and economic claims seems required. Alternatively, some assert that the regulations contained in FDAMA further limit the dissemination of potentially useful health care economic research. In restricting what types of claims may be promoted, and by limiting to whom such claims can be made, the Act further extended the FDA's regulatory authority (Figure 13-1).

DEVELOPMENTS IN ISSUES RELATED TO FREE SPEECH

The FDA permits promotional drug claims only for indications approved by the Administration. Non-approved, off-label uses cannot be promoted, even when supported by sound clinical evidence. Some argue that this restrictive position impedes the flow of information that may potentially improve therapies and save lives.[61] Though recognizing this argument, the FDA has maintained its prohibition on off-label promotion by reprimanding offenders through warning letters and other penalties.

The FDA is concerned with drug off-label promotion for several related reasons. Most importantly, the Agency is concerned about the use of medications that have not been deemed efficacious through the standards maintained by the approval process. Studies supporting off-label drug use may be nonrandomized or not controlled. Companies may be inclined to distort research results to further encourage an unlabeled use. Recognizing the potential for such information to mislead, the FDA prohibits the promotion of off-label use in accordance with its responsibility to protect public health.

Solutions for protecting users from information that could misleadingly convey safety or efficacy have been described. The use of a disclaimer has been suggested, indicating the lack of safety and efficacy requirements as required for FDA approval.[11] Another approach is the implementation of a credentialing system, with an evaluating body indicating if the research conforms to accepted principles and methods.[55]

Prescribers are free to use medications for unlabeled indications. Therapies for diseases such as cancer or AIDS often incorporate regimens that have not been approved. Though the FDA strongly encourages manufacturers to seek approval for additional indications, incentives for submitting supplemental new drug applications are absent when off-label uses become the standard of care. Gaining approval for an indication requires expensive clinical trials that may conclude shortly before patent expiration. Drug companies would be less inclined to seek FDA approval for an additional indication if off-label use could be encouraged through promotion in a less expensive and more timely manner.

The FDA's restriction of off-label promotional claims has recently been challenged.[62] Both pharmaceutical manufacturers and practitioners have argued that limiting the dissemination of truthful information is unconstitutional, regardless of whether such information pertains to an FDA-approved use. Representing this position was the Washington Legal Foundation (WLF), a nonprofit organization describing its mission as "to defend and promote the principles of free enterprise and individual rights."[63] The Foundation's activities are funded by a nationwide constituency of individual and corporate donors.[63] In 1994, the WLF initiated a suit against the FDA, charging that FDA prohibition of off-label promotion violated free speech provisions of the First Amendment. Specifically, the Foundation asserted that the FDA could not restrict the dissemination of information that was neither false nor misleading. Additionally, they argued that scientific knowledge about the safe and effective use of medications often precedes FDA approval.

The FDA recognized the importance of off-label drug therapy, but maintained that incentives existed for promoters to manipulate research to influence prescribing. It was further argued that conduct, and not speech, was being regulated. The FDA claimed to be regulating the sale of products that were not approved for the intended off-label use. During its defense, the FDA also claimed that speech was not restricted, but permitted if in accordance with regulations contained in the FDAMA.

The FDA's arguments were dismissed in 1999 by Judge Royce Lamberth, who ruled that the Administration was bound by the First Amendment and could no longer restrict promotions regarding off-label drug use. Judge Lamberth summarized the court's position, noting that "the First Amendment is premised upon the idea that people do not need the government's permission to engage in truthful, non-misleading speech about lawful activity." Manufacturers could now promote off-label uses of medications, providing that the drug has an FDA-approved indication for at least one condition, that promotional claims are not false and misleading, and that the information has appeared in a peer-reviewed, published article. The FDA quickly moved to appeal this decision, maintaining the position that the regulation of potentially misleading off-label claims was legally warranted.

With the regulatory authority of the FDA successfully challenged, stakeholders began to consider potential ramifications. The Lamberth ruling had important implications for regulation of health care economic information as described in the FDAMA. Specifically questioned was the FDA's authority to prohibit the promotion of off-label health care economic information. The ruling potentially eliminated the need for the FDA to clarify the distinction between outcome and approved indication as previously discussed. Further, FDA regulation restricting the audience of truthful health economic claims may be considered a violation of free speech. Such claims, if accurate and non-misleading should be disseminable to all, according to principles established by Judge Lamberth's ruling.

The FDA's appeal of the Lamberth ruling was heard during January and February of 2000.[64] In a change of strategy, the FDA argued that off-label promotional claims were evidence that a manufacturer was attempting to engage in the distribution of drugs for an unapproved use. The Administration claimed regulatory authority over the sale of products for an unapproved indication in interstate commerce, and considered off-label promotional materials suggestive of such intent.

The US Court of Appeals for the District of Columbia accepted the FDA's position, acknowledging that it is illegal for a manufacturer to distribute a drug with the intent that it be used for an off-label indication. However, the District Court's ruling remained in effect; the FDA could not "prohibit, restrict, sanction, or otherwise seek to limit" the promotional claims made by manufacturers. However, the Appeals Court ruled that the FDA could use such claims as proof of intent to distribute a drug for an unlabeled use in interstate commerce.

IMPLICATIONS

By considering off-label promotion evidence of intent to distribute a drug for an unlabeled use, the FDA has circuitously regained control over off-label promotional claims. However, it is uncertain how aggressively the FDA will enforce this authority, since specific warnings could result in new litigation. Further, other FDA concerns such as direct-to-consumer drug advertising and Internet pharmacy regulation have appeared to consume much of the Agency's resources as of late. Nevertheless, stakeholders await guidance from the FDA regarding the types of promotional claims that can be made, and to whom such claims can be promoted.

Several other important issues related to the FDAMA linger. The need for distinction between clinical and economic claims remains, including the degree of substantiation required for demonstrating cost-effectiveness. A clearer interpretation is required of other FDAMA clauses, such as the "competent and reliable" evidence requirement for economic claims and the "qualified committees or groups" responsible for evaluating supporting evidence. Finally, to what degree do cost-effectiveness outcomes need to be related to an approved indication? Clarification of this point becomes important in the wake of the FDA's successful appeal of the Lamberth ruling.

In the interim, both drug company promoters and the intended users of health care economic information are wise to adhere to generally accepted scientific principles of health economic research. Such tenets include the use of good methodology, employing valid instruments and with appropriate scoring and statistical methods. Transparency of costs is essential, with the inclusion and description of all relevant economic effects. Adhering to such practices can decrease the potential for health economic research to be considered inaccurate or misleading.

CONCLUSION

The demand for health care economic information will continue to increase, with decision makers attempting to maximize value obtained from drug expenditures. Strong competition among firms seeking formulary approval creates the need for distinctive, convincing promotional materials that demonstrate superior clinical and economic outcomes. Firms that can provide evidence of superiority for a promoted product can achieve a significant market advantage.

The FDA is responsible for ensuring that promoted health care economic claims are neither inaccurate nor misleading. The Food and Drug Administration Modernization Act of 1997 provided revised criteria for the substantiation of promoted health care economic claims, establishing different standards for clinical and economic promoted information. Future interpretation of key components of the legislation will eminently determine the impact the regulations will have on the dissemination of health economic materials.

The FDAMA and the WLF case were significant actions in facilitating the flow of important and useful health care economic information. However, certain sections remain subject to interpretation that has yet to be provided. Future guidance from the FDA is awaited, particularly in light of the continued controversies regarding off-label promotion. Meanwhile, manufacturers must adhere to currently accepted research standards.

REFERENCES

1. Anis AH, Rahman T, Schechter MT: Using pharmacoeconomic analysis to make drug insurance coverage decisions. *Pharmacoeconomics* 1998;13(1 Pt 2):119–126.
2. Bakst A: Pharmacoeconomics and the formulary decision-making process. *Hosp Formul* 1995;30(1):42–50.
3. Detsky AS: Using cost-effectiveness analysis for formulary decision making: from theory into practice. *BMJ* 1995;310(6986):1028.
4. Grabowski H, Mullins CD: Pharmacy benefit management, cost-effectiveness analysis and drug formulary decisions. *Soc Sci Med* 1997;45(4):535–544.
5. Hatoum HT, Freeman RA: The use of pharmacoeconomic data in formulary selection. *Top Hosp Pharm Manag* 1994;13(4):11–22.
6. Langley PC: Meeting the information needs of drug purchasers: the evolution of formulary submission guidelines. *Clin Ther* 1999;21(4):768–787; discussion 767.
7. Sanchez LA: Pharmacoeconomics and formulary decision making. *Pharmacoeconomics* 1996;9(Suppl 1):16–25.
8. Larson LN: Cost determination and analysis. In: Bootman JL, ed., *Principles of Pharmacoeconomics*. Cincinnati: Harvey Whitney Books; 1998; 45–59.
9. Koopmanschap MA, Rutten FF: Indirect costs in economic studies: confronting the confusion. *Pharmacoeconomics* 1993;4(6):446–454.
10. Thwaites R, Townsend RJ: Pharmacoeconomics in the new millennium. A pharmaceutical industry perspective. *Pharmacoeconomics* 1998;13(2):175–180.
11. Luce BR, Hillman AL: When is a cost-effectiveness claim valid? How much should the FDA care? *Am J Manag Care* 1997;3(11):1660–1666.
12. Baugh DK, Pine PL, Blackwell S: Trends in Medicaid prescription drug utilization and payments, 1990–97. *Health Care Financ Rev* 1999;20(3):79–105.

13. Braden BR, Cowan CA, Lazenby HC, et al.: National health expenditures, 1997. *Health Care Financ Rev* 1998;20(1):83–126.
14. Hensley S: Prescription costs become harder to swallow. Providers and payers get a big dose of reality with explosive spending and patient demand for new drugs. *Mod Health* 1999;29(34):30–34.
15. Mehl B, Santell JP: Projecting future drug expenditures–2000 [In Process Citation]. *Am J Health Syst Pharm* 2000;57(2):129–138.
16. Copeland C: Prescription drugs: issues of cost, coverage, and quality. *EBRI Issue Brief* 1999(208):1–21.
17. Johnson JA, Bootman JL: Pharmacoeconomic analysis in formulary decisions: an international perspective. *Am J Hosp Pharm* 1994;51(20):2593–2598.
18. Glennie JL, Torrance GW, Baladi JF, et al.: The revised Canadian Guidelines for the Economic Evaluation of Pharmaceuticals. *Pharmacoeconomics* 1999;15(5):459–468.
19. Mitchell A: Update and evaluation of Australian guidelines. Government perspective. *Med Care* 1996;34(12 Suppl):DS216–DS225.
20. Dickson M, Bootman JL: Pharmacoeconomics: an international perspective. In: Bootman JL, Townsend RJ, McGhan WF, eds, *Principles of Pharmacoeconomics*. Cincinnati: Harvey Whitney Books; 1998, pp 25–26.
21. Kane NM: Pharmaceutical cost containment and innovation in the United States. *Health Policy* 1997;41(Suppl):S71–S89.
22. US Food and Drug Administration Milestones in US Food and Drug Law History, 1999. Rockville, MD: FDA backgrounder #BG99-4.
23. Sonnedecker G: The rise of legislative standards: Food and Drug Law. In: Urdang C, Kremers G, eds., *History of Pharmacy*. Philadelphia: J.B. Lippincott Company; 1976: 220–221.
24. 21 U.S.C. §501(b).
25. Janssen WF: America's first food and drug laws. *Hosp Formul* 1976; 11(8):434–437.
26. Mandell G, Sande M: Antimicrobial agents. In: Goodman L, Gilman G, eds., *The Pharmacological Basis of Therapeutics*. New York: Collier Macmillan; 1985; 1115.
27. Hare R: The birth of penicillin and the disarming of microbes. London: Allen & Unwin; 1970.
28. Wienstein L, Madoff M, Samet C: The sulfonamides. *New Engl J Med* 1960;263:793–800.
29. Ben-Zion T: The food and drug regulations. In: Tuber F, ed., *Proving New Drugs: A Guide to Clinical Trials*. Clinton, MA: The Colonial Press, Inc.; 1969:60.
30. 21 U.S.C. §353(b)(1).
31. Kucukarslan S, Hakim Z, Sullivan D, et al.: Points to consider about prescription drug prices: an overview of federal policy and pricing studies. *Clin Ther* 1993;15(4):726–738.

32. Taussig H: A study of the German outbreak of phocomelia. *JAMA* 1962;180(13):80–88.
33. 21 U.S.C. §§321, 331–332, 348, 351–353, 355, 357–360, 372, 374, 376, 381.
34. 21 U.S.C §505(d).
35. Woodcock J: Comparing treatments: The role of the FDA: safety, effectiveness and cost-effectiveness. Masur Auditorium, NIH, March 23–24,1995.
36. Boston Consulting Group: The contribution of pharmaceutical companies: What's at stake for America, September 1993.
37. Comments of the Staffs of the Bureaus of Economics and Consumer Protection of the Federal Trade Commission. In the Matter of Pharmaceutical Marketing and Information Exchange in Managed Care Environments; FDA Public Hearings, 1996: Docket No. 95N-0228.
38. Working Agreement between FTC and Food and Drug Administration, 4 Trade Reg. Rep. (CHH) 9,851 (1971).
39. Kessler DA, Pines WL: The federal regulation of prescription drug advertising and promotion [see comments]. *JAMA* 1990;264(18):2409–2415.
40. 21 C.F.R. §202.1
41. Brehany J, Cohen P, Sax MJ: The drug formulary decision-making process. *Healthplan* 1999;40(3):85–92.
42. Fine A: Increased direct-to-consumer advertising driving pharmaceutical costs, trends. *Exec Solut Health Manag* 1999;2(1):2–3.
43. Baylor-Henry M, Drezin NA: Regulation of prescription drug promotion: direct-to-consumer advertising. *Clin Ther* 1998;20(Suppl C):C86–C95.
44. Paul H. Rubin PDJEC, Ph.D. Department of Health and Human Services Public Health Services Food and Drug Administration: FDA Public Hearing Direct-to-Consumer Promotion, Department of Health and Human Services Public Health Services Food and Drug Administration, 1995.
45. Udvarhelyi IS, Colditz GA, Rai A, Epstein AM: Cost-effectiveness and cost-benefit analyses in the medical literature. Are the methods being used correctly? [see comments]. *Ann Intern Med* 1992;116(3):238–244.
46. Russell LB, Gold MR, Siegel JE, Daniels N, Weinstein MC: The role of cost-effectiveness analysis in health and medicine. Panel on Cost-Effectiveness in Health and Medicine [see comments]. *JAMA* 1996;276(14):1172–1177.
47. Siegel JE, Weinstein MC, Russell LB, Gold MR: Recommendations for reporting cost-effectiveness analyses. Panel on Cost-Effectiveness in Health and Medicine [see comments]. *JAMA* 1996;276(16):1339–1341.
48. Luce BR: Cost-effectiveness analysis: obstacles to standardization and its use in regulating pharmaceuticals [editorial]. *Pharmacoeconomics* 1993;3(1):1–9.
49. Kaplan NM: Pitfalls in the interpretation of pharmacoeconomic studies. *Pharmacoeconomics* 1992;1(5):303–305.

50. Food and Drug Administration Division of Drug Marketing, Advertising, and Communications: Principles for the Review of Pharmacoeconomic Promotion (draft). Rockville, MD, March 20, 1995.
51. Byford S, Palmer S: Common errors and controversies in pharmacoeconomic analyses [see comments]. *Pharmacoeconomics* 1998;13(6):659–666.
52. Robinson M: Should the FDA regulate pharmacoeconomic studies? *Health Aff (Millwood)* 1996;15(3):54–71.
53. Freemantle N, Drummond M: Should clinical trials with concurrent economic analyses be blinded? [see comments]. *JAMA* 1997;277(1):63–64.
54. Perfetto EM: FDA reform: implications for health economic research and pharmacy practice. *J Am Pharm Assoc (Wash.)* 1998;38(2):118–120.
55. Neumann PJ, Zinner DE, Paltiel AD: The FDA and regulation of cost-effectiveness claims. *Health Aff (Millwood)* 1996;15(3):54–71.
56. FDA hears opinions on need for regulation of pharmacoeconomic information [news]. *Am Fam Physician* 1996;54(1):353–358.
57. Sanchez LA, Lee J: Use and misuse of pharmacoeconomic terms: a definitions primer. *Am J Health Syst Pharm* 1995;52(17):1871.
58. Pharmaceutical Research and Manufacturers of America: Re: Promotional Use of Health Care Economic Information—Recommended Approach for Implementing FDAMA Sec.114. FDA Docket 98D-0468: Health Care Economic Information, 1998.
59. Food and Drug Modernization Act, Pub. L. No. 105-115, 111 Stat. 2296 (codified at 21 U.S.C. § 343(r)(3)(C) and (D)).
60. Sarpong D: Application of pharmacoeconomics and outcomes research in formulary decision making. *Drug Benefit Trends* 1999;11(8):53–57.
61. Burditt G: Court Again Nullifies FDA Policies Restricting Health Care Information, Washington Legal Foundation, 1999.
62. Henney et al. *v*. Washington Legal Foundation, in Civil Action 94-1306 (RCL). United States District Court for the District of Columbia, 1999.
63. Washington Legal Foundation: Mission and Goals. http://www.wlf.org/mission.htm. accessed 1/22/2000.
64. Washington Legal Foundation *v*. Henney, in Civil Action 99-5304 (RCL). United States Appeals Court for the District of Columbia, 2000.

Index